Advance Praise

"Linda Blachman and her mothers h₂ ... ut
coping with cancer. These are deepl, ... iov-
ing told as only mothers 'up against ...uiner Morning is
a wonderful book, a gift of the huma ... ii response to great challenge
and ultimate concern."

Charles Garfield, PhD
Author, *Sometimes My Heart Goes Numb: Love and Caregiving in a Time of AIDS*
Founder, SHANTI, and clinical professor of psychology, University of California
Medical School at San Francisco

∞

"Stories are true wisdom and these stories, especially, are great gifts. In a
culture that doesn't recognize or value wisdom, these stories are rare and
profound offerings to the survivors, to the next generation, to those of us
who are left behind here. Because of these stories, we will be sustained. We
will know, even in our loneliness and loss, how to live our lives."

Deena Metzger
Author, *Entering the Ghost River: Meditations on the Theory and Practice of
Healing; Tree: Essays and Pieces; Writing for Your Life:
A Guide and Companion to the Inner World*

∞

"*Another Morning* is the best oral history of the experience of cancer that I
have ever seen. Linda Blachman has written an essential documentary resource for clinicians and health researchers, and she offers those living with
cancer the companionship of generously shared experiences."

Arthur W. Frank, MD
Author, *The Renewal of Generosity* and *The Wounded Storyteller.*

∞

"The powerful stories in *Another Morning* take us from the stark truth of
illness and fear to the light-hearted laughter and hope that we all deserve
in times of duress. These narratives are valuable reading for anyone who is
caring for themselves and their children through a journey of healing and
uncertainty."

Debu Tripathy, MD
Coauthor, *Breast Cancer: Beyond Convention*
(with Mary Tagliaferri, MD and Isaac Cohen, MD)
Professor of internal medicine, medical oncologist, University of Texas Southwestern
Medical Center

"This book brings hope and courage not only to mothers with cancer going through the experience, but to anyone who doubts the mettle of the human spirit. It is an important resource to [ill mothers] and to all of us who share in their pain and fear, and marvel at the way they can respond, especially when they get to tell and appreciate their stories and not feel alone. This is a beautifully written book and made me feel more a willing part of humanity for reading it."

Martin L. Rossman, MD, Dipl. Ac. (NCCAOM)
Author, *Fighting Cancer from Within*

"This book bubbles with existential energy, giving voice to women who are both nurturing life and facing death. Linda Blachman has gathered and provided collective wisdom from women who are urgently sorting out what matters in life."

David Spiegel, MD
Willson Professor, Stanford University School of Medicine
Author, *Living Beyond Limits*

"In a culture in which families shy away from talk of cancer and death, and the medical world offers treatment while remaining oblivious to patients' lives as mothers and partners, Blachman's book has much to teach us. I laughed and cried at the insight and humor of these women as I read their living stories. This book holds valuable insights and models of coping—for parents and grandparents, for anyone who has been touched by illness, and for health and mental health professionals who care for patients."

Carolyn Pape Cowan, PhD
Department of Psychology, University of California at Berkeley
Author, *When Partners Become Parents: The Big Life Change for Couples*

Another
MORNING

Another MORNING

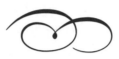

VOICES OF **TRUTH** AND **HOPE** FROM MOTHERS WITH CANCER

LINDA BLACHMAN

SEAL PRESS

Another Morning
Voices of Truth and Hope from Mothers with Cancer

Copyright © 2006, 2000 by Linda Blachman

AVALON
publishing group incorporated

Published by Seal Press
An Imprint of Avalon Publishing Group, Incorporated
1400 65th Street, Suite 250
Emeryville, CA 94608

ISBN-10 1-58005-178-2
ISBN-13 978- 1-58005-178-1

9 8 7 6 5 4 3 2 1

Library of Congress Cataloging-in-Publication Data
Blachman, Linda.
Another morning : voices of truth and hope from
mothers with cancer / Linda Blachman.
p. cm.
Includes bibliographical references.
ISBN-13: 978-1-58005-178-1
ISBN-10: 1-58005-178-2
1. Cancer in women--Psychological aspects. 2. Cancer--Patients--Family
relationships. 3. Mothers--Mental health. 4. Self-help groups. I. Title.
RC281.W65.B53 2006
362.196'994--dc22
2005027120

Cover design by Gerilyn Attebery
Interior design by Megan Cooney
Printed in the United States of America by Worzalla
Distributed by Publishers Group West

In memory of my parents
Ruth Brenes Blachman and Max Louis Blachman

For Shira

We never know how high we are
Till we are asked to rise
And then if we are true to plan
Our statures touch the skies—

—*Emily Dickinson*

CONTENTS

INTRODUCTION

PERHAPS YOU'RE A MOTHER, a mother whose life seems to stretch out before you like a purple ribbon waving in the breeze. Everything appears possible for you, for your family. But one day, life changes without your permission. Suddenly, you can no longer rely on your beliefs about the way things are. You can no longer promise your children a secure world and a positive future.

It might be a diagnosis of cancer, heart disease, multiple sclerosis, or some other disease that alters your world. Or your marriage ends. You get a pink slip with your paycheck and there isn't enough to cover next month's rent, or you wake up one morning so depressed you can't get out of bed. Whatever the cause, you are a mother, you will do anything to protect your children from suffering, and you feel responsible. You tell yourself you're only human—vulnerable and scared. But mothers are supposed to be strong. Your story isn't supposed to turn out this way, and that is really hard to talk about.

Maybe your life hasn't been disturbed by a personal crisis. Maybe you heard one too many stories about a child abduction, a school massacre, a mother your age who became critically ill or died, and all of a sudden, you can't shake off the tremors of anxiety. You realize how tenuous life is for all of us, and you can't shield your kids from that knowledge. When one of them asks, "Mom, that won't happen to us, will it?" you reply, "Of course not!" but certainty fled a long time ago.

It might be that your own mother died before you had a chance to know her, before you thought to ask her the questions that would unlock the secrets of her life and yours. Perhaps you were young when she died and you've never stopped wondering what she went through, what she might have said had someone just asked. Why didn't anyone ask her? The ache of being motherless is compounded by another loss that few speak about: the loss of her story.

The story of motherhood has holes in it, the holes of unanswered questions: How do mothers go on living and loving with shattered illusions? How do they help their children feel protected when their own security is threatened? How do they "get back to normal" when they no longer know what normal is? Can mothers ever be seen as both strong and fallible, as whole human beings? Why do we ask so much of mothers and so little about them?

The mothers you will meet in this book have lived with these questions. They have grappled with two of life's greatest challenges—mothering and mortality—and have done so in a culture that avoids talking about death or acknowledging the underside of motherhood. They are ordinary women who have had to respond to every mother's nightmare: a cancer diagnosis while raising children. Seriously ill mothers know what it's like to feel betrayed by life. They also live with the knowledge that they might default on the promise to care for their children until adulthood. As one mother said, "To raise a child while living with cancer is to have your heart break. We have to learn how to live with broken hearts."

Sooner or later, all parents have to learn how to live with broken hearts and teach their children to do so too. Mothers with cancer have wisdom to offer those coping with turbulent times from any cause. Their experiences are equally valuable for those who love or support a mother who is going through a life-altering illness, and for those whose mothers died early in their lives.

Why cancer? Because it seems that we all know someone who's been diagnosed with it. Because cancer still carries greater fear and stigma than most diseases. Because people driven to the edge of existence can be our best teachers, giving us new perspective. These are the women who have inspired this book—mothers living with cancer while raising children. Each one has a story, a voice larger than her embattled body, and an important message to deliver. But often, it is difficult for others to listen.

For the past decade, stopping to listen deeply has been the task of the Mothers' Living Stories Project, a nonprofit group that I founded and direct. Mothers' Living Stories brings attention, compassion, and support to ill mothers by helping them record their life stories as a healing process for themselves, and as a way to open communication within families and to create cherished legacies for their children. For many of the women, speaking to a listener in the presence of a tape recorder is a freeing and helpful, though sometimes challenging, experience.

When I founded the project, I did not have a life-threatening illness, but I had developed a condition that threatened my way of life and sense of self. An inoperable back injury led to three years of disability and uncertainty about whether I would walk again. During that time, I lost my job, my mother died, and my daughter graduated from high school and left home. My world collapsed along with my spine.

As my recuperation dragged on, I wondered what it must be like for women with younger children and more serious diseases, like cancer, AIDS, or MS. This line of inquiry was a logical continuation of my public health career. The theme of both my professional life and personal life has been mothering—its meaning, challenge, and opportunity—in a culture that sentimentalizes mothers while undermining their work. For twenty years, I had been a researcher, educator, consultant, and counselor specializing in family health and parenting. My primary interest was in maternal mental health, especially in how to provide care for the primary caregiver, who, in most families, is still a woman. I had worked on behalf of couples over thirty deciding to have children, pregnant and postpartum mothers, mothers who abused children, mothers who abused themselves with substances, and those who were impoverished. I was particularly drawn to issues that are stigmatized and silenced.

It was not a great stretch from mental health challenges to medical ones like cancer, from the wonder of birth to the mystery of death. But most of us do not go willingly into the land of sickness, and I was no exception. Illness changed me. I saw what living in chronic pain and isolation can do to a person, how devastating dependency is. But I also learned how a serious illness can lead to positive changes. Like children, many American parents need to be forced into a time-out to slow down and think about their lives. As difficult and life shattering as illness may be, it is one of the few experiences that can offer that opportunity.

As I lay in bed questioning everything, my mind kept returning to women living with cancer and children. If, as Joan Didion writes, "[we] tell ourselves stories in order to live," I wanted to understand what stories these women were telling themselves. How were they reconstructing their lives after trauma? What would it mean for a woman to let go before her mothering work was done?

In 1995, I expected to find numerous academic studies, popular books, resources, and services, but instead I found silence, especially the silence of mothers' voices. No one knew the number of mothers with cancer locally, statewide, or nationally; mothers were not counted by tumor registries, which collect and publish disease data.[1] I was stunned by registry representatives and researchers who explained that "Do you have children?" and "How old are they?" are not "medically relevant" questions. I knew that numbers talk. A constituency that is not counted is discounted—invisible and unserved.

I had assumed that children would be a crucial factor in their mothers' treatment decisions and would have a profound effect on their will to live and on medical outcomes. I could hardly imagine any group more in need of attention and support than critically ill mothers struggling to raise their children. Why so little interest? Where were the mothers' voices?

After my back recovered, I invited two colleagues to help me convene focus groups of mothers living with cancer in the San Francisco Bay Area. I wanted to ask them about their experiences parenting through serious illness and to better understand their needs. I wanted to get their endorsement for the kind of program I hoped to develop, one that would meet some of those needs in a meaningful way.

That's where it began—listening to the women, their isolation, their hunger to talk. Initially, I was the only person recording the stories. Later, I trained a group of volunteers in deep listening, being present with illness and dying, and methods of documenting oral history. I also instructed them about the project's four-part process for recording mothers' narratives: a guided life review or autobiography; an in-depth interview on mothering through illness; an ethical will or legacy of spirit, meaning, and value; and personal messages for children. Mothers receive either an edited manuscript or a gift box of audiotapes. Volunteer listeners learn how to offer a valuable service while exploring their reactions to illness and death and gaining an appreciation for their own stories. They also participate in a Listeners' Circle, an ongoing group to support each other in the work.

Ten listeners, most of whom have remained with the project for more than seven years, have recorded seventy life stories. I also interviewed each mother about the story of her illness, specifically her experiences while mothering during cancer. Selected stories form the core of this book. It has been enriched by mothers in our focus groups, support groups, and writing circles, and by informal conversations with mothers, family members, individuals who lost parents during childhood, and health care professionals across the country.

While the stories were recorded, all of the women were living with cancer, the majority with breast cancer. Although many of them would survive for years, they were all facing the possibility of death at an early age: twenty-four to fifty-five. And each of them was raising children under eighteen. They were Asian American, African American, Caucasian, Hispanic/Latina, Native American, Near Eastern, citizen and immigrant, low, middle, and high income, well-educated and not, religious and not, single parent and partnered, adoptive and biological parents, heterosexual and lesbian. They were mothers of infants and toddlers, elementary school children, adolescents. They differed in parenting styles, personal styles, political beliefs, and attitudes toward illness.

Some of them were newly diagnosed and had just completed treatment. Some believed that they were cured and would only need periodic check-ups. Some were holding on tight through the roller coaster ride of each new treatment for aggressive cancers or for metastatic disease—cancer that had left its original site and migrated elsewhere in the body. Some knew that they had only a short time to live. A common desire led them to the Mothers' Living Stories Project. More than anything, they wanted to live long enough to fulfill the parental contract and see their children grow to self-sufficiency. They chose to review their lives and record their stories, as one mother said, "to tell my children how I feel and the things that are in my heart, all the things that I wanted to teach them." Each wanted to be sure that her children would know who their mother was and how she felt about them. They wanted to create a tangible gift that might help their children in the future. They wanted to be remembered.

The mothers' voices are sometimes filled with anguish, but there is far more than that. They have found ways to live with courage, dignity, humor, and joy and have taught their children to do the same. Now, through this book, they can teach all of us.

None of us escapes illness, loss, or grief. For those of us who become parents or have other important relationships with children, both wounding and healing can be especially complex. Part of the collective story of parents is to walk the wire of life with children in tow, trying to keep them from seeing too much too soon or from slipping off. This is hard to do in the best of times. After cancer, divorce, or other major loss, the equilibrium is challenged. Sometimes parents topple, and the children fall, too.

Today, when I think of parents doing their balancing act, I no longer focus on the kinds of questions so common in parenting parlance, as important as they are: How to balance paid work and family obligations? How to create "quality time" for kids and for adult relationships and for ourselves? How to juggle all the responsibilities without feeling exhausted or guilty? Mothers living with cancer struggle with these issues exponentially; their special perspective is illuminating for all parents. But, after witnessing these women's lives, I ask other questions. I ask whether we are willing to see and hear the whole of life—not only its beauty but also its brutality. What, besides a major crisis or loss, will force us to take a good look and to think about what we see? How can we learn to speak responsibly to each other and to children about suffering and death? And what is the price we pay for choosing our blindness, deafness, and silence?

The events of September 11, 2001, have made these questions urgent for all of us who feel responsible for future generations. Terrifying acts have shattered the illusions of the temporarily well and provisionally safe, pushing all of us to the edge and forcing us to address many of the same issues ill mothers have been living with in isolation. For the parental task is dual: to shelter children's psyches with necessary illusions during their long dependency, and to foster their ability to live in the real world by a process of gradual disillusionment. The real world contains health and sickness, life and death, hope and despair, strength and weakness.

Even with a grave injury, healing can take place. We may not be able to cure a physical disease or erase psychological damage, but, even in our final moments, we can strive toward wholeness. We can be parents who have open eyes and surer footing. How does healing occur? First, by accepting the truth of the wound. By experiencing the pain rather than running from it, and that includes letting our children have their own pain. Healing also occurs by imbuing the facts with meaning, texture, and voice—creating a story.

Story is at the heart of the project's work because I am convinced of its healing power. Stories can save us and can change us, transform the way we think about the injury. As healer and breast cancer survivor Deena Metzger says, "The story of the wound is not, 'I am wounded,' which has become the mantra of our victim-oriented culture. The story is, 'What does it mean to be wounded in this way? How do I carry the wound?' Sometimes the terrible wound can become the terrible gift."[2]

In telling their stories, the mothers in this book have transformed their terrible experiences with cancer into offerings. Arthur Frank, physician and cancer survivor, explains in *The Wounded Storyteller* that turning suffering into testimony is a moral act: In telling a "good story," one that has "narrative truth," the ill person becomes a witness and "rises to the occasion."[3]

The mothers have risen to the occasion by allowing their stories to be published in order to bring attention and support to parents living with any disease or major challenge. They also wanted to educate all those people who know someone who is sick or dying and would like to help more effectively but don't know how. Only a few mothers were initially motivated to record their stories as a way to heal themselves. Yet, that is what happened for each woman. Telling the cancer story helped to tame the trauma and to integrate it into the larger life narrative.

These are teaching stories. They teach by revealing what it's like to raise children with an awareness of mortality and by posing the big questions that confront us all at some point. They offer both positive and negative examples. You may resonate with one, not be interested in another, and feel repelled by a third. There can be learning in each instance. If you are ill, you may find that some stories speak to you now and others do not; take what you need.

This book is for those who are curious about the process of recording life stories, or how the limits of life can enrich living and parenting, or how the stories of ill mothers can reveal distortions in our cultural narratives of motherhood and of death. This book is also about the work of listening and how stories can heal those who receive them. Arthur Frank says: "One of our most difficult duties as human beings is to listen to the voices of those who suffer. . . . Listening is hard, but it is also a fundamental moral act." At the same time, "in listening for the other, we listen for ourselves."[4]

We listen to these women whose lives have been cracked open to see what really matters. We listen to them because each word counts when you want your children to know everything you understand about life, when you're speaking after you have been silent and are poised to be silent again. We listen to the mothers' words because they care so much about the world they will have to leave to their beloved children, because they have struggled to offer them, and us, a vision of hope and faith.

When I began recording mothers' stories, I realized that we would be engaged in holy work, holy in the way attending a birth is holy, coming close as it does to life's mystery. To honor the time we would spend together, I wrote a blessing to read at the beginning of recording and another to read at the very end. Similarly, when I began writing each day, I would ask for guidance to serve these women and their stories well as a faithful witness and messenger.

Each story, ranging from twelve minutes to twelve hours of audiotape, is worthy of a book. Indeed, the majority of transcripts were initially more than one hundred single-spaced pages each. My task was to whittle each down, discover its essence, and sculpt it into a chapter. I have tried to maintain the integrity of each woman's voice and her intent as I understood it. Occasionally, I add a word or phrase in brackets to define a term or clarify the mother's intention or emotions.

The publisher and I shared a commitment to bringing these women's stories to the community. For both of us, preserving the integrity of first-person voices while presenting easily readable texts was not an easy task. In order to honor and preserve the emotional immediacy, integrity, and singular music of each voice, we chose to maintain the authenticity of each mother's original speech.

Although almost all of the mothers agreed to have their identities disclosed, I have disguised them out of respect for the privacy of their families. Names of hospitals, medical practitioners, and other individuals are also fictitious. Responsibility for the selections, the editing, and the commentary is mine.

Preceding each of the three parts of the book is a chapter giving an overview of my personal and professional observations about the prior set of stories and introducing the next set, along with new themes. Within each story, my questions and reactions usually appear in italics. My reflections in no way suggest that I fully understand what individuals living with cancer endure. Nor am I comparing my own difficulties in parenting to the mothers'. But I hope to show something about the challenges and gifts of listening. To be fully present to another's experience is to open up to one's own. The willingness to face what another's story elicits in us, including the fear and pain, is a key requirement of being a good listener. It is worth the risk.

—Linda Blachman
Berkeley, California, November 2005

part ONE
Breaking Silence: Living with Primary Illness

ONE: "WATER IN A DESERT"
A CHORUS OF MOTHERS

SEVEN WOMEN CROWD into my home on a sunny Sunday morning. At my invitation, they help themselves to tea, bagels, and fruit and then find seats in the living room. They exchange tentative smiles and shy glances in greeting.

All are mothers living with breast cancer who have given up three precious hours to attend a focus group I have convened.

Just as we are about to begin, the eighth participant, Jude, hobbles to the door on crutches. Jude is thirty-eight and lives with two children under five and her husband, who is recovering from a heart attack. When I told her about the focus groups, she started sobbing, then explained, "I've been through three cancer support groups already and have been the only woman with young children. It's just been so lonely. I've broken my leg and my husband is on disability, but I'll pay for a taxi to get there."

That telephone call was my first clear indication from ill mothers of how invisible they feel, invisibility I had noticed during the year I spent exploring the resources available for parents with cancer. I looked forward to finding out if other mothers with cancer shared Jude's experience.

All eight mothers are now present; the group is ready to begin.

Dr. Carolyn Cowan, a project advisor and my co-facilitator for this group, opens with introductions. We had decided that Carolyn, a twenty-five-year breast cancer veteran, would ask most of the questions, allowing me to observe, take notes, and follow up as needed.

"All of you are mothers living with cancer. Why don't we start by going around the circle, and you each say your name, perhaps the age

of your child or children, and a little bit about what brought you here today?" Carolyn turns to the woman immediately to her right.

Mabel: My name is Mabel. I have a twenty-month-old son. I just finished treatment about four weeks ago. I'm a little in denial, I think, like the last eight months happened to someone else. I had a baby last year. When I was starting my treatment—I had a very aggressive tumor—I was thirty-two years old. I've really been healthy my entire life. I was considering having a breast reduction and saw a plastic surgeon who, just on routine examination, found a sizable lump. I had a mammogram, and three days later, I had a lumpectomy. Five of eighteen nodes were positive. I was shocked! They couldn't believe it because there's no history in my family, and I'd just had this baby, and everything was great in my life. . . .

So, going forward, you know, I think all the time about living a long time. *[Tearfully]* And we're not going to have any more kids. I kind of keep things in perspective, remember that each day is a gift, and try to not be overwhelmed by the fear. Because I think it's terrible to live in fear. I mean, I don't want it in my house. So I wanted to meet younger women to know how to deal with the issue of possible recurrence and what's going to happen down the line if it happens.

Carolyn smiles at the next woman, pale-skinned and blond, whose face is lined with pain.

Jennifer: I'm Jennifer. I have twin girls that are ten. It's going to be hard for me to talk. *[Choking back tears]* My husband died from cancer about two years ago. We went through three years of his being ill. I was trying to keep everybody together. So, when I was diagnosed last year, when the doctor first came out that I might have it, I just said, *I'm sorry, I don't want to know. If I have it, I'm going to die, so forget it, I'm not going to deal with it.* Fortunately, my lymph nodes were clean and [the cancer] was slow-growing, so the prognosis is reasonably good. I've just been trying to deal with it.

I went to a support group, and all the women that were talking to me had raised their families and had grandchildren. I couldn't identify with them. I just wanted to talk about kids. This is the first time I've talked to so many mothers with cancer.

Jennifer smiles tentatively, looking around the room. We all smile back and then study our hands while taking in the tragedy behind this mother's abbreviated story.

Lisa: My name's Lisa, and I have two children, a twelve-year-old daughter and a nine-year-old son. I'm two years out from my cancer, so they were ten and seven. I came to this group because I'm concerned about how to deal with this in the future. My mother had breast cancer, although she's still living, but I've been doing a family history and realized that with my great-grandmother, there was cancer on her side of the family.

My son was young enough that I don't know [if] he actually knew what was going on. I'm really concerned about my daughter. She would throw up every night before she went to sleep. That was really hard for me because I didn't know what to do for her. It seemed so physical. She would work herself up and throw up, and I felt so helpless not knowing what to do. It was, as everybody knows, crazy enough for yourself, and then trying to figure out how to support your children, too . . . God! It's so hard to be a parent regardless of whether you have breast cancer or not.

Since I've been diagnosed, she's been really scared, wanting to sleep in our room and not able to go to sleep at night. She kept saying everything in the room was moving fast. We have a little meditation room in our house, and so we went in there, and I tried to be with her as she was breathing and feeling scared. Then, all of a sudden, all this stuff started coming out about a couple of her friends at school that she was really upset with. They were making fun about her breasts because she was getting so developed. She said, "You guys are making fun about me, and you know that my mom had breast cancer and that I might get it!"

Then she said to me, "Grandma had it and you had it, and now I'm going to get it." I'm, like, *whoa*, 'cause I had no idea that was going on for her. No matter what they're saying or not, they're thinking so many thoughts.

She's doing well now. She's so grown up, I can't believe it. She came to me the other day and said, "Mom, I have this lump in my chest." At first I just sort of tossed it off and said, "Oh, it's just a breast bud." Then I realized I don't know what a breast bud is. *[Laughs]* So I had to call the doctor, and she said, "Don't worry, it's perfectly normal." But I'm concerned about how to prepare her for the very good possibility of developing cancer. I was even thinking about should I have her tested. So that's why I'm here.

Lisa exhales loudly, breaking the tension. Everyone laughs. She pulls her feet up and sinks into the overstuffed chair. Mabel slips off her shoes and stretches her toes. The women are settling in. Heads turn to Sandy, a tall, very thin woman who is next in the circle.

Sandy: I'm Sandy, and I was diagnosed with breast cancer—it will be two years in October. At the time, I had a fifteen-year-old who now is almost seventeen, and she to this day, can't discuss it. The first day, we sat down and I said, "I need to let you know that I have breast cancer," and she burst into tears and jumped up and said, "Well, it's early, isn't it?" Oh, boy.

Her father and I separated three years ago after twenty years of marriage, and it was kind of ugly at the end, and I got very depressed, and she became the parent for a while. Then, the next day, you find out you have cancer.

It's really affected our relationship a lot. It's so painful for her that she's kind of stepped away. Sometimes I think I'm not firm enough with her. At the same time, it's like you overdo. I think the hardest [thing] to deal with about being a parent was how guilty I felt. You have a child, and you are responsible for them, and this isn't what it's supposed to be. You're not supposed to make them scared, number one, and you're not supposed to die, number two.

She's relieved to see I'm doing better but still doesn't want to deal with it. It's something *I* have to keep dealing with every day. I am being treated for cancer—it's not gone. So, it's difficult. In our support group, there are two women with young children. When anybody says they're parents of young kids, everybody in the group just automatically cries—women who don't like children, women who've never had children. Everyone in the group will weep and change the subject.

Sandy shrugs her bony shoulders, sighs, and sits back. We pause for a minute to consider what she has said. Carolyn smiles at Sara, a short, plump redhead, who is next.

Sara: My name is Sara. I have two sons, almost four and twenty-one months. I'm in a support group that does address some of the issues because there are a few mothers in the group. But few of them work.

I work a full-time job. And I have always been looking for the mix of small kids, cancer, and work. But the most important issue to me is being a mother of young children and having cancer. And also being a child of a mother that died of breast cancer. So I'm grateful to have the opportunity to talk to other moms about that, and I would love to see my grandchildren. I'd love to get to my sons' bar mitzvahs. You know?

Everyone knows. Sara turns to Rose, a Chinese American woman with intense brown eyes. The pace picks up.

Rose: My name is Rose. I have a boy who just turned five and a girl who is two-and-a-half years old. I wanted to come to this group because I have been going to support groups on and off, but there wasn't anybody who was a mother of young children. So many of these groups—even new projects for younger women with breast cancer—don't take into account that people have young kids and some kind of accommodation needs to be made. It's like, we *do* have kids.

Everyone nods in agreement. A few murmur "Yes" and "That's right!" Irene, a petite woman with a dark mass of curly hair setting off an angelic face, begins to speak.

Irene: I'm Irene. I never thought I would get cancer. Never, ever, ever. I still think some days it can't really be possible. I was diagnosed in December with breast cancer. I have a three-year-old daughter. And the first thing I thought was: *I don't want this to affect my child.* It caused me such pain to think that Mia had to go through this.

We had already been dealing with having two years of surgery for a birth defect. Dealing with the medical field and finding them unsupportive, and trying to get child life services and the fact that there's nothing for three-year-olds. Even groups for kids having cancer start at five.

So, three months after her last surgery, to get the diagnosis felt like, *How could this be true?* Not just for me, but how could I ask this little girl to go through anything else? My first thoughts were about her and how to help her.

We had been planning to get pregnant again, but we waited—the medical stuff had been so intense and draining. Then I got my diagnosis. She had talked a lot about wanting a sibling, and when I got the mastectomy, she burst into tears and said, "But we were going to have lots of babies." I think maybe she made a connection between not having a breast and not having babies because she proposed we could warm up bottles of milk. "We could do that, Mom, we *could.*" She had a lot to say. "How can we be a family without brothers and sisters?"

I just sat and sobbed. And she cried. I tried to contain myself and said, "Well, we're not going to be having a baby right now. We're going to do *this* right now." I tried to be honest with her and support her. I wanted to tell her enough so that she understood but wasn't frightened. For a three-year-old, she's very articulate. She would say things like, "I'm worried that you're going to die from this," which was really hard. *[Chokes up and pauses]*

I feel like things are starting to settle down again. I just wish that there was more information. Especially for little kids. I really get frustrated that people seem to think either that a three-year-old doesn't need to know anything or she's too young to talk to about it. The books I was finding weren't great. You know, books about a mom having chemotherapy or in the hospital for a bone marrow transplant. It was hard to find something that was general enough but talked honestly about what is cancer, what does that mean? *[Turns to Lisa]* There wasn't a book to say, we'll go in the meditation room and we'll just be there—we'll see what comes out. Nobody gives you those kinds of ideas.

So, we just slogged through as we have with everything. I worked very hard because I wanted to be there for her, and I wanted to take care of myself. I've been doing more things for myself, going to two different support groups, and so sometimes I've been away from her more than I've ever been. That's been a challenge, to find that balance of being there and keeping things regular for her and focusing on myself. Having cancer and going through all this has been a humbling experience.

Irene stops and turns to the mother next to her, who has yet to speak.

Jude: Okay! My name is Jude, and I have two small children, boys, ages three and four. When I was diagnosed, I was thirty-seven. They were two and three. I am in a very long treatment right now because I had been misdiagnosed. So, I'm getting treatment which is taking a year, a solid year, and raising these two children. I've been in and out of a lot of support groups, and I had not met anybody with small children. *[Gesturing to Rose]* Except I met her one time, and she never came back. *[Both laugh]* I'd been looking the whole year to find women with breast cancer who are raising little children, you know, because the issues are so *[Points to heart]* right here. They dominate every day of my life. And it was *very* important to get to this project because I want to hear how women deal with an illness and children and survive.

Like the rest of us, Jude has been hanging onto every word as stories have begun to unfold. I note that mothers living with cancer want to tell the tales of mothering through illness, not unlike the desire most women have to exchange pregnancy and birth stories.

Carolyn comments on the range of life experience among the mothers, as well as the striking commonality of feelings and concerns. She suggests: "Perhaps we can continue with what your immediate concerns as a parent were at diagnosis for yourself and for your kids, how that's changed over time, and also what kinds of help you've needed and received." She turns to Jude, who quickly picks up where she left off.

Jude: In order to tell you a little bit about what I was feeling when I was first diagnosed, I have to give you a little domestic history.

I was always kind of physically overwhelmed with the two kids. My husband was working constantly, and my husband is also an alcoholic. Our only family is on the East Coast, so we have no familial support whatsoever, and we're very stretched economically. And then I found this lump. I went to my medical practitioners, and they went, "That's not a lump." The main practitioner told me that it was hormones. And it was a painful lump! She told me to go chart it for six months. She said it would go up and down and that would prove it was hormones. And I foolishly believed her. I was so overwhelmed just changing two kids' diapers, you know? And six months later, the lump was so big and my breast was so painful that I had to go in there and demand to see someone else. I said, "I will *not* see that woman who told me it was hormones."

Jude saw a surgeon who treated her for an infection for another six weeks. She was told that cancer rarely presents with pain, and her initial mammogram showed nothing, which is not surprising. Mammography can be unreliable for the dense tissue of young breasts leading to false negatives and, in some cases, to false positives and unnecessary procedures and anxiety. Or young women may discover suspicious signs of cancer on their own and then find that their concerns are not taken seriously. By the time Jude had a needle biopsy and double lumpectomy, seven months had passed and the tumors had grown. No one explained to her how large the tumors were; she discovered it by seeing her pathology report.

Jude: Then they told me, "We have to take your breast off immediately. First you'll have to have chemo, then you'll have to have radiation, and you have to start tomorrow." All of a sudden, this is an immediate emergency. And I couldn't understand. By that time, I was so disillusioned with the medical community that I wouldn't listen to a word they said. The doctors were working to save my life, but I didn't trust them anymore. I was so angry. I was like, "Excuse me? For seven months you said this was nothing." I was like, "Hold the phone here. I've got two little babies at home." And they were like, "Well, you know, yada, yada, it's a very aggressive tumor, yada, yada."

I had to force my doctors to put something else on the table than instant mastectomy. I said, "I cannot go spend weeks in the hospital. You put something else on the table right now while I research this and figure it out." I said, "I want more tests." You have to be your own advocate. It's unbelievable how they'll just shlep you around!

So, with very few economic resources, I had to become like a computer and start programming as much cancer information as I could, searching for a second opinion and doctors that I trusted. And you're scared. You don't know what will happen in treatment. The most important thing was functioning. How could I take care of my kids every day and go through cancer treatment? And the only person I met who had any word about that was Rose here. She said, "Chemo's pretty rough. I don't think you're going to be able to take care of your kids." She said it very honestly. "I think you should look for some help." That scared me, but at least it was somebody I knew and trusted 'cause she had kids.

From that point, I wanted to find good treatment and stop being so scared and try to resource a network to get through treatment on a daily basis, changing those diapers, dealing with those kids. We had no support network for daycare or anything at all. Since then, I have found subsidized daycare for both my children and gotten a second opinion and gotten into treatment.

I am now on my second course of chemo, okay? I started the Taxol a month ago. What happened, unfortunately, in between the Adriamycin and the Taxol is my husband—who was all of forty-one—had a heart attack. So I guess we're under a lot of stress.

Then I took a break. I had to care for the kids while he was in the hospital, and I couldn't have done it on the second chemo. I find I'm much better when I listen to myself instead of just doing what these medical people push me into. We're living on disability right now, his. And he's going back to work next week. The best thing about my husband's heart attack is it sobered him up. And things are calmer for my children—there's not as much fear around trust and life and death.

I had to learn how to tell my four-year-old, who was very cognizant that I was sick, about the disease. The three-year-old, he's not that clear. So I would tell him, "Mommy has a lump in her breast. Feel her breast. This is bad, the doctor's going to take it out. They may have to take it off." Then he said, "But, Mommy, I don't want you to not have a breast." I said, "Well, then they could make me another one." He got that. "Could they make you another one in two minutes?" [Laughs]

Okay. So we got through that, but that was after getting the emergency-fear-death thing out of the house. I had to learn from social workers not to let that out verbally. I was terrified that I was going to die immediately and my children were going to be raised by this alcoholic man, you know. So I had to go through support groups and find other ways to learn that women *will* survive cancer and treatment—just get a doctor you trust and a program you trust.

After we got the fear out of the household, my four-year-old came to me one day—he had picked up on my fear of dying—and he said, "Mommy, I'll never forget you." My biggest fear was that I was going to go away immediately, the way the doctors were talking, and he wouldn't even know who his mother was. So he comes over to take care of me by saying, "Mommy, I'll never forget you." That's his little caring way to say, "It'll be okay, we'll get through this, and I'll always have you in my heart." He's only four years old, and he says that to me.

Jude bows her head to cry a little and blows her nose. We all wait in silence. Rose reaches for the box of tissues, takes one, and passes the box to the others.

Jude: It's very important not to make promises to him that I can't keep. I want to let him know there's treatment and hopefully we have a future. I want to *express* hope. So I taught him that they're taking my lump out and giving me medicine that's making me sick. And when I get sick, my hair will fall out. And, after treatment, I will get better.

It's nice. Now we're living with cancer. We're not crying and dying and afraid of cancer. We get through it one day at a time, and things are calmer and better. And I'm very glad to know other women with children because if you guys can do it, I can do it. We can all do it.

By now, the mothers need no prompting. Lisa jumps in as soon as Jude makes it clear that she's done.

Lisa: I was diagnosed when my children were ten and seven. Obviously, with children that young, the biggest issue was survival, getting them to a stage where they could know that if anything did happen, they would be okay.

I can remember going to the oncologist the first time, and I barged in and said, "I need ten years. I don't care what you have to do." We were debating at that point whether chemo was necessary or not, and I was set on having it. I said, "If I don't do every possible thing I can do to get these ten years," which would have gotten both of them into college, "I won't be able to live with that." He said, "I really think that radiation would be fine." It was a small tumor, very early. I said, "No." Clearly *I* could have lived with it. But I couldn't live without knowing that I had done everything to get those ten years. The whole focus was on time. It wasn't on living and getting through this and being cancer-free. It had to be ten years. Nothing else was acceptable.

Sandy has been nodding vigorously and picks up where Lisa left off.

Sandy: When you said you want to get your kids older, since the day I got this diagnosis, it's been, "I need to have her in a good college and grounded, and I'll know then that it's okay." I say, "Well, at least she's in high school." You know, you always bargain. So now my bargain is next June; she'll graduate from high school. But I know that's to dampen my guilt. I keep saying, "If I keep getting her to the next step and then I'm not here anymore, she'll have a little more security, or she'll have more skills."

But then, in the support group the other night, a woman said, "Well, you need to wait until she gets her PhD. Knock off this negative

thinking! This is crap, you're still young! She's going to go to graduate school, and you need to keep being around." It was a good reality
check. At seventeen, she still needs her mother. I realize that there's no
ideal time.

Jennifer looks thoughtful as she addresses Lisa and Sandy: You
said that you did chemotherapy because of your children, and I decided
not to have chemotherapy because of my children. Had my husband
not gone through treatment, I probably would have done it. But I knew
that I couldn't. With my kids, you see, we had watched their father's
demise. My husband was okay *until* he did chemotherapy. Chemo for
him was useless, his cancer metastasized, he just went down. I couldn't
do it because of my kids.

Irene: The issue about getting these kids older is so important.
Before I went for my mastectomy, I had to find some peace around that
because I felt that it was one thing if I tried to accept my own death; it
was another thing to leave my child. That is excruciating. It wasn't just
that I wanted to be alive, but I want to be alive for *her.* How can I leave
this tiny person to deal with my death?

I really wanted to be rolled off to surgery and just have some peace
that my daughter would be fine. And I had to trust that she was going
to have her own path in this life. I don't know if I always believed that
at every moment, but that was the only way I could find any peace—
somehow she would be loved and supported and cared for, no matter
what. I don't want to leave her with the loss of her mom at such a
young age. And I think it also comes up in day-to-day parenting. I feel
like I want to be this more-perfect mom. I don't want her to remember
her mom yelling at her. I think it touches more guilt in me.

When I first thought about doing reconstruction, I thought, you
know, I can't do anything more that's going to get in the way of my being able to be a parent to her. At first I said, "No reconstruction at all,"
because it felt self-indulgent. But she kept asking when I was going to
get a breast. I did do reconstruction. She was actually happy about that.
[Looks around the circle] If you all would get a nipple, everything's
fine. *[Laughs]*

Rose: I'm trying to think how it was. I don't know that I ever felt
that way, that I needed to live longer for my kids. I'm sure I must have
at some point. But thinking back, it's almost like this big lesson of just

being present in each day. I hated chemotherapy. I didn't want to do it. I wanted to quit. I threw away the last week of pills. It was my only rebellion. And sometimes I think that if it comes back, there is no way I will go through chemotherapy again. I almost feel that I was really selfish. But it's okay, too, because that's how I needed to be during the whole thing. I gave myself total permission to be however I was and to feel whatever I was feeling. I also focused on day-to-day, being there with my kids.

We're overdue for a break. Over half of our time is gone; the women have begun to talk to each other, ignoring Carolyn and me. As I replenish the food, I listen to the excited voices of young mothers getting to know each other. Their stories trace the familiar paths of modern motherhood—love and commitment alongside ambivalence, guilt, and perfectionism, difficulties in balancing care for self with care for others, fear of being called "selfish"—all deeply furrowed by the encounter with mortality.

Anyone receiving a diagnosis of cancer or other life-threatening disease experiences a welter of emotions: shock, anger, terror, pain, grief. And the desire to live. But we differ in what makes us want to live so much that we will subject ourselves to brutal surgeries and treatments with side effects that are often harder to endure than the disease.

For each of these women, the fear of leaving her children without a mother seems to surpass the fear of death itself. Not every mother directs her fear into undergoing extensive treatment in order to buy time. But the basis for making decisions about treatment appears to be the perceived welfare of the children, even when the mother's personal needs vie for attention.

When we reconvene, I invite the mothers to say more about their experiences, especially as parents, with healthcare providers and with community resources.

Mabel: After you've gone through treatment, every time you go to the doctor, you wonder, *What's he going to tell you?* My big fear for my children is that I'm going to go to the doctors and they're not going to find something until it's too late. I've discovered a lot of women have to struggle to get people to listen [when they say] that there's something wrong.

Rose: I had very intense effects from the chemo and radiation.

I was already working too much when I was diagnosed—about sixty to seventy hours a week. My doctor didn't know I had two kids under five at home and was working like that. When I started treatment, he said, "Oh, you don't have to change your life." My husband said, "Great." So I only missed one day of work during the whole year I was getting treatment. I fell apart when it was all over. I was very, very sick for a long time after. So I've refocused my life. But I didn't find any written resources about what to tell the children.[1] Very few medical practitioners even asked, "Do you have children?"

Irene: I agree. Nobody ever asked me, "Are you a mother?" That question never came up from the medical people or even the complementary practitioners. Who will take care of your child? What will happen if you have chemotherapy? How are you going to get to treatment? Who's going to come with you if your husband's taking care of your daughter? People need to wake up and realize this disease is happening to many younger women with younger children.

Sara, the redhead who has said very little up to now, seems fired up.

Sara: From medical professionals, I wanted compassion. Partly as a parent, partly as a woman with an illness that was potentially long-term, I needed to be able to talk to somebody. I needed a doctor who understood that I had kids. When you're making decisions, that they would understand about that. I envision a very small thing: *Ask* the moms what is it that they need. Ask the moms. But I think the medical profession thinks: *People are going to be intimidated, and people are going to do what we say.*

I come from a counseling background, and I see that professionals are setting their boundaries because it is very stressful. I feel like they need to open their boundaries up a little bit. I do my own exit interview and tell them, "I hope that when other patients come in here, you will ask them about their lives." I understand they have to deal with a lot of people. But it feels right to me that doctors see the people behind the cancer. Not just the doctors. It's the technicians taking the blood. It's the nurses. It's the schedulers. It's everyone.

It has to start with the frontline people, who are the schedulers. They're, like, big people in your life. They're just doing their job, you know, they have millions of people that have cancer coming to their door every day: "This is urgent!"

I remember the radiation oncologist was fabulous, the technicians were fabulous. They asked me about my kids. The radiologist said, "Is there anything I can do for you?" I said, "Yes, find a cure." *[Prolonged laughter from the group]* And he said, "This is the cure." Of course, he was bullshitting me. But I felt good that he was being positive.

But the scheduler was the problem. She said, "Okay, you'll come Friday at six PM. You'll come Tuesday at twelve-thirty." And I said, "Excuse me? I can't do that. I have kids, I have to pick them up, I have to go to work." I'm working part-time now, so I'm really scrambling. And she goes, "No, we can't do that." Then I melted down—I was screaming. I had to get a social worker to intervene to get me the time that I needed. But I had to fight. All the energy . . .

I'm always amazed by the way that people treat you. There's an automatic assumption that if you're having radiation, then there's nothing else in your life but this, and it offends me. It would be so simple to say, "What's going on in your life? Is there a time that works for you?" They need to know that we want to empower ourselves, we want to be with our kids, we want to be at our jobs. It's not being in denial. It's *we want our whole life as much as we can.* They don't always get that. I don't feel like they're trained. It's not their fault. But someone should say, "Be sensitive. These women are on edge."

Jennifer: Right! I got a little wiggy, so they sent for the social worker. *[Laughter]*

Voices: Yup, they do, they do. Get the shrink!

Jennifer: The radiation got a little old. You had to go thirty-six days. My whole back is burned, you figure they're frying your heart, so I started yelling at them. They kept saying, "Wouldn't you like to see someone?" *"No! I'm fine!"* So one day they said, "We've sent for the social worker." We had a long talk, and she said, "You seem a little stressed." *"What do you mean?"* So we reviewed the seven hundred things I was doing, and she said, "Well, you could go on disability." I didn't think that was the answer, but it was funny. It's like you don't get permission to be mad.

Voices: Yeah!

The mothers have been nodding, laughing, and wiping away tears.

They recognize that anger, action, and sometimes a well-timed melt-down can demand attention and be antidotes to frustration and terror. Failing to get their needs met, these women may act in ways that are immediately effective but are also exhausting and sometimes get them labeled as "aggressive" and "demanding."

The drive to stay alive for the children and the fear behind it quickly translate into the desire to be taken seriously by medical practitioners, which becomes another fear: that their doctors will fail them in some way. Certainly, women have positive experiences with some physicians, but doctors often minimize the effects of a cancer diagnosis and treatment on the family, in part to try to make everyone feel better. The lack of attention to the complexities of ill mothers' lives can have disastrous medical and emotional consequences, as Rose testified.

The possibility of misdiagnosis, delayed diagnosis, or simply not being listened to is magnified for low-income and uninsured women, uneducated women, and women of color, all of whom face additional barriers to healthcare. These barriers may contribute to the disproportionately high death rate from breast cancer for African American women.[2] I mention these concerns to the group and invite their thoughts.

Rose: There are all these women out there who are getting nothing. They don't have resources, they don't have time, they don't have child-care, and who is helping them? A lot of people get treated at the county hospital, and if they have doctors that are busy . . . it's like they're slogging through this on their own. So much of what has gotten me through this is having friends and resources, and knowing how to work my way through the medical profession.

Mabel: Women need to learn how to negotiate, and they need to learn how to yell at their insurance companies at a time when they have no self-worth and no energy. A skill as important as talking to children is knowing how to fight the system. Some of the women I know have had terrible experiences with doctors. There have been major errors, they've been disrespected, no returned phone calls, insurance companies canceling surgery the day it was going to be, saying you're not eligible, so that's a thing that women need a lot of help with.

Irene: I know some people don't make it to treatment because they don't know where the bus is, or the bus didn't come, and there's nobody to take care of their kids. There should be drop-in childcare in all treatment centers.

Jude: You ask us what women who are living with illnesses and children need. I hear everyone saying we need resources for functioning with children and a disease on a daily basis. What we need the most isn't there.

When I first got the diagnosis, I found out that there were these huge networks of cancer support groups, and the women I called were all so wonderful. So I thought, well, *of course it's going to be out there for women with children and cancer.* And there was nothing. I called cancer support networks, I called the American Cancer Society, and the women in the cancer organizations go, "I'm so sorry. We don't know anything like that. We don't know who to refer you to. Call the Red Cross." I called the Red Cross, I called the Salvation Army, I called Catholic Services. *There are no comprehensive resource organizations to help mothers living with chronic illnesses raise children.* There are no resource directories, there are no resources.[3]

My biggest fear after the doctor told me I wouldn't be able to care for my kids was, what happens when we cannot afford for my husband to take off from work on the day or two after the chemo, when I'm so sick that I can't get up and change my child's diaper? What's going to happen? Is Protective Services going to come and take my children away because they're not well fed? I want a phone number where I can call someone and say, "Is there some kind person who'll come a day or two a week after the chemo treatments and help me on the days I can't stand up? Is there someone else who could come on the days that my children have to go to daycare?"

We have to have some resources. And the emotional is just as important as the physical. You know, getting referred to therapy is just as important as getting somebody to bring a meal. It's all happening at the same time. It's not like you can go, "Okay, emotions wait, diapers now. Okay, emotions on, diapers off." I've had to learn to take it one day at a time, one diaper at a time, one meal at a time, one temper tantrum at a time, one chemo treatment at a time.

Sara adds: And you can't ask your family if you have one. I mean, you *can*, but I don't want to keep asking and asking. It's hard to say, "Can you help me again?" You use up asking. It's better to be able to go to someplace that would understand from the professional perspective. If there was such a resource, it would at least acknowledge that this is part of what happens when women are ill and have young children. And you wouldn't have to struggle with yourself and ask, "Is it bad enough today for me to ask someone? Maybe it'll be worse another day, and I'll wait. I'll see if I can stand it."

Jude: You have to learn that it's okay to start reaching out, and then the resources have to be there. But the mother has to not feel guilty about not doing her job and realize it's time to get help. Where I'm getting my counseling, they have a sign up that says, ASKING FOR HELP IS A SIGN OF STRENGTH. But the woman has to be able to do that instead of sitting there scared and overwhelmed. If I hadn't done that, I might still be in emergency hysterical mode.

Cancer is becoming chronic.[4] We're talking about a chronic epidemic, where women are raising kids and living with it every day. Surgeons are very nonverbal. Their bedside manners are horrible, okay? But one thing the surgeon did say at the time I was sitting there in shock after he finally used the C–word on me is that cancer's really changing for women. He said, "There's a lot of it out there, but what's happening now is women are living with it. Just because they use the word 'cancer' doesn't mean women are all dying any more."

It's so important to change that emergency keyword. Instead of being *"Terror! Fear! Die!"* it's "We're going to deal with it, we're going to cope with it, and we're going to do it one diaper at a time, one treatment at a time, one support group at a time." It's very important to get that out into the world: It's turning into a chronic disease where we're living with it, not dying with it. And that's what the title of your project is about, and that's what the stories will do. *[Voices agreeing]* Stories of *living* mothers. Because you *are*—you're living with it. You're always going to be living with it.

Several voices: Yeah. Right!

By now, the women have spontaneously begun to talk about their relationships and people's reactions to their illness. Carolyn asks: "What about your relationships outside the healthcare system? What kind of help have you wanted? How have others responded?"

Mabel: There have been a lot of very pleasant surprises. The people that have trouble dealing with it, that's just how they are. A lot of people really were there in a nice way. It's helpful to feel that you're not so alone in this whole situation. People showed you sides that you didn't know they had.

Voices: Yeah. That's true.

Lisa: My husband and I were fighting. We got in a huge argument the night before my mastectomy. But he was incredible. He was the best there was, and he was the worst there was. God!

Mabel: [Laughs] When I was first diagnosed, I think I worried more about my husband and how he would deal with the kids if I died!

Sara: Although my husband loves me very much, I have not found him to be the most supportive person in this situation. He can't be—it's too much for him. I'm not giving him an excuse. I've got lots of anger about it. I've known that I need more things like this group and my friends. I can't rely just on him.

Work has been my salvation. It's made me feel competent. My job covers my insurance. That's why I keep my job—I'm afraid not to have insurance now. But the other neat thing that I've found is my boss. I've heard bad stories of people losing their jobs. But my boss took a different approach, and if I was to die at some point soon, she can feel really, really great about how she treated me. Because she went so out of the way to be compassionate: "Take care of yourself, leave early, don't worry about it." She was the person that got all my donated sick days for me. And she continues to say, "Whatever it is that you need to do, your job is not an issue. All the things that you're scared about are not an issue. Maybe your kids are going to be sick, it's okay. These are *your* sick days now, and you are to use them how you're going to use them."

My sister called to give me a phone number of a support group, and she said, "You really need to be in one of these groups because otherwise your friends and family will get tired of hearing." I knew what she was saying. She didn't want to have to listen to it. But at the same time, when I went to get radiation, she had made all these arrangements with the hospital. So I've decided to let people help in any way they want. Guess what? Everybody can have a job.

But, boy, people get angry at you or avoidant because it's so scary. They love you, and they're afraid. You wanna say, "God, it's not catching!" I always thought it would be awful to have AIDS. After having cancer, I realize how truly awful it must be to have a disease that there is no cure for and that people blame you for having and also feel they'll catch. People are so uptight.

Kindnesses shown during hard times make lasting impressions, as in Sara's story about her boss. But for every positive story, there is usually a negative one, sometimes within the same relationship. These experiences linger, too.

Mabel: I work for a small public relations agency, mostly women, about forty or fifty employees. And they were all really great in action. They cooked meals and did this and that. But I found that when people came over and talked, a lot of times they wouldn't really want to hear it, they couldn't deal with it, as much as I think they wanted, in their hearts, to help out. I wish that there were more people who would listen to us when we're hurting inside and we don't have anybody to talk to, to pay attention and give us a few minutes of their time, give us moral support and encouragement. That's what we want.

Jennifer: I'm amazed at how much I have to do to help people deal with me. My boss was horrible, just horrible. I said, "I'm going to need some help. I can't do these long hours." And he looked at me and said, "Jennifer, everybody's got their own private radiation. You're not the only one. Do you want to keep this job or not?" Here I'm trying to support my kids, my house. So I ended up doing it. But it was horrible. So what I find I have to do is not only keep it inside myself, but I have to support them, sort of "jolly" them to make them feel okay. It's like you're Typhoid Mary—"We'll get it." Or like you're a disaster—"Don't come too close." I got really depressed.

Other women jump in and respond to Jennifer:

"Because then they have to feel the feelings that it brings up for them about you dying or their own dying. You're so vulnerable, and you're bumping up against people's vulnerabilities."

"People are scared of cancer. It's pretty scary. You can deal with it if you have to and it's in your world, but you don't want to know about it. I used to be that way too."

"People are so bad if they don't know how to deal with it, so instead they make you the wrong person."

"It's their own fear."

"They either get angry or avoid you."

Cancer is not contagious. Fear is. And fear is epidemic where it concerns disease, disability, and aging. Whether senior citizen or young parent, physician or patient, we're frightened when it comes to serious illness and loss invading our own lives or the lives of those we love. However well intentioned we may be, our fears infect our relationships with those who are living with illness and loss. Fear determines whether and how we offer help. It informs our judgments about the ill and our projections onto them. It influences whether we invite an ill person to talk or whether we let her know by our distance, comments, or facial expressions that we don't want to listen. The issue is not fear: We all have it. The issue is how we carry our fear and bring it to a manageable level. Will we come forward with compassion and hang in there in spite of the fear?

The entrance of mortality into the mothers' consciousness opened up a hornet's nest of their own fears. In each group, the passion of the stories that poured out indicated just how much had been bottled up, how much terror the women were living with, how hungry they were to listen to each other, how alone they had been with their experience. As one mother said: "I loved hearing everybody's stories. It was like water after being in a desert."

As I prepared for writing this book five years after the focus groups, I listened to the tapes again and was reminded of something that I hadn't been able to get a handle on earlier. It had to do with the way the first group was scheduled for two hours but the women didn't want to leave, so we scheduled later groups for three hours, and the women still didn't want to leave. It had to do with the way the sounds in the middle and end of the sessions were completely different from the awkward, reserved beginnings. It was the way hushed, respectful listening to a story would be followed by peals of laughter or shared tears or a chorus of voices interrupting each other to talk at once. It was the sound of silence being broken.

TWO: HOLDING PATTERNS

A CANCER DIAGNOSIS enters a home like a powerful force of nature. It pushes things aside, takes up residence, demands attention. Everyone in the vicinity is affected, whether or not emotions aroused by the invader's presence are expressed.

Jude's doctor was right in saying that many cancers are now chronic illnesses rather than precursors to an immediate or inevitable death. Advances have been made in medicine and in cultural attitudes and language. The word "cancer" has gradually replaced familiar euphemisms—the "C-word" in speech, "a long illness" in obituaries.

Nevertheless, certain diseases—cancer being one of them—automatically raise the specter of death and, therefore, fear. Buddhist teacher Pema Chödrön says, "All fear is fear of death." Fear is a powerful emotion that can mobilize action and speech or invite denial, paralysis, and silence. In our culture, the latter prevail. We now have a hospice movement, a death-and-dying industry, and scores of books and television specials that portray the experience of dying. But death and its handmaidens, illness and aging, remain the elephant in America's living room.

What do we do with the elephant? Generally, the ill and well alike try not to think about it, try not to talk about it. We certainly don't prepare for it. Seventy percent of American adults have not made wills, much less recorded their ethical wills or legacies.[1] Why plan for that which we can endlessly stave off? All of us have been exposed to the culture's emphasis on mastery and control, buttressed by extended life expectancies. Most of us have internalized the message that we should be able to cure all illness and overcome all odds, even—especially—death.

Listening to the mothers talk about their fears, I understand why we can learn so much from them. They do not have the luxury of denial. The invader is already in their living rooms. So are the kids. As Jude said, "It's all happening at the same time." The whole catastrophe is right there, inescapable. Living with cancer and children means sharing space with death and continuing to embrace life, both under the same roof.

The women in this and other focus groups were pleased to be in a place where they could openly express their feelings and discuss the complexity of their experiences. They talked and talked. And, as they did, they answered some of the questions my colleagues and I had formulated, while raising others.

First, they helped us begin to identify the many needs of ill mothers: talking with the children about sickness and death, having an array of supportive services and information easily available, and finding others with whom they could speak about the issues closest to their hearts. Mothers with cancer loved being together, but they also wanted to be acknowledged outside the cancer circle. They wanted to be seen as alive as long as they were alive.

Second, the mothers had found neither services nor literature specific to their needs. Nor had they heard about the few resources I had located. They were too overwhelmed with medical decision-making and treatments to seek them out, and the scarce resources were difficult to find.

Third, mothers did not feel seen and had found few opportunities to be heard *as mothers*, whether by their physicians or by representatives of most organizations serving the ill. The invisibility of their particular concerns, coupled with the lack of support, heaped additional stress on them.

The mothers also validated what I had assumed to be obvious. Their children were their first thought at diagnosis, the driving force behind treatment decisions, and the source of their greatest anxiety and anguish as well as of their joy. If mothering hadn't been central before cancer, it was now.

The centrality of the children made the lack of attention to parenting concerns in the community even more apparent. Even when childrearing is shared with a spouse or partner, a mother's incapacity compromises the functioning of the entire family. Under the best of circumstances, mothers need support in raising children. It seemed logical that during illness, their needs would be greatly intensified.

Back in 1977, when I gave birth, long before mothers' support groups and parenting education proliferated, I thought, *What could be more obvious than a first-time mother's need for some loving care, basic information, mentoring, and help?* When I founded the project, I wondered, *What could be more obvious than a seriously ill mother's need for resources and support?* And yet, in the mid-1990s, the needs of these women were as unacknowledged and unmet as those of most mothers twenty years earlier.

Why was there so little curiosity or consciousness about the plight of mothers with cancer? These women were having to hold their children against chaos and terror, often by themselves. What was holding *them*?

Following the focus groups, I met with project advisors to discuss our direction. The project initiated Mothering Through Cancer support groups, which became an important resource for some San Francisco Bay Area mothers, as well as a laboratory for our learning. With the volunteer effort and initiative of one of the mothers, we also published the Bay Area Resource Guide on Parenting Through Cancer to spare the mothers and their families countless hours of research about how to help their children.

But I couldn't shake the bigger questions. Why the magnitude of the silence? Why were mothers hidden, even within the breast cancer community?

I assumed that fear of cancer and its association to death were partially responsible and that the stigma and invisibility borne by ill mothers was similar to that of other sick and disabled people, especially cancer patients.[2] Yet, cultural attitudes had not stopped the proliferation of cancer support groups, research studies, books, articles, associations, and agencies serving individuals with a range of medical issues. Why were most new studies of young women with cancer during prime childbearing years neglecting to ask about mothering?

The silence seemed to go beyond what some representatives from tumor registries called "the difficulty of adding new data elements," what some medical practitioners described as "the lack of time to focus on anything but disease and treatment in the HMO era," and what some in the cancer community insisted was "the focus on older women because breast cancer has been an older women's disease." It even went beyond what several researchers called "the invisibility of certain women's health issues."

Something was terribly wrong with the picture. Denial and fear of death is a necessary but insufficient explanation for ignoring mothers living with cancer. I began to suspect that the fear-based reactions to the women in the focus groups had as much to do with our cultural confusion about motherhood as with mortality. The reactions had to do, more accurately, with the combination of both, which meet in the lives of these mothers. If being sick is generally depressing and frightening, if cancer raises the specter of death, if death is to be avoided at all costs, then seriously ill mothers of young children strike an emotional chord on an altogether different scale.

Friends and colleagues agreed. Edd Conboy, psychotherapist and member of the project's steering committee, said, "Very few can think about the mortality of our own mothers, even as adults, because for the child to think of being without a parent is unbearable. There is a healthy unconscious delusion about the permanency of mother. The world can't exist without her."

When any of us hear that a young mother is sick, our hearts may go out to her, but we tend to identify more with the frightened or bereft child. A rift in the most primal bond threatens all of us. As Sandy found in her support group, and as I was beginning to discover, when mothers with cancer talk about their experiences, "Everyone in the group will weep and change the subject."

We cry. We don't know what to say. We run in the other direction. Mothers have always been the screen upon which we project our greatest longings and worst nightmares, often missing the imperfect human being underneath. The cult of motherhood, with its assignment of total responsibility and inflated expectations to one ordinary woman raising children, doesn't help.

Mothers give us life and are supposed to create the conditions in which life can be nourished and sustained. Mothers are supposed to protect children from pain, sorrow, and loss. Mothers are supposed to be strong, reliable, resilient. Mothers must not become ill or dependent. Mothers are not supposed to die. This is the mother we all want. This is the mother a woman hopes and expects to be. Anything else is unthinkable.

Mothers with cancer are living the unthinkable. The individual narratives of these women were being played out against the backdrop of a much larger story involving our worst fears. The denial of mortality and the denial of the dark side of motherhood intersect in the lives of ill mothers, who then bear the unfortunate burden of our projections.

Our culture's narratives are not generous enough to hold these women's experience. The stories we tell ourselves about mortality are too narrow to include the possibility of our mothers' deaths, much less our own. The motherhood myth, which has changed far less than we'd like to believe, is similarly constricted. It does not recognize the possibility of death, or even the possibility of human limitation, fatigue, or failure.

Like all mothers, a mother living with cancer can be dependent or despondent, crave rest and relief, struggle with failings and desire and temper. But, unlike most mothers, these women cannot dissemble. Cancer cracks open their stories, forcibly enlarging the range of life experience to include illness and the threat of death. Critical illness creates a motherhood in which a woman's flawed humanity cannot be ignored.

Another question had become increasingly urgent: While the mothers cared for their children, who was caring for the mothers? This question, I came to realize, was related to one I am frequently asked: Why, of all the needs mothers living with cancer have, did recording life stories become the core of my work?

First, I have used writing through most of my life as a way to release emotion, explore my thoughts, and better understand myself and my surroundings. This led me to study the health benefits of oral and written narratives and to train in oral history methods. Numerous studies demonstrate the therapeutic effects on the immune system of writing about personal trauma and emotions.[3] I also knew that listening to ourselves tell our stories and having them empathetically witnessed and responded to is the basis of most counseling and psychotherapy.

Second, over the years of my work in family health and parenting, I had taken as axiomatic that what is done for children must also be done for primary caregivers. I wanted as much to create a healing process for the mothers as to prepare a tangible legacy that would help their children. The project offers mothers a "holding environment" made up of two elements—a caring relationship and the midwifing of story within that relationship. These are two of the things children need in beginning the precarious human journey. The ability to create meaningful narratives of self and world develops within a secure human attachment.

Ultimately, I put story at the center of our work because I was convinced of its healing power, reflected in the statement attributed to Isak Dinesen, "All suffering is bearable if it is seen as part of a story." All of us suffer, and all of us live through story. Barbara Meyerhoff, anthropologist and author of *Number Our Days*, also said it well: "People everywhere have always needed to narrate their lives and worlds, as surely as they have needed food, love, sex, and safety. . . . *Homo narrans*, humankind as storyteller, is a human constant."[4]

In childhood, we begin creating narratives of our lives. We take the threads of parental messages, family stories, religious beliefs, ethnic and national tales, cultural myths, experiences, dreams, and imaginings, and we weave provisional answers to our questions about ourselves, others, and the world into a coherent and, we hope, durable fabric. These answers become sustaining stories.

Stories fulfill two of our deepest human needs: meaning and connection. They connect us to our own experience, to each other and our communities, to those who came before and those who will come after. They give us a notion of identity and place, make sense of events, and allow us the feeling of control, however illusory. Stories, in other words, are conceptual structures, containers that make us feel secure by taming chaos into meaningful patterns. They also have transformative aspects. Our stories, like our lives, are not immutable. They are works in progress, offering the possibility of revision and change, and of hope.

Things are always happening in life to shake up our life narratives. Sometimes, change happens through conscious choices to write our lives differently. We may add new characters, new events, new roles, or new chapters. A woman may, for example, choose to become a mother. A prospective mother has to make room in her psyche, as well as her body, to welcome a new being, role, set of ideals, and expectations. Motherhood poses questions: What kind of mother do I want to be?

How will my life change? How will I hold onto my self? New questions and roles demand new stories that expand and alter the previous narrative. The revised story of "myself as mother" will be constructed from the experience of being mothered, the desire to repeat or change that example, the experience with other maternal figures, familial and religious expectations of mothers, private fantasies and hopes, and messages about motherhood in the media and the arts. A young woman takes all this in and crafts a working model of herself as mother, a story about who she will be. From all the warring impulses and images, she struggles to find a way to be "good enough."

As a mother shapes her own narrative, she simultaneously creates a holding environment to cradle her infant's vulnerable psyche. She teaches her children values and essential lessons in living by example, by daily tasks of care, and by implicitly or explicitly telling stories.

The first stories are preservative and conservative, addressing protection, the most basic responsibility of motherhood: "I will always be here for you." "I will protect you and keep you safe." "The world is a trustworthy place." A mother needs other powerful stories in order to fulfill a second critical task—to facilitate the growing child's development. "I want a better life for you or, at the very least, as good as I've had." "I want opportunities for you to develop your potential." And still other stories fulfill a third maternal imperative, to socialize children into the prevailing culture and subculture. "I want you to behave well, to fit in, to be accepted and acceptable."[5]

Our lives and, therefore, our stories are always under construction, being revised against experience. Stories of protection, growth, and socialization continue to evolve, trailing the evolving consciousness and choices of both mother and child.

But sometimes, we are not the authors of change writing our lives— rather, we are written upon. We construct a story-shelter on sand, and then something unpredictable comes along and blows the house down: a divorce, the death of a loved one, the loss of a job, an accident, an earthquake, a diagnosis of cancer.

Uninvited changes seize us, threaten our sense of meaning and control, undermine security and trust. Suddenly, the stories we've told ourselves about who we are, how the world works, and what matters no longer hold. We're shaken, disoriented.

Arthur Frank states that illness "wrecks" stories because the "present is not what the past was supposed to lead up to, and the future is scarcely thinkable."[6] The big questions of identity, value, and faith reopen: What does it mean that I am now disabled, ill, dying? Who am I if I can't do the things I used to do? Where is God? How do I live in a shattered world?

When our lives are rent, how we go on depends in some measure on how, in Rainer Maria Rilke's words, we will "live the questions." The psychological and spiritual tasks in the face of a fractured narrative are to find new answers by assigning meaning to the event and somehow enlarging and adapting our story to accommodate it. As Frank says, storytelling is "repair work on the wreck."[7]

For a mother facing trauma, the questions and the tasks are doubled. When a mother's universe is threatened, so is her children's. Even when children seem unaware, the mother carries for them the dangers, the pain, and the fear. She must rebuild her own sense of coherence in order to present them with a tolerable reality. Like Jude, she has to get the terror out of the house or, at least, bring it down to manageable proportions.

This is where the mothers were when the listeners and I met them—in the midst of their torpedoed stories, striving to make sense of what had happened to their lives, to understand who they were becoming through the illness, and to find ways to contain their fear and communicate safety, sanity, and hope.

And this is what the listeners and I have tried to offer the mothers, what each of us can learn to offer others in need: the opportunity to review a life, to find a voice, to share suffering, and to seek and tell the true stories. How? By asking open-ended questions and by compassionately holding the answers: Tell me your story, tell me what it's been like for you to parent through illness, tell me what you want others to understand about what you're going through, tell me what you want your children to know.

The mothers in the focus groups introduced many common themes. Now, it is time to listen to the story of a single life over time.[8] The following chapters show how individual mothers at different stages of illness are revising stories for themselves and their children in light of cancer. Each story includes enough personal history to provide an understanding of the impact cancer had on a mother's life. We start with three women who are living with a first-time diagnosis of primary breast cancer: Diana Loew, Marge Schmitt, and Lorraine McKinley.

THREE: "SECRETS MAKE YOU SICK"
DIANA LOEW

A BROWN-SHINGLED HOUSE deep in the woods. Uneven stone stairs that lead to a long front porch strewn with toys and tools. A robust man in a plaid flannel shirt chopping wood near one end of the house—Diana's husband, Timothy.

She greets me with a hug after ushering me into a modest L-shaped living-dining room filled with comfortable furniture. Children's arts-and-crafts projects are displayed everywhere—on the walls, the refrigerator door, the living room floor.

Diana Loew is a small woman whose short, black curls frame her face. Dark brown eyes crinkle and disappear when she laughs. She laughs often—at the mess in the house, which she apologizes for, at the newly adopted black kitten, which knocks over a lamp, and at herself for forgetting to put the kettle on. As I set up the tape recorder and Diana prepares tea, I suggest that if it feels comfortable, she might consider creating a small ritual to begin each session, such as reading a prayer or poem or lighting a candle. Diana chooses a small, multicolored candle she and her children made almost a year ago. "It's funny that I never lit it. I guess it's been sitting around, waiting for the right time."

The right time for Diana is now, at forty-four years old, four years after ending her treatment for primary breast cancer. Life has returned to something like normal. Her hair has grown back, and her energy, natural optimism, and love of good food have long since returned. She is working again full time as a primary school teacher.

Diana wants to record her life story mostly for her two

daughters, Katie and Lorna, but also for herself. She wants to reflect on the place of the cancer experience in the entirety of her life and to share what she's learned with others: "I got so much from other women who were going through breast cancer at the time that I was. I think it's just one big circle of people receiving and giving, and this is a way of giving back."

Diana was the first mother whose story I recorded. I chose to begin with her because she had already passed through the cancer crisis, she had both a professional and personal perspective on children's needs, and she was eager to share her story.

Although she complains of being overworked and juggling too many responsibilities, Diana seems to manage it all without excessive conflict. Her priorities are clear. "Just working with kids and being a mother has been very fulfilling for me. That makes my life have purpose." Her children attend the school at which she teaches, in the same tight-knit rural community where her family lives. "I'm just one of the cogs. That's a good place to be—taking care of my little corner." Art, nature, and social justice are also among her passions.

The words "safety," "protection," and "comfort" are sprinkled throughout Diana's story and her philosophy of child rearing. She considers herself fortunate to have grown up with economic ease in a loving family, surrounded by a community of adults with social and political commitments, people who served as strong role models. Her childhood was unblemished by serious illness, loss, or trauma.

Diana set out to create the same safe, comfortable world for her daughters, and, to a large extent, she has succeeded. The story she intended and the one she lives with her family are congruent. She and Timothy feel blessed with a strong marriage—"We keep working at it," she says—and two "easy kids."

But no matter how idyllic a life looks from the outside, we cannot presume to know the internal reality. As my father used to say, everybody's got their little bundle of sorrows.

As an adult, Diana experienced several deaths in her extended family, which had a big impact on her. "I don't know if I was afraid of death, but I don't think I ever really had to face it. In our family, we had rather toodled along and made it many years without a close death. Then, nine years ago, my sister had a baby who lived only eleven days and died in her lap. There was an illusion of innocence and good fortune before that, and it took down that curtain. My only aunt and her husband died within two years of each other, both of cancer. She was just fifty-two. Those deaths and others have contributed to my feeling that a life is a life is a life, however long it is. It can be a day or eleven days or fifty-two years or ninety years, and there is no saying when a life is complete."

Although the intrusion of mortality temporarily exposed an alternative view of reality, none of these losses threatened Diana's belief that life made sense, until her father, without warning, left her mother after forty years of marriage, exploding the happy-family myth. The divorce dismantled her beliefs about "the way things are" and left her angry with her father, who was shocked that adult children would be so upset. Her father didn't know that divorce tears apart the story of safety and continuity upon which even grown children depend, especially when they are parents trying to create a similar story for their own youngsters.

The divorce reinforced Diana's belief that "a child grows up needing to believe their parents." She had just struggled to explain Grandma and Grandpa's divorce to her children when her cancer diagnosis imposed yet another narrative line, another set of concerns about truth, lies, reality, and responsibility on herself and her children. It didn't help that her father was diagnosed with lung cancer during the same year. This time the curtain stayed down. But rewriting her post-divorce family script and pondering the big questions had to wait while her illness took over.

Immediately after a cancer diagnosis, the questions a woman asks herself are sharp, fear-driven queries concerning survival. Diana describes what those early months were like.

DIANA

Late in the fall of '92, I started feeling very anxious, and I couldn't explain it. Normally, when I get depressed or anxious, I don't have a difficult time pinpointing what it is. This time, it was just sort of a free-floating anxiety. I decided to call a therapist. It had been a very difficult year. My parents' divorce went through that fall, the school was in upheaval, and work was so stressful that, while I had done pretty regular breast exams, I lapsed for a number of months. But something in January made me check again, and I found a lump in my right breast. And, like so many women, I put off calling the doctor.

I finally got around to having an appointment in early February. I was coming for a regular checkup, and I was so anxious about the lump that I didn't even tell them. I think I wanted to see if they would find it, hoping they wouldn't and then, of course, it wouldn't be there. But they found it instantly. The nurse practitioner found it first, and then the doctor came and checked it out, and she did what I now know to be absolutely the right thing and said, "You need to get to a surgeon immediately" and got on the phone herself and made the appointment for me.

I had had a mammogram maybe only a year or so before that; I was turning forty-one that year. [Sighing] I think I saw the surgeon within a couple of days, and she said she needed to do a needle biopsy. I remember sitting in her office, anxiously waiting for this appointment, and seeing a flyer for a newly forming breast cancer support group on the wall, thinking, "Oh, my goodness, that *can't* be me, *won't* be me." In fact, I joined that group a couple of months later.

I wasn't going to tell Timothy when I first found the lump, but he could tell there was something wrong the minute he walked in the house. He was there the day I came back from the doctor the first time, and from that point forward, he went to every doctor's appointment and every treatment with me. In fact, I think it was hard for him after I got through all the treatments, letting me go by myself.

The surgeon, Loretta Brown, did a needle biopsy. It wasn't completely conclusive, and the mammogram that I had right around that time didn't show anything. So she decided to do a surgical biopsy. She took out a two-centimeter lump. I went to school the next day. I called her from my office, and she gave me the news over the telephone that it was cancer, and I was devastated.

I know when I got that news, my kids' faces were right in my line of vision. At the time, they were four and not quite seven. Lorna was in preschool, and Katie was in first grade.

When I first got the diagnosis, like a lot of people, I equated the word "cancer" with death. It was going to be sooner or later, but now it was going to happen within not so long a time. I was pretty convinced that I wasn't going to live long, even though I knew women who had lived many years with breast cancer. I think one of the first pieces of information for a woman to learn when she gets a diagnosis like this is that it doesn't necessarily mean death.

Timothy and I went to Lorctta Brown's office, and she sat us down and took a long time. First she said, "Yes, this is cancer, and I'm going to treat you, and you are going to live a nice, long life." I mean, she couldn't have been more reassuring, whether or not it was true. Really, she has no guarantee. But it was her manner; even her words were the right thing to say at the time. She is a young mother herself. I intuitively feel that the doctors I've had who are parents of young children understand in a very visceral way what this means.

It took a while for that to sink in. I kind of read it as, "How very nice, she's being so kind." She guaranteed me she would cure me of it, and I know she can't do that. That *was* being kind, but, the more I read and understand about the disease, I know that she was being more than kind. That can change the whole tone about how you deal with a disease like this in terms of your parenting. Are you making quick arrangements for everything to be taken care of, or are you taking a slightly longer view?

We started talking about what my options were between lumpectomy and mastectomy, and I felt instantly that I would do whatever I needed to do. I needed to beat this. I had no intention of not living through my kids' childhoods, if not much longer. But, at that moment, I was focusing on their childhoods.

She said, "I think if the lump is removed, we'll have to go back in and get the margins, whichever you decide. And we'll have to test the lymph nodes." She explained all that, none of which I had yet understood. I guess there was a little bit of time to make the decision because I consulted with at least one other doctor about which way to go. The final decision was to have a mastectomy. My breasts are very small. They would have had to take out so much of a small breast that it would have been disfiguring. I really didn't care—I'm not attached to my breasts in that sort of way. I had just nursed two children two years each, and we didn't plan to have more children. I felt like I had been lucky, and they had done the job. I wanted to live.

I also was not clear enough on all the options at that point. I think I still had hope that I could just have the surgery and that would take care of it. I started to do lots of reading and talking to people and spent an awful lot of time on the telephone. My mother came around the time of the surgery. Our therapist, Martina, was enormously support-ive. Everybody was. I felt like I could talk about it and that there was community around me, both family and friends.

Some of the best support I got was from other women who were breast cancer survivors and mothers. I knew them through my school community. One was a parent of two former students, who said to me, "Look, chances are you've got at least five years. Think about how much older your children are going to be, and you're going to have this much more time with them, at least." I can't tell you how comforting that was to hear. It was like she'd thrown a warm blanket around me.

On March 28 of '93, I had the mastectomy. It was like being in an altered state. Suddenly, all the little, nitty-gritty details of your life melt away, and you have this incredible focus on what you need to take care of.

I stayed in the hospital only overnight. It was painful at first, but they gave me some anti-inflammatory drug and I was very comfortable. The drains were probably the worst of the surgery. And now, looking back on it, the surgery doesn't seem to me to be so terrible. It wasn't like losing a major organ. Once I looked at myself after they took the dressings off, I wasn't frightened of it any more. But then, news came within a few days that I had seven out of seventeen lymph nodes with cancer. That was probably the worst moment.

Then, I had to start a whole new round of deciding what the next treatment should be and finding the right doctors to do that. It was a rainy day when we went to see Dr. Foote. There was a high window in the room, and I remember sitting [and] looking out the window at the rain, and this very steel-eyed, gray-haired woman comes in, very busi-nesslike, dressed very smartly in expensive clothes. I felt she was talking about me as a mechanical body with cancer. She never asked one single question about me as a person. She talked about her horses. I remember looking out the window as she left the room at one point and thinking, "I am going to die of this."

She said I had a garden variety of cancer. The practice had a patient they were trying a new chemo on, and she thought I should try it. There had been no studies done on it. It was experimental. You have to make so many decisions just then, and you don't know what you're doing.

The protocol Dr. Foote recommended sounded horrible. She said they had a patient who was in her twelfth week on it and she was doing fine, and she would call the woman and see if she would be willing to talk to me. The other patient called me, and there was lots wrong with Dr. Foote's description of her. First of all, she was the mother of a three-year-old and she was in her fourth, not twelfth, week of treatment. She was so sick she couldn't get out of bed except to go to the treatments. She was depressed and felt Dr. Foote had no idea, never asked her how she was doing.

Diana decided to see a different oncologist, Dr. Shukla, at another medical center much farther from her home.

He said, "This is totally unnecessary for you." Of course, I wanted to hear that. He said what he thought I needed, and I went home and thought about it. By contrast, he's a gentle, kindly man who didn't take a huge amount of time to find out who I am, but certainly I felt like more of a person and that I'd get good care there. The whole thing felt more right to me.

One of the ways I dealt with my anxiety was by making conscious decisions all the way along about the treatment. The way I live my life in terms of my health, I probably wouldn't have chosen poisoning my body with chemotherapy. But Martina, my therapist, made me make a conscious decision about it and not just decide to do it because everybody said you should. We went through a couple of weeks of trying to intuitively figure it out, really sitting there and going through the exercise of "What do you feel like on your deathbed? What do you want to look back at and feel about yourself and what you've done? What do you want out of your life? What's really important to you?" And not do that from my forty-year-old standpoint, thinking *for sure I have another forty years to glide through* and *I'll get to that, I'll get to that.* But really having to face the possibility that maybe it'll be now.

Timothy went with me to all these sessions, and all of us felt intuitively that the surgery probably took care of the cancer, but what I finally decided was I needed to do chemo for myself because of the kids. Because if it ever came back and I *hadn't* done the chemo, I would never be able to resolve it. I am fully cognizant chemo is not a be all and end all, but I had to take care of it in every way I could. Being a mother was really *the* major guide of my decisions, how I was during the treatment, and how I think about it afterward.

I had a fair amount of cancer in my family. I used to wonder who would be the next person. Well, I was. When I first got the diagnosis, I was furious because it was almost exactly a year since my parents' divorce, and I had a lot of mixed feelings about my father. I said to my sister, "Shit! It wasn't supposed to be me! It should have been him."

He had a lung cancer lump while I was in chemo. He would talk about how he and I had this experience of cancer in common. It was very hard for me to hear. He has a very good doctor who saw this little lump and got it out of there. The whole episode must have lasted a couple of weeks; he is fine. It was scary for my father. I would never diminish that. But I didn't feel it was an experience he and I had in common. He was no longer parenting kids at home.

If Timothy and I hadn't had the children—it's hard to remember not having the children—I might have made different choices about treatment. I know nothing for sure, of course, but I would have been much more accepting of the disease. While I certainly wouldn't have wanted to have left him, a spouse relationship is replaceable in people's lives. This is not to say that I wouldn't have fought the disease, but I don't think I would have felt this physical surge that was going to make me climb out of that hole because I wasn't going to let that happen for the girls. Losing your mother or father is a trauma for a child that you don't get over.

I do believe with everything in me that the mind-body connection is strong and that healing has a lot to do with a will to live. Which is not to say that if you get sick and die it's because you had no will to live, as one doctor indicated to my uncle, who was dying of lymphoma. That, I think, is a cruel hoax. But I do believe that it's very possible that having children helped. I feel like my kids were my north star throughout this thing and still are, in a way, and that that's a good thing to have.

I had chemo—Adriamycin and Cytoxan. I could have chosen a slightly milder treatment, CMF[1], which didn't have the Adriamycin in it. There was definite hair loss with Adriamycin. Dr. Shukla said they were just starting to find that if you treat it aggressively up to a point [during] the first round, the long-term results are better. He said, "I'm also thinking about the effects on your life in the long haul. You're a young mother, let's get you through this."

I ended up having four treatments, one every three weeks. We talked about a fifth, but I was very sick from the chemo. I had it in the morning, and by five o'clock, I started vomiting. I got in a cycle of vomiting, and it's very hard to break out of it. I had to let it run its course.

My will was so strong that I was going to get through this. What I presented to the children was that, but when I was flat on my back and couldn't get out of bed, it was pretty hard on them. I think most children experience one of their parents being ill as a very frightening time. Their very Rock of Gibraltar is yanked out from under, and they need a lot of coddling. For the fourth treatment, we had friends who offered to have the kids stay with them, and although the kids had hardly spent any time away from home without us, Katie grabbed at the chance. She stayed away, I think, four days. She wanted to come back when I was fine, and she couldn't be around me when I wasn't. It was really devastating for her. Lorna was younger. She didn't really understand all of it, I don't think.

I think there is a way in which it was more normal for them during the treatment to go off and be with their friends, to be in other people's houses. At one point, Katie said about one of her friend's mothers, who is like me in some ways, but is extraordinarily athletic which I am not in any way, shape, or form, "I wish you were like Nancy," and I said, "Excuse me! What do you mean?" And she said, "I don't really wish you were like her. I really wish you were just you, but without cancer." [Sighs] It was hard to read them all the time and not just be able to collapse when you wanted to, where you wanted to.

I lost all my hair within the third week, before I even had the second treatment. The actual losing of the hair was dreadful. Having clumps and clumps come out. Once it was gone, I was really okay with it. It was just a different reality. "Well, here I am with no hair." Of all the things that happened, it wasn't that bad. It became, honestly, kind of fun to get up in the morning and think of what to put on my head.

It was uncomfortable for Katie to see me or have anyone see me without hair. I would walk around with nothing on because the truth is I don't like anything over my ears, and I'm not a hat person. I had chemo from April through June, and it was warm. One time, one of Katie's friends, who was very curious about what I looked like anyway came over before I was entirely dressed. I came to the door with nothing on my head, and the poor child stood there with her mouth open, and I had to apologize and go get something. *[Laughing]* My therapist assured me how healthy this was that Katie was worried about herself—that's what a seven year old should be doing—rather than worrying about me.

For me, being sick was the hardest part—not sick from cancer but the treatment is going to kill you if the cancer doesn't. Chemo was postponed twice because I couldn't withstand it. I had a white blood cell count of less than five hundred, and so I had to take these extraordinarily expensive injections of a drug called Neupogen. It builds back up your resistance. [But] I ended up with very low resistance in general.

The last treatment particularly was hard. I guess it just builds up in your body. There were women in my support group who went through exactly the same treatment and could get up the next day and go to work. It became a pattern that the first week of the treatment was an "out week" for me. My mother came for each of those treatments, and she made me egg custard, and that was the first thing that I could eat, and I would slowly get back to eating food. And there is nothing like a good meal after a time like that. Then, I had two weeks of feeling quite well before the next treatment.

It was hard and frustrating for everybody for me not to be able to do in the way that I normally do. I'm a very energetic person, and I do a lot for everybody in the family. Food is so much a part of our family's life. For the months of my chemo, we didn't cook a meal. The school community organized themselves and brought food over every other night for three months. While the food that was brought was absolutely delicious, after a while Katie was saying "Mommy, when are you going to cook our food again?" It wasn't normal having all these people attend to us in this way, and my kids didn't like not being able to choose what they wanted. For me that was great. And my mother coming and cooking for the kids was like what they ate. But also having Grandma around meant that I was going to be sick. So that was a mixed bag.

She probably would have been here even more, but it was hard for Timothy to have her in the house. There were conflicts to work out about who was doing the caretaking. Mostly, I had her come for Katie and Lorna. I didn't want Katie to actually take care of me. I wanted them taken care of in the way they were accustomed to being taken care of, and really, only my mother and one of my sisters knew how to do that besides Timothy. Timothy was taking care of me and trying to work. So I convinced him that I needed to be mothered then.

My mother was pretty remarkable. She just carried her mothering right on. I hope she fell apart with somebody else, but she held it together for me. I've talked to a woman whose mother couldn't handle it, doesn't want to talk about it. It's still hard for my mother to talk about the ultimate possibility. If I'll talk about the possibility of a recurrence or another cancer, she'll quickly say, "Well, let's just hope that, if that happens, by then they'll have a cure." And that's the end of it. The subject is closed.

I got a lot of what I wanted and needed. I needed details that I couldn't handle myself taken care of so life would be as normal as possible for the four of us, but specifically for the kids. Little errands. People were very generous in offering to take our kids. It became an issue because they didn't understand how much what we needed was to be home and safe and normal and together. I almost felt like they thought I was putting them off or not taking the offer seriously when I refused them. My kids didn't want to go to people's houses all the time. The only houses they wanted to go to were the ones that they went to very regularly. The worst thing for them would have been to be shipped off all the time, even though, at times, it would have been better for me. But we were all hanging on by a fairly delicate thread, and that would have tipped it over.

People try to be generous and don't always understand the ways in which they can. People often say, "What can I do to help you? Call me for anything." Then you have to come up with a way, and sometimes it's just too much work.

What would you want them to say?

"I'm going to the market. What can I pick up for you?" Or, "Don't think about dinner." Or, "What days can I bring your kids home from school?" Say something specific.

I appreciated most the friends and family who would talk about it directly and not just circumvent the issue: "I'm so sorry." But it's a tough subject, and most people don't have the skills or don't know what to do. But I can think back to a couple of friends who said, "How does it feel to have your hair gone?" And "What is this like for you?" And they really wanted to know. They were really listening, and I appreciated that a lot.

Almost all my friends have children, and I imagine them to be just like me in that their greatest fear is not surviving their children's childhood. I can't think specifically of anybody who asked me, "What is this like when you have kids?" I was able to talk to some people. I brought up how scared I was in terms of my kids.

Were they able to hear that?

They were, in varying degrees. If they were parents themselves, they could absolutely relate to it. But there isn't a whole lot to say. People say that when you go through a crisis, your friends are there for you for a while, and then they get tired of hearing about the subject, and they're ready for you to move on. When my sister lost her baby and had run through all the friends and still needed to process it, what she said is she didn't need me to say anything, I didn't have to give her suggestions or advice. She just needed me to listen. That's what she appreciated the most. Some people can't have a conversation without offering help; they feel that if you're talking to them about it, it's because you're asking for something. Just having a listener is enormously valuable.

It felt good to get back to doing whenever I could. But I also pared it down to what was most important. There were some things that were hard for me not to be able to do. When I was so sick that I couldn't read the kids a story. You know, lying in bed and thinking about getting up and going into my bathroom, which is what, ten feet? The last treatment, I remember lying there and I couldn't stand having music on, couldn't stand any input. I was so sick, and I remember lying there and just staring at the veins in my hands, thinking, "If this is what my life is reduced to, this isn't worth it." If I ever get to be this sick all the time, then I will be able to let go. Because I'd have lost all my relationships. The kids would be gone from my life. There was nothing I could have done for them . . .

I was glad the kids weren't in the house because there was pressure to look and feel better than I actually did if they were there. On the other hand, I was depressed and angry that it was so bad that they had to leave home in order to get through the few days. That was tolerable knowing that it was because of the chemotherapy and that it was finite. If it ever gets to a place where it's because of the illness itself, that will be a different story. They'll be older, and I have no doubt that we'll find ways to deal with it. But I'm very conscious that was the closest I've ever felt in my life to being that ill and knowing what it must feel like to be dying. I've done enough reading about death and dying now to know that I could get to a place of letting go. There would be the time for that.

I got in a mind-set finally of accepting that this is what's happening, and I just have to succumb to it. It was what I needed to do, and I had to drop everything in the way. Some of that anger that I experienced at first is partly what propelled me into taking care of myself. There was a serene sort of clarity once all the decisions were made that I knew what I had to do. I was on a program—chemo and then radiation. I was going to therapy. I was getting a massage. I didn't even allow myself to think about what the long-term prognosis was. I was just on that path and I was doing it.

I've never been a successful meditator. Going out and taking a walk by the mountains or ocean works for me. I took walks when I felt well enough to do it and was reading more. In a bizarre sort of way, it was one of the more peaceful times in my life. I wasn't worried about a lot of the peripheral things. My school was in absolute turmoil, and I couldn't do anything about it. I had to take care of myself, and I did. It was the job I had at that time.

By the time I got to radiation, I was pretty well rested. Typically, they give you a few weeks to recover from chemo before starting radiation, and I think I had a four-week break. We needed a vacation, the four of us, and we went to Hawaii. I came back and started the radiation, every day for six weeks. The radiation oncologist is a truly wonderful doctor, extremely compassionate. I'm now seeing her once a year, and I can't believe what she remembers from one year to the next, like details about my kids. That is smart doctoring. She's a good healer.

For me, radiation compared to chemo was nothing. I was showing up there for fifteen minutes a day, listening to music of my choice. The staff was fabulous. They made it a decent experience. After three weeks of radiation, the school year started, and my doctor told me I was crazy to go back to work, but I really wanted to at that point. She felt I should only go at the most fifteen hours a week, but pretty much I went back in to my job.

As soon as I had enough hair, which was probably like a quarter of an inch all over my head, I stopped wearing hats, a little sooner than Katie was ready for. My hair came back initially in these tight, little, corkscrew curls, so it actually was kind of fun. It was a relief to be past the treatments.

Cancer and the need to stay alive for her children gave Diana permission for unprecedented self-care: illness as a vacation from maternal duties. It was only later that she learned that "it was okay to want to survive not just for their sake but for my own sake." But, of course, this was no holiday. In the midst of chaos Diana also had to create a coherent container for the children. I wondered how she met the challenge of talking about cancer at home and at work and what role communication played in her healing.

People feel like pariahs because they've got cancer. You didn't do anything to deserve this disease. I don't know how I got it. I didn't ask for it. None of us asked for it. There is no shame to it. I work in a child-oriented environment, so people tend to be much more sensitive. Most teachers are mothers. I was given the freedom basically to work when and as much as I could. I could choose when to return. They were paying me anyway.

And I didn't have to hide it from anybody. Not only that, I ended up writing a letter to the whole school community because I couldn't handle having to tell every person the story. One parent had given her child complete misinformation. At least, the child came away with misunderstanding about cancer, thinking that if she came near me, she would catch it. She was one of the students I worked with, and it prompted me to write the letter, telling people in the school community what Timothy and I were saying to our kids and encouraging people to say something similar should the subject come up. It was good for me, and it was good for them, too. There I was, walking around looking fairly normal, and the next time the kids saw me, I had no hair, and they were going to wonder.

To me, it was easier to have it out in the open. It seemed much worse to have it whispered about and have an error going around. Not everybody is like me, comfortable talking about it. Some people are much more private. And I recognize that, too.

One of my friends said, "Secrets make you sick." It's bad enough that you're going through it. Having to walk around and hide it from everybody is . . . I can't imagine. I was lucky enough not to have to do it.

I was careful about conversations around the kids because I was always feeling like someone might go into territory that I hadn't yet talked to them about or perhaps wasn't going to talk to them about. There were whole arenas of this that they were not old enough to appreciate. People were pretty good about that. But sometimes, there are adults who talk around children as though children aren't there.

We told the kids about the lump before I had the surgical biopsy. They knew something was going on because I was on the phone all the time and a lot of it was behind closed doors. Or Daddy and I would go off and have a conversation, and there was crying. So we didn't wait a long time to tell them because it was too obvious there was something going on in the house.

We told them that I had a lump in my breast, and that if it was left there it would make me very sick, and so it needed to be taken out. I don't think the first time we talked to them we called it "cancer," but one friend said, "You need to use the word with your kids because if you don't, other people will, and you better make sure that it's coming from you first." That was such good advice.

Soon after the diagnosis, I remember very clearly sitting on the living room floor and telling them this news. I was holding Katie in my lap, and Timothy was holding Lorna, and Lorna said, "Well, Mommy"—bouncing up and down—"Mommy, you have to have it taken out because if you don't, you could die." No one had said anything about death or that it would make me sick at all. And that was that for her. She sort of toodled on through it except that she needed a lot more sitting in her teacher's lap that spring. When she was frustrated at my not being up and well, she took it out on Grandma—you know, she was kind of snippy. And, as soon as the treatments were over, that disappeared. So Lorna had a very indirect way of dealing with it. She was kind of skipping through. She's open about talking about it, doesn't remember a lot, I don't think.

Katie, being older and a more private person, worried more. She got much more cranky and temperamental and touchy; she went through a time when you could say "boo" to her and she would cry. Katie held it together probably too well all through the treatment and had a little collapse at the end. But that was fine. At least she collapsed. It would have been more worrisome if she hadn't.

It's hard to tell how much information is enough. We didn't tell them absolutely everything. Like, we didn't tell them how many women die of breast cancer every year. We tried to read along the way how much was just enough information. With Lorna, you could tell because she changed the subject. [Laughs] It was clear that we'd gone far enough. It was a little harder to read Katie and give her enough information. As we keep talking about it and she gets older, I'll be able to give her more.

I think being able to talk about it openly was important. They had teachers who were my colleagues and friends, and if they needed to talk, they would. You know, they like to feel my prosthesis—which is the real one and which is the not-real one. They'll lie on me. Katie wants to make sure that it's not left around in case a friend is over; she doesn't want anyone to see it. I undress in front of them all the time, so that's probably a good thing. I'm not sure how open they'll be now in front of their friends, but I'll talk about cancer very openly all the time because we'll read something in the paper, know someone else who is going through it.

One thing we haven't faced yet is their own risk because they're still young girls. Katie's getting closer to menstruation age, and I probably will face that around that time. I know that statistically, only five percent of breast cancers are genetically based or have a genetic connection.[2] So they have as big a risk as anyone else. None of us know what these risks are. I guess I'm conscious about doing things in terms of their health. I always was careful, but I'm more careful now about what they eat. What we all eat. I will talk openly that I eat an even lower fat diet than the rest of the family because I don't want cancer to come back and eventually that'll be important for them. Maybe. I qualify all of this when I say it to them.

I don't have any illusion that if I don't eat cheese for the rest of my life it's going to be a guarantee that I won't have cancer again. But I'll feel better about myself because I'm not doing it. *[Laughter]* I get on Tim's case because a lot of times I don't feel like he's taking care of his health well enough: "It's bad enough they have a mother with cancer, but you're not exercising and you're not . . ." I mean, what a nudge! It's terribly annoying, it's probably a little neurotic, but I can't help it. We consciously brought them into this world, and we owe it to them. I'll accept that neurosis as what I need to do to feel okay.

But I did something truly terrible once. *[Laughs]* Someone gave them each a makeup kit with nail polish in it for Christmas. Lorna was delighting in putting on the nail polish and then taking it off with nail polish remover, which a friend of mine has said has carcinogenic stuff in it. It was really bothering me. I said to her, "I don't want you to use this because the stuff in there could cause cancer." She never touched it again. So they have that fear.

It became obvious over time that Katie had, still has, this aversion to vomiting. It can be a cat, it can be a person. She has to get out of the way. Lorna got sick a couple of times and had to throw up, and poor Katie was terrified. We were in an airport waiting room. Lorna felt nauseous, we made it to a bathroom, and Katie was stuck in the stall with her. It was like you had put her in there with a python. She was just crawling out of her skin. She was as far away as she could possibly be and still see me because she couldn't stand to be there.

I finally figured out that it came from some other cancer experience she had even before mine. Archie, who was this family friend, died of lung cancer. During our last visit to him, he was pretty ill. He was sitting at the dining room table and choked on his food in front of the kids. Lorna was two and Katie was four, and, see, that's where the throwing-up aversion started. It started there and went into mine. Throwing up meant dying. Because Archie died. That was the last time we saw him. And, no matter what I could say to Katie, that it wasn't related, that people could throw up and have the flu, people throw up when they're pregnant, I did. . . . She said at one point, "You know, Mommy, how will I ever get over this?" And I said, "We just have to keep working at this, every time it happens, we have to keep talking about it." So.

Each of those times where someone has gotten sick and Katie has had to deal with it, it's been an opportunity to go back and talk about cancer again. And each time we've had to do that, she's been enough older and we could talk about it on a new level. The last time, which has been within the last year, Lorna was sick and lying on the couch, and Katie wouldn't leave my side. She followed me all around the house. I was in the kitchen doing something, and she was sitting up on the counter right next to me, and she said, "Mommy, could you have died from the cancer?" We talked about it at the time. She was eight and a half, probably, and I said, "Yes, but that's why I had all the treatments." She said, "Well, what would happen if you did die?" And I said, "Well, people who love each other hold each other in their hearts, and they hold each other forever, and I have you forever, and you have me forever, even if I'm not here." That's all I can do for them, take care of me and make sure I'm here as long as I can be here. *[Choking up]*

I see it's still so emotional for you.

You know, in a way, I hope it always will be. It's so big. I hope the bigness of it, the enormity of it, doesn't go away, that I don't slip back so much into that unconscious state that I forget that it feels like this.

Do you talk to them as if you still have cancer?

No. We talk about that I *had* cancer. The same day Katie asked me if I could have died of it, she said, "Will you ever get it again?" I would never say "no" because I can't promise that. I said, "I certainly hope not, and, if I do, I know I did everything I could to not get it back the first time, and I will do everything I can to treat it again." No one can guarantee those things. I think you talk about it like you're a recovering alcoholic. Because it would be cruel to them to promise them that it's totally gone. See, that's what they've had to face. But the good thing to face in this life is that we *don't* know, and life is fragile and precious, and you don't blithely go along taking it for granted.

I think there are ways in which cancer has affected my whole life. While I don't think about it with quite the frequency that I did for a while, I don't think that there's a day that goes by that I'm not conscious that it's happened. In the last year or so it's settled to a background noise, a dull wondering.

Like anybody who faces a terminal illness, especially when you are the parent of young children, cancer is the biggest eye-opener and turner-around that you could possibly have. We didn't go into this parenting period of our lives thinking that this would happen. Nobody does. The assumption is that you will be there all the way through. I think your worst fear as a mother is that you won't be there for your children in some ways. So, to have created these two little beings that I love as much as I love myself and to face that possibility of dying prematurely was pain beyond description. The terror of cancer recurring or metastasizing is about that.

As one of my friends says, the whole thing was sort of a cruel gift. I have to honestly say at this point, I'm not happy I got cancer, I could give this experience up happily for anything else, but I'm not sorry that this has happened to me.

The cruel part is obvious. What's the gift?

The wake-up. Understanding what's important. There is a time close to the diagnosis, and it can last for quite a while, where things become incredibly clear, and a lot of what absorbs us in our daily life sifts away, just the garbage that we deal with all the time that's unavoidable. During that time, I understood very clearly what's truly important. That my children are one of the most precious things in my life. I knew that before I had cancer, but it heightened it and opened me up so that everything seems a little more sacred and precious.

Before cancer, I always felt the frustration of how fast time is going with them, but now I am taking those moments to stop and ingest what this feels like right now at this moment. What does this child's body feel like right now, at seven years old?

Which is not to say that I have avoided being anxious about relatively petty things since then. As someone in my support group said, "I thought when I first got this that I would never again fight with my husband, never yell at my children—you know, all those nevers." Of course, you revert, but you do it with a new understanding, try to hang onto that clarity and not lose it. I think that's why I'm drawn to helping cancer organizations.

The gift part of cancer is that melting away of the illusion that you have control over a lot of things. The big things. We don't—and so learning to sit in comfort with that. Cancer's made me face what I feel about death and that we all have to do it some time.

There are tragic deaths, there are tragic lives, but death itself is not tragic. It would be tragic for my children to lose their mother at even this age, but they would survive it. So I think I have more confidence in all of our ability to survive it and understand that it's a common experience. Certainly, death is the other common experience we all have, besides birth, and I'm grateful for the chance to face it at this time in my life, not later, and to be able to talk about it and read and think about it more, feeling more and more comfortable that I'm being a truly conscious mother.

I grew up in a family where death was taboo. It was something you protect children from. Because of my illness, it's become something that we talk about a lot more openly. In my school, we're in our eighth or ninth year of putting up a Day of the Dead altar, a Mexican tradition that falls on November first. It's a chance every year not just to honor the dead in our lives but talk about that as a natural part of life. Well, this is easy for me to say when I'm sitting here feeling very healthy and alive. *[Laughter]* I was sick from the treatment, not the illness, so I imagine I have places to go.

I guess what I do now is just let it be there. Live with it. Every year, I feel better that the kids are solid, and should something come up again for me, we lived through it once, we'll do what we need to do again. I also know that whatever comes along, I have the strength to be able to deal with it, that maybe people who don't go through that don't always know about themselves.

So many people have said to me throughout the whole thing, "You handled it so incredibly!" "You did such a job, you're so strong! You just went through the whole thing!"

What do you think I would have done? *[With some irritation]* I had two kids at home. What would the alternative have been? To just plain succumb to it? To whine my way through it? Other people will say to me, "I don't think I could do that." I disagree. I think that you could if you had to—if you have children and care about being their parent and care about your own survival.

I believe that each of us has a deeper well of strength from which to draw than we know. It's amazing what we can face if we have to. I've had to dig deeper than I ever knew I had available to me, and I'm kind of amazed. I'm grateful to know that about myself. It's a dubious gift, this disease, but there are many ways in which I feel much richer and wiser and more knowledgeable about myself.

And it's been a gift for my children. I was the sort of mother when they were very tiny who wanted them to have a fairy-like, magical kind of childhood. I didn't want them to have to experience terribly tough things. I'm not overly protective. It's not like I won't let them do anything physical or I don't want them to struggle. But I think I'm logically protective; I wanted to cushion their young lives. Even after all these years of working with children, I was taken aback that they would have to struggle with something like this so young.

My thinking has changed through these several years of cancer, probably to take a 180-degree turn. It's not like I'm out there looking for tough things for them to do, but I'm grateful in a bizarre way for them having had to go through this. And I'm eagerly pushing them in places now that challenge them a bit, pushing against the places that are harder for them. Katie being the shy kid that she is, I think it's great when she has to stand up in front of the class and give a talk or go to someone's house that she hasn't been to before. What's been wonderful to watch is she might go in kicking and screaming or terrified and anxious, but she'll do it. They both are learning something about having to push themselves through something that's hard.

Life is an ongoing lesson. Every day there are lessons. Like the Buddhists, I think in some ways, suffering is inevitable. It's a part of life. It's probably out of the times when we suffer the most that we grow the most. I think that's what it means to be human, the constantly striving and learning and growing, not staying complacent. Although Timothy and I joke, it feels like we've earned a gliding period. It would be nice if nothing happened for a while. Absolutely nothing. People who have been through tough times and come out the other end have more than wisdom. There's a beauty in the acceptance of the ups and downs of life, and suffering is very much a part of that.

But I'm really referring to a more normal course of life suffering, which I consider mine to be. I would never pretend to understand anybody else's suffering. I think that I've been lucky. I think the kind of suffering I've been through pales in comparison to living in Sarajevo, or during the Holocaust years in Eastern Europe, or in Cambodia. It's nothing like that. I've managed to do this in a relative lap of luxury. But I do think it's made me much more empathetic to the kinds of things that people go through in their lives. I also think that each of us suffers in our own way, and while we can somewhat understand the suffering of others, the truth is we do it alone. My experience can only be generalized to a certain extent. But the most important thing any of us can hold in our lives is the love we have, to hold it dear and take good care of it, to take it and give it.

I was struck by the number of times Diana mentioned that she didn't have illusions anymore: about the magical power of a healthy diet, or her ability to perfectly protect her children, or her cancer-free status. Cancer wrested Diana's story from her hands, thrusting her into a state of discontinuity. Slowly, as she began to reconstitute a plot that incorporated suffering and mortality in a different way, Diana became better equipped to introduce her children to life as it is rather than as she wished it to be. Eventually, she expanded her story of mothering to include adversity as inevitable and even potentially beneficial.

It seemed that Diana's healing began as she surrendered to the new reality and then found ways to take back her own story, rather than just reacting to cancer. In reaching out and talking openly about cancer with her family and community, she not only received the help she needed but also prepared others, including her children, to accept her new perspective. Her choice was to cope with the cancer experience with as much consciousness as possible, to confront her worst fears, and to keep the lessons of facing mortality visible as a reminder, like a bright line stitched into a sampler.

Telling her story was part of the healing. Diana said, "I've always wondered, where's the end of the story? I've always wondered that, even when I was a child. At the point of treatment, I wasn't thinking forward very much. Cancer is a wake-up call to stop in your tracks and take stock. Recording the story helped me to be more connected to the future again. Telling it was one of the steps along the way over the last four years."

FOUR: "CANCER SAVED MY LIFE"
MARGE SCHMITT

THE CANVAS UPON which Margaret Schmitt paints her concerns about life is larger than most. As a woman in her support group once said, "When Marge talks about saving the world, she's talking about the *world*." This world is based on a web of connections for which everyone is responsible, in which no one should be left out. Marge lived the saying "It takes a village" before it became a cliché.

We first meet at a breast cancer conference. At the end of my presentation, I pass around a sign-up sheet for project participants or volunteer listeners. Marge signs up for both. She reaches out and takes my hand. "I'm Margaret Schmitt—call me Marge. I want to get involved." Later in the day, she approaches me again and tells me she has just been diagnosed, but also that she is a sociology researcher and professor with skills that could help the project.

A few weeks later, as we begin recruiting listeners, I call her. "I've just started chemotherapy, but I'm doing very well!" Marge's voice has more buoyancy on chemo than mine does after a good night's sleep. Nevertheless, she has had only one treatment, and I am cautious. The disease and reactions to medication are unpredictable. I urge Marge to postpone taking on a volunteer commitment, and she reluctantly agrees. But her eagerness to record her life story overcomes my reservations: The reflective process is more helpful and the story more cohesive once medical crises have abated.

Before we meet again, I try to visualize the woman I had met at the conference: tall, eyes that notice everything, a flow of highly intelligent words and ideas punctuated by peals of laughter, often directed toward herself. We complete our brief intake visit as Marge drinks her blended nutritional breakfast and jokes about "having the energy of a slug," her main side effect from chemotherapy.

As I get to know her, I develop slug-envy. Marge is a full professor of sociology (the first woman in her department and later the first female chair). She lived for eleven years in Africa as researcher and teacher, stood up to power on behalf of the poor, and gave expert testimony at a White House conference ("My brief moment of fame"). No less important to Marge are her husband, Preston, and twelve-year-old son, Todd: "Motherhood really changed my life. It's been amazing!"

Marge wants to record her story in part because she's "hoping this research will help other mothers with breast cancer." She understands that, along with providing services, we are learning in order to educate others. She wants to assist, if only by being interviewed.

Marge records some stories about her family of origin for Todd, describing her father as "interesting, smart, innovative, curious," with great ambitions for his oldest child. But he was also "a very frightening person" who flew into rages from post-traumatic stress disorder that began after fighting on the front lines during World War II. Marge clearly doesn't want to dwell on her past or on anything negative. "I think we've talked enough about my childhood. My adulthood was much more interesting than my childhood." Adolescence is given even shorter shrift: "I made it through!"

Beyond some gentle suggestions, I always want to allow the mother control of her story, especially when so much control is lost during serious illness. I don't understand why Marge wants to skip over her formative years, but she is clear about the stories she wants to tell and the stories that carry energy for her. "I've done lots and lots of interesting things, like jumping out of airplanes. I love to sing, and I've always sung in choirs. But the things, other than my upbringing, that I think really made me who I am are three, maybe four."

Marge distills her life into an outline that includes the major experiences that shaped her development and a number of enduring passions—including mothering—that are sustaining her through cancer. The first defining experience was the Vietnam War. "The lesson of the Vietnam War was that you had to bear witness to what you believe when something wrong was happening, no matter how afraid you are. And I've done that all my life as a result."

When Marge finished her master's degree, she "wanted to do something useful, something real." She joined VISTA, a domestic version of the Peace Corps, as a welfare rights organizer. Confronting real poverty among the working poor in the United States was a second major influence. "One of the things that I learned in VISTA which has informed my practice ever since is giving away my skills so that other people can have them and speak for themselves.

"The third *really, really* important thing in my life was going to Africa." Marge spent five years in Tanzania and four in Botswana. She married Preston in Kenya and spent a year there with him, and they also lived in Zimbabwe. Todd has already spent almost two of his twelve years in Africa.

"My master's was in international development, and I wanted to save the world. I thought that we had all these wonderful things to take from America and save the world with. When I got to Tanzania, there were some very good people in USAID but most of them didn't speak Swahili. They didn't understand the culture, the economy. I saw people who were living really, really well and who were very arrogant, causing havoc in the lives of poor people. So I understood at a gut level for the first time the whole notion of colonialism and imperialism, even in the name of doing good. With my own students, nobody goes in the field until they speak the language, and everybody is instructed about who's bearing the consequences of what they're doing."

The fourth major influence was the "intellectual intensity and seriousness about theory" that Marge found when she began teaching at a major university. "It changed the way I taught, and it changed some of the ways I went about doing my research. I just made full professor, so I'm really happy."

Marge begins her story by describing the experiences that have made her who she is at fifty-one.

MARGE

I didn't want children, and I got pregnant by accident. I hadn't been at all prepared for motherhood, and I was very ambivalent about this event, but I took very good care of myself, did all the right things. He was born by cesarean section, and I remember the surgeon lifting him out. I fell in love. That was it. Before he was born, I was thinking, "We'll never go to a movie again or get to do this and that," all of which was absolutely true. But it didn't matter. Watching this child grow is just a miracle!

I was overwhelmed by the joy of it and by the connection that it gave me to mothers everywhere. People say, "Oh, you've done such a wonderful job raising Todd, he's such a wonderful kid," and I say that a lot of people helped raise Todd—daycare people and friends. I'm proud of the fact. It *does* take a whole village to raise a child, hokey as that's become.

What I try to teach my son has to do with being respectful of everyone and kind to everyone. We always work at our church's homeless dinners. First, we were doing the cooking, and I said, "No, no, no, we want Todd to see real people and serve them with his own hands!" It's about connections again, about how we're all connected.

Other passions have to do with my profession. I love the life of the mind. I am a klutz, so the life of the body is not for me. I wanted to be doing research, working with data. Those *Ah ha!* moments, when you suddenly see the pattern, when you say, 'Oh, I get it. Oh, my gosh!, when you know you've got something that's bomb-proof, that it makes a difference. That's a passion.

The jumping off place for my work is poverty. How do people who are poor make a livelihood? What happens to women who have no rights to the land? I think about the babies. I was in Bangladesh, we were out in villages, and Todd was about seven months old. I knew what he weighed, how he felt when I picked him up, and so I knew in a visceral sense when I picked up these Bangladesh babies how emaciated they were even if they looked healthy.

Social justice and being politically active has been a major theme. A lot of it came from graduate school, from the Vietnam War, from VISTA, and then going overseas and *really seeing*, really seeing. My driving questions have to do with: How can you do something about it, trying to get other people to think about this. I mean, we can't even do something about poverty in this country, which is one of the richest in the world.

The other passion is teaching, which is exhilarating and scary and humbling, particularly at my university, where three-fourths of your students are smarter than you are. *[Laughs]* When you teach, you hand on. I have a rule that you always take the data back to the village. Always. If they fall on the ground laughing, you know you've got it wrong. And it's their information. In Zimbabwe, it's the same thing as in VISTA—to hand on the skills to the people who work with me so that when I leave a village, they can do the same things for themselves. Any research I've done, I stay connected.

A life theme is neighborliness and sharing. Wherever I lived, building community, bringing people together, opening your home. Part of it came from my mother. Part of it came from living in Africa. Politeness is so important there. For example, when you see somebody who's on crutches in Tanzania, you would say, "*Pole sana*, I'm sorry." When you meet somebody, you say, "Good morning." I remember running into the university once, to my secretary, and I said, "Mr. Parkipuni, I need blah-blah." He grabbed me by the shoulders, he said, "Professor Schmitt, first you greet. You say, 'How are you? How did you sleep? How's your family? How's your house?'" You always greet people because every time you greet somebody, you're helping to weave the fabric of society, starting in your family, the neighborhood.

For Marge, spinning these tales from her rich experiences of travel and work is central to her mothering. She is teaching her son values and connecting him to the larger world: "I think it's kind of joyous to say, 'Oh, here are all these stories I can give to Todd. Here's something of who I am which is different from the photos or articles.'"

I imagine Marge sitting in the middle of a web she has consciously executed, connecting all the strands into a whole. The weave of her life story is so tight that it seems as bomb-proof as her data. I find it hard not to be swept along into the drama of her experiences. Yet, I can't help wondering whether it all looks a bit too good to be true. Sometimes, what is left out of a story is as important as what gets included. And Marge has not yet talked about cancer. We record her cancer narrative just as she completes treatment.

I was actually diagnosed with cancer in South Africa. I was going to a conference to lecture for two weeks and work with students, give a paper, and then go back to my field sites in Zimbabwe and

Mozambique. The story of my illness is ironic because I'm sort of a hypochondriac. I never caught this, and the signs were absolutely clear.

I got to Germany, and my right nipple retracted and I thought, "Oh, it's cold," but of course my left nipple hadn't retracted. Then I got laryngitis, and I was totally fixated on my throat because I had to give public lectures and I couldn't talk, so I just thought, "Nipple, *schnipple*."

Then I got to Capetown, and it was still retracted, and I said, "Oh, no, this is not cool because it's summer in Capetown in January." Somebody from the conference was going to the doctor, and I thought, "Oh, well, I'll go and see, it's probably a blocked milk duct or mastitis or something. I just need some antibiotics."

So I went, and the guy was a total idiot. But he was smart enough to see . . . He said, "You don't need antibiotics," and called his buddy, who was a breast surgeon. He took a fine needle aspiration and said, "You know, it looks like a tumor," and whipped me down the hall to have a sonogram and a mammogram, and by six o'clock, I had a diagnosis. I was a beneficiary of South African racism. I was incredibly lucky because I could bypass this waiting that everyone else has to do.

When the doctor told me, the first thing I said to him was, "I'm going to beat it." I was upset, but I wasn't hysterical. I was mostly mad. Here was this trip I'd been waiting to make, and I had to come home. And then, the thought of my son, Todd . . . I said, "I'm not going to leave him without a mother." That I could not bear.

I immediately moved into list-mode. I had to call Preston [and ask him] to call the gynecologist and the people who were expecting me and tell them I'm not coming and explain why, and could they get to the villages and tell [the people there.] I know people do this differently, but I said, "The only thing I'm doing from now on out until whenever is to get well." So, one of the lists I made was all the things I was going to cancel. I was absolutely ruthless. My students had to see another professor. I resigned from every committee. I told the places where I'm an editor, "Don't send me any manuscripts."

The word spread because there I was with my suitcases, and people came up and hugged me and said, "You have to get well because we need you." That was so important because it meant there are places where people see my work is making a difference.

I flew home. My mother was very upset. But I said, "You know, Mom, the minute I had that diagnosis, I said I'm going to beat it, and I started to fight, and I certainly learned that from you." My mother has had many serious illnesses in her life, and she's always had her chin up and fought. I wasn't terrified because I was going to fight the cancer. That's probably the most important thing I've said.

My husband met me at the airport with a bunch of roses and drove me straight to the hospital, and they did another mammogram and said, "Oh, it will be a miracle if you can get a sonogram today," and I walked straight in and got a sonogram. This doctor said, "This is probably Stage II." Friends brought dinner the night I got home, and one of the husbands took Preston and Todd out. There was this being enveloped, which was so good.

So I had surgery, then chemo—Adriamycin—lost all my hair, and radiation, and radiation burn, and here I am on the other side.

Todd was just twelve when you were diagnosed. How did you initially talk with him about your illness?

I had called Preston, and he said to Todd, "Mommy's sick, and she's coming home," but Todd knows there are enough diseases you can pick up in Africa, it could be anything. We were concerned because one of his teachers, Joanne, had died of pancreatic cancer the week before, and his friend Sam's father had metastasized prostate cancer. So Preston called Sam's mother, who's an adolescent social worker, and said, "Zena, how do we handle this?" Zena asked Sam, "What did we say that was right and wrong?" and Sam said, "Well, the most important thing is to know how uncertain it could be."

When I got home, we had dinner, and then we sat down on the sofa and, holding our arms around him, said, "You know, I have cancer. It's not the cancer Joanne had. It's a kind of cancer that we know a lot about, but you never know what's going to happen. I'm going to have surgery, and probably going to be very sick for a while, and I think I'm going to get well." He took it really, really well, I think. He probably said, "Oh!" *[Laughs]* He didn't cry.

Very shortly after I got sick, my brother and sister gave us a VCR—we'd never had a TV—so I could watch funny videos. You can tell what a techno-peasant I am. As a result, we saw this video of Todd when he was three that we'd never seen, and they were singing, "When My

Mommy Comes Back" in it, so I started singing that around the house all the time, particularly before the surgery. I wasn't sure whether I was singing it for him or for me: "I'm going to be there for you."

I sort of went into training for surgery, walking every day and eating miso and all this stuff, which I think actually did help 'cause I whipped through surgery. I would walk halfway and meet Todd coming home from school because I wanted him to see me as well as possible. I'm a very energetic person—it's probably not obvious at the moment—so I wanted him to see I still had that energy, I wasn't falling into a thousand pieces.

We made a joke out of my hair falling out. We had a contest, and the entrants were Todd and his friend and Jubili the dog *[Laughs]* to guess what day my last hair would fall out. The person who won could choose their prize. In the end, not every hair fell out, so everybody got a prize. I had to show them my hair every day, and he thought it was kind of cool, you know, I had this little baby mohawk. We tried to make all the things that might be scary unscary. But still he knew Joanne had died. Sam's father died, and then another girl's mother died of breast cancer.

There were only two times I saw him really react. One was when I was in the hospital. Preston brought him to see me, and there I am, I'm gray, I've got tubes, I was on oxygen. He came into the room, walked up, gave me a kiss, and walked straight out onto the balcony. I asked him to make me a picture that I put up in the hospital room. I was drinking sixteen ounces of carrot juice every day. I asked him to make that for me every day so he had something that he was doing to help me get well.

The other time was with chemo. I had these foggy moments. Todd was on Netscape, and if you pick up the phone, it cuts you off. He said, "I'm going on Netscape, Mom, don't go on the phone," and I said, "Right, okay, I won't," and I walked upstairs and picked up the phone to make a call. I mean, it was like thirty seconds. I couldn't remember. And he was irate. He started to cry. He just lost it. He has a very strong sense of justice, so if you do all the right things, then the right things should happen. And he couldn't believe I couldn't remember for thirty seconds. I'm the person who keeps the house organized, I remember lunches. . . . That was the straw that broke the camel's back: Mom was not Mom. Though I was trying my best to be perky, you can't do it.

There were two kinds of issues. One was trying to help him understand that I really didn't have a brain at that moment. So I would say to him, "You know, this is the drug—I'm very, very sick, and you have to accept that. I didn't choose this, but we all have to live with it, and it's hard for all of us."

The other was that it doesn't matter how upset you are, there are behaviors you can't do. There were business calls, and Todd got on the phone and was totally obnoxious. I had to go downstairs and say, "You can't behave like this. Go to your room. It doesn't matter how aggravated you are, you cannot behave like that."

Todd and Preston had to do a lot more chores. I asked Todd to do something one day, and he said, "No, I don't want to do it, I'm tired," and I said, "Well, we all have to do more because I'm sick, I can't do what I used to do," and he said, "But I *am* doing more." He started listing, and he wasn't belligerent, and I said, "You're right. Okay, you don't have to do that." So trying to show him that I understood. I thought he needed to be cut a little slack 'cause it's hard. It's hard.

I missed the whole spring soccer season. It was right in the middle of the chemo, and I could not get up. The amount of time I spent sleeping is really astonishing. *[Laughs]* It wiped me out, so there were a lot of things I just wasn't paying attention to. Like, I know Todd is growing like gangbusters and must have eaten a lot of junk food and odd meals 'cause I wasn't on top of it. I just couldn't. I'm not going to beat myself up about it. You can only do what you can do.

I'd have these little bursts of "things Mother wants you to remember." *[Laughs]* We'd gone out to Inverness for one night earlier in the spring, and we were walking and talking, saying hello to people, which is part of what I learned in Africa, and I said to Todd, "You should always greet people because it's weaving the fabric of society." I was kind of making up [for lost time]. Deferred mothering—you get it all at once.

What does it mean to be a parent? Of course, it varies with the age of the kid and how sick you are. What are the parts of parenting that are most important to the kid? What parts are most important for you? How do you hand the parenting over to the other parent during the time when you're so wiped, and what can you drop?

For me, it was maintaining the physical presence—walking to

school, meeting him, kissing him goodnight every night, and then going, "Oh, my goodness, I forgot to tell you all these rules for living. Pay attention. I'm going to give you twenty right now." "Eat your vegetables" is what I dropped. If I'd known I was dying, I would have been at the soccer games because of what it meant, but I said, "There'll be another soccer season."

Now, we're moving into adolescence. One of the most helpful things was a mom with cancer who said, "I've got teenage kids, and mostly they're mad because they have to do more chores." *[Laughter]* Just knowing that's what was coming was helpful.

We all could use help with parenting, God knows. That's why I organized the sixth-grade mothers of sons at our school. We had lunch and got ready for adolescence. We said, "We should not go through this alone." There were so many mothers who said, "Oh, I thought it was just my kid. I thought I was alone." I didn't think that; I'm a sociologist!

The times when Todd talks, I try to make sure I'm there. I always put him to bed. What he often does is call out, "Hey, Mom," and then I'll go back in. I don't care what I'm doing. You have to wait for the moment, and then, when it comes, you go with it.

Every day of chemo, we watched videos together. We put the TV in our bedroom. The only place to sit was on our bed, so we all sat on the bed watching the video, which meant that Todd could, without it being a big deal, cuddle up, which he did a lot, particularly in the beginning. You know, he's twelve, he's supposed to be separating, but it was a space in which everyone could be physically close together.

How do you talk to your kid? How do you go on talking to your kid and keep that space open? Once isn't enough. It goes on being an issue. And with a twelve-year-old boy, what could be more embarrassing than to have a mom with breast cancer? I called every single one of Todd's teachers and the parents of all his friends so they would be listening and be there if Todd needed somebody to talk to. So, I had a whole team out there. My surgeon said if we wanted to bring Todd in, we could. Todd didn't want to. The radiation therapist said, "You know, bring him in, we'll show him the machines." I thought he would think that was cool, but he didn't want to see it.

How do you know when they're scared? When Todd walked out

on the balcony in the hospital, that was a no-brainer. But what if you are dying? What do you do? We all have this little cloud: It could come back. I believe that I've beaten it, but I have night terrors like everybody else. What if it comes back before he's out of high school? I think *[Knocks on a wooden table]* it's going to be okay. He's a very good kid, a stable kid, he has a good sense of values, and I think having gone through this experience together is kind of awesome. But listening more, talking more, trying to keep those spaces open—that's hard.

When I was going through chemo, Todd discovered a lump in his nipple and it hurt, and I said to him, "I can tell you that if it hurts, it's not cancer, but I'm going to call the advice nurse right now." I called the advice nurse, and she said, "Oh, yes, this is very common in boys," so I told him, and about a week later he said, "But it's still there." I called his pediatrician, and I said, "Todd has got to see you. I know this is nothing, but he's got to see you." This guy is a specialist and has an incredibly crowded schedule, and he made room. We went in, and John climbed up on the examining table with him, examined him, put his arms around him, and explained this isn't cancer. And that was so important. Of course, when we came out, Todd said, "Well, why did we go see him? We could have just called." *[Laughs]*

This cancer does have implications for him. I said to my oncologist yesterday, "I know in my heart of hearts I've beaten this. What do you think of that?" He said, "I think that's a very healthy way to think." I also asked him, "I know what it means for a daughter. What does it mean for a son, for Todd? And he said, "Well, I'd recommend that he not have a sex-change operation."

But it may be that the sons of women with breast cancer have a higher incidence of prostate cancer.[1] There's going to be a point at which he probably should be checking for that. So, it's not just my mortality, but it's his mortality, and that's very upsetting to me.

What has been the hardest or the most frightening part for you in all this?

It's the fear of dying and leaving him. Even to say it, to think that I wouldn't be there to be giving him my love, protecting him, rejoicing in his growing—that would break my heart. I've been so lucky—well, I've been sick as hell, let's not forget that, but I haven't been debilitated in the way some are. But to have him see me really, really sick and not be able to do anything about that. . . . Because you want your kids not to be frightened. And realizing, "Wow, I've spent a lot of time when I should have been mothering but couldn't." That's the hard thing. But the thought of leaving . . . How do you hand over if you're dying? Where else can the parenting come from? I know that people would be there for him, my family and my friends, but you are not replaceable. It would be the same thing if Preston were to die. Preston is not replaceable. When my father died, that was my *father*. I don't know how you make peace with that.

Until now, Marge had related her cancer story, even the parts about Todd, with the same exuberance and ease as her other adventures. In fact, she seemed to have been sailing through the cancer experience, announcing her arrival at the next port, "Here I am on the other side." Now the wind shifts.

I don't know why, but I always had a sense of building memories for him so that if something did happen, he always had these things to hang onto. Sometimes, it sweeps me away—the fear, the fierceness of that love. I started making a cookbook called *Todd Can Cook* several years ago. Every time we would cook something together, I'd put in an entry. I always tried to make it a little funny. To leave him many tangible tokens of my love.

That hasn't changed, but when you're face-to-face with your own mortality, I'm much more conscious of the values and lessons that I want him to have articulated very clearly, and I think I'm doing that—like this sudden "weaving the fabric of society" speech. It's given me opportunities to talk about neighborliness. There are things that we have always done as neighbors, but now we have been big-time recipients. And about colleagues. All these cards would come in—we get calls from all over the world, and talking with him about who was calling and how this helped. That whole thing of thanking people, really being aware of the teams of people that go into healing.

I think some very good things have come out of it. He's experienced the love of friends and neighbors and family, people pulling together. He's learned that no matter how scary something is, it's never a forbidden topic of conversation. I think it's really important that people should be out front with the fact that they have cancer. When people are ill, taking care of them helps the community. I really feel that. Right now, I'm in the receiving mode, and I've been in the giving mode, and I'll be in the giving mode again. You know, some people hide it. I find that incredible. Man, I was out there. I wanted everyone in the world on my team!

He's learned that you can make carrot juice for somebody. You can help heal other people. If I've been brave, he's known what bravery is. I now realize I don't know what "bravery" means because everyone I know with cancer is dealing with cancer, so I guess we're all brave. And he's learned you don't have to collapse in the face of it. You still tell jokes. You still go for walks. We had my husband's fiftieth birthday party right in the middle of my chemo.

What keeps you going when things are hard?

Celebrating. Cancer, for me, has been a thousand tiny celebrations. "My drains are out two days early. Yippee." "Look, I can get my arm over my head." "Look, my hair's falling out, it means the chemo's working." "Now chemo's over. We're going to have a no-cancer dancing party, date to be announced." I have to be able to stay up until ten and dance. Making the celebrations for him, too.

You know, he'll tease for candy or potato chips, and I don't answer, "No, you can't, you'll get cancer and die," or "Grrrr, this is terrible, you can't have that, you can have health-giving broccoli." When we were out at Point Reyes, I started singing—I have no idea why this popped into my head—the U.S. Marine Corps hymn, "Semper Fidelis." I just started laughing. I realized that it was such a relief for everybody to be laughing. And being silly. And that it was over. Of course, I have six appointments that have something to do with cancer this week. Never mind.

Do you think being a parent has helped you to cope with cancer?

I think being a mother absolutely gives you something to live for, and it gives you something to do. You've got to be there for that kid every day. You have to be present—not just awake, present. That love is always there, so you've got that coming in. Todd's been like a lodestar for me.

I really believe that all that love and caring from friends all over the world, but most particularly from Preston and Todd, have helped me get well. I have come through this so lightly. It has been awful, but compared to a lot of people, I've been very lucky. Some of that's biology,

I'm sure, but some of it's having that incredible support. This disease binds you to anybody else who has it. People I wait with in radiation—I know all of their stories. We're all in this together.

The humor has gotten me through it. I can't say whether my faith has gotten me through it or not because my faith is so complex. I mean, I'm not criticizing anybody for crying all day if that's how they get through cancer, but I think that it's better not to be crying all day.

I've said to people, "Cancer saved my life"—which sounds very odd—because before the diagnosis I had been, over a period of eighteen months, suffering from depression. It had become quite severe in the fall, and I had gone on Prozac at the end of October. It was making a difference, I was starting to see myself again. But with the cancer . . . whereas before that, every day I'd been saying, "I wish I were dead, I wish I were dead," I was now saying, "I'm beating this, you're not going to kill me, forget it." So, the experience has been not only recovering from cancer but recovering from depression. I've had a chance to get well from two things. So that's been sort of ironic.

My guess is that the cancer is probably easier for Todd than the depression. Because with the cancer, he could *do* something. He could make the carrot juice. He could cuddle up. I mean, I was *really* depressed. I had trouble with insomnia. I taught three classes right through it. It was like being on autopilot. But it was coming to a point where I was getting very close to being non-functional. It was scary. I would sit in the back of my closet—it sounds embarrassing and stupid, but you know about depression—crying, and I didn't know why. I remember driving [home] one day from work and crying and saying, "Nobody cares about me," and Todd said, "I care about you," and I had the wits about me to say, "I know you love me, Todd. I love you, too."

Watching somebody unravel in front of your very eyes, I think, was more frightening. With cancer, I spent so much time sleeping, I didn't look my best, but there was never a day I didn't get out of bed and get dressed and do stuff, meet him at school. So, I suspect the depression was probably worse for him.

Have you talked with him at all about these changes you've been through?

I haven't. No. He's a very private somebody. He's one of those, "How's school?" "Fine." "What did you do?" "Stuff." With the cancer, I had no choice about being open about how I was in a hard place. Actually, during the depression, once I did say to him, "Sometimes Mommy feels really, really sad, and it's not your fault." It's this terribly delicate balance. Kids aren't there to take care of you. I needed to be more willing to share when it's tough for me without it being: "And therefore, you should do something about it."

In spite of my earlier skepticism about Marge's airtight story, her sudden disclosure shocks me. I thought we had arrived at a place where the cancer experience seemed well integrated into her larger journey surprisingly soon after treatment. But with one sentence, "Cancer saved my life," Marge alters course and steers us into less charted waters.

At first, it is difficult to put Marge Schmitt and depression together. "Unraveling," "non-functional," "suicidal," and "isolated" are unlikely descriptions of this confident, connected, life-loving woman of action. But "Mom was no longer Mom." Such is the power of depressive illness, which, like cancer, does not discriminate. Depressed mothers can also be physically ill, and, as in Marge's case, the two conditions can interact in surprising ways.

Depression, not cancer, was the pivotal event that unraveled the web Marge had created, ripping up connections, especially to her own life force. That long-awaited trip to Africa must have been terribly important for her, offering a way out of depression and back into the world. The subsequent cancer diagnosis might have literally shocked her back into herself. At the very least, the diagnosis had mobilized anger that had been suppressed. It had also reminded her that she had something to live for—her son.

Cancer helped Marge go from "I wish I were dead" to "You're not going to kill me." But, in many ways, she is still in the middle of the illness crisis—and a torn-up story—in spite of her repeated announcements to the contrary. As Marge continues to talk about the factors in her healing, including her "complex faith," I feel as if the tape of her cancer story has been rewound and restarted. Now, a different singer and song begin to emerge.

Cancer has been, for me, a very spiritual kind of thing. Maybe I should talk about that.

When I was diagnosed with cancer, I didn't ask, "Why is God

doing this to me?" 'cause I know about distribution curves. *[Laughs]* The academic life and spiritual life are kind of mutually exclusive. I always found it hard to find that somebody I knew to be really smart was also deeply religious. It seemed inconsistent. One of the things about cancer, maybe also just growing older, is finding a spiritual part of myself I never knew before.

The only really spiritual experience I had before this was at home working one day. All of a sudden, the garden—I can't say it was filled with light, but there was this moment when I said, "If there really is a God and it's a loving God, this is what God's love is like." I've never had a spiritual feeling in a Christian church. I find most ministers have no sense of spirituality. It's just another profession.

But I wanted to go to communion. I was afraid. There's such a mystique around cancer. I always thought it was something you died of. In my hotel room in South Africa, I wasn't exactly afraid. But I was. It was very complex. I thought, *I've done bad things in my life, none of which were all that horrible, but they sort of loomed large, I'll go to hell, whatever hell is, exactly.*

We had a horrible experience at church. Preston was afraid he would cry if he asked them to pray for me, so he told the pastor. There's a time in our service when people say "Peace of the Lord" and shake hands or hug everyone and go and talk. But after the pastor announced my cancer, everybody avoided us. We were just stunned. Because in South Africa, there I was with two hundred and fifty strangers, most of whom came up and hugged me—the word kind of spread.

Marge received communion in her home from an "amazing" minister she knows, and she continues to explore other avenues of spirituality and healing. I wonder how she balances these practices with her work and home life.

There are conflicts. One is trying to keep the balance that cancer's allowed me to have. I've been able to be off work spending a lot of time with Todd and Preston. I said from the beginning, "I'm not sacrificing my family on the altar of tenure," and I never did. But giving myself permission to take care of myself, which I think is hard for a lot of women because we were raised to take care of other people. So, one of the reasons for staying on sick leave is practicing that. I've been working on a twenty-year sleep deficit. I'm still saying, "No, no, I won't do that. You can see me in my office hours when they start in January. Go away, leave me alone."

I've learned so much. I think cancer has taught me to calm down, be more focused, be more contemplative, trying to weed out the stuff that isn't going to make a difference. I've discovered that I love doing art. It's a kind of creativity, an outlet. I've learned the practices of yoga and meditation, and I'm pretty faithful. They're profoundly spiritual. They're about connection and also more about openness and living in your body. Well, now I have a different body.

And I don't think you can ever forget how fragile the thread of life is and how there's so many things that don't matter. So, you're bald? You're alive! [Laughs] I stood in front of seven hundred people and sang with a bald head. A lot of that stuff doesn't matter.

I sang in a chorus two weeks ago, and they had all these potato chips and all this stuff, and I ate carrots, and it wasn't even a choice. One day, I just had to say, "The most important thing I have to do is fight for my life." It would be a hell of a lot easier if you were out with a sword. But you do the soy, eat organic, get rid of all the plastic in the microwave, take your medicine. It means those things for Todd, too, that it's serious. It's easier for me to change my diet than to change his diet—I haven't done it perfectly—but I'm working on it. So, that has changed my mothering.

I'm going to be there for Todd. Whatever it takes. I always think, "Todd didn't ask to be born." It's really important to be there for him. You can't give it to him when you're eighty and have enough time.

The big question for me is how I'm going to use my work time so it makes the biggest difference in eliminating injustice—well, not quite, but making a dent. But I have to have the other things because they sustain me.

I ask Marge if she thinks differently now about saving the world.

Spirituality has come to me to be a series of connections at many, many levels, and I guess I only started to think about that with the cancer. But I believe you have to take action. Just accepting everything is not part of who I am. I guess spirituality has always been wrapped up in the ethics in my life and in social justice issues. There are gifts God gave us, and we should use them to make the world a better place—a place where there's no suffering, no injustice, no one's living in poverty, where we're taking care of the environment, not poisoning it. We have to figure out ways to stop cancer. I firmly believe it has to do with pollution of the environment, with over-consumption. Each one of us, myself included, needs to work on making "enough" a bigger part of our vocabulary. We don't need more, more, more, more of this and that. I think that also means paying attention to violence, both in its physical and its non-physical forms. And decent housing, enough clean water and food, and clean air. We need to have shorter work weeks. We're such workaholics. It's so enormous. We have to *do* something about this!

Given the gifts I have and the time I may or may not have, what are the things I absolutely have to do? How to hand on what I know how to do, and how to do stuff that's going to make a difference? That's a big one. I don't know. I do not know. Is writing where I should be putting my time? Is it research in Zimbabwe? Should I be spending more time on teaching? *I've got to choose.* Because I want to do too many things. Some things I've done that made me important are also things that have made a difference, but some of them are just, I'm embarrassed to say, ego-stroking stuff. That's out. I am returning to obscurity. I intend never to be as stressed again, knock on wood. At least I will never be triple-booked again, says Scarlett O'Hara. *[Laughs]*

Is there a change you can make to bring more healing into your life right now?

The Buddhists talk about softening around things that you can't change. So, with the cancer, it's fighting against it but also softening around the experience. That, to me, has been a very profound insight. Softening toward myself, being more forgiving, giving myself more time, and softening towards others. I am in a very judgmental profession. That's something that I try to be: less judgmental.

If I have dreams, I'm fighting with somebody or arguing with somebody. Now, when I wake up, I re-do the dream so it has no fighting. Yeah, trying to get rid of anger, kind of letting that stuff go. You know, if you're doing social justice stuff, it's real easy to get incredibly self-righteous. That's kind of obnoxious. Let that go, too. I try to do my yoga every day and meditation, so the practice supports that softening. Actually, I never thought that you can be strong without being angry. You *can* be strong and be gentle. That's what I'm learning.

The role of anger during serious illness is complex for Marge. Anger helped pull her out of depression, but it is exhausting to fight all the time. I wonder what she's taken away from having close friends, some quite young, die from cancer.

What do I take away from that? An enormous sense of unfairness. I have not been able to soften their deaths. They were too soon, and they took wonderful people out of the world. I guess the one thing you take out of it is that you can die at any time. You and everyone around you is precious.

Do you feel that your own situation is unfair?

"Unfair" somehow means that you deserved something and you got something else, and I don't think there's any sort of deserving.

One of the things about art therapy for me was that it is a brain bypass. It just comes out of the fingers, whether I'm sewing a quilt square or drawing. As a result, I learned a lot of things that I couldn't articulate in words. I didn't even know they were there. One was my rage at having cancer.

I have not chosen cancer. It's not a gift. If it is, I want to find the return counter. *[Laughs]* It's not original, I'm sure you've heard this a thousand times.

I made a square for the breast cancer quilt, and I sent photocopies to my mother, my brother, and my sister. It had a poem with it which was about what they do with all the breasts. It was a fairly enraged poem, and my brother said, *"Never send me anything again."* My sister loved it, and my mother said, "Well, I'm glad you were able to get rid of some of your resentment. All my friends are coming to see your quilt square, and I want to know what symbolism there is."

I was blown away that she had accepted this thing which was enraged and wanted to know about it. So, I think my relationship with my mother has really been healed and deepened by this—my whole family. We've always been a fairly close family, but the tensions, particularly with the depression, were higher, and all of that has healed.

My mother, like my son, is a very private somebody, and she always has to live by rules, and it's allowed her to say how much she cares, and it's allowed me, because I've had the time to work on the depression, to forgive her for how I was treated when I was a child. That forgiveness was very important. Cancer gives you a permission to say "I love you" to people.

And what do you most hope for yourself at this point?
I hope that I do not have a recurrence. I know that if I have one I will deal with it bravely, courageously, and with grace. But I don't want to, thank you. *[Laughs]* And then the other hopes are that I'll be a good mother to my son, and he'll grow up to be a good and wonderful person, and that my work will make a difference. From recording this story, I came up with a rather fierce little slogan. I met with my students last week, and we all toasted: "May our research be a thorn in the side of those who do evil and a spear in the hand of those who do good." That's a pretty big hope. *[Laughs]* Pretty big.

I never asked Marge about what had led to her depression or explored in depth the interaction of the two illnesses and their impact on her mothering. Part of my reticence stemmed from timing: She had just completed chemotherapy, and the material might have been too raw to pursue.

Marge hadn't wanted to dwell on the negative or on her formative years. Perhaps, like her mother and son, she is a "very private somebody," at least in certain areas of her life. She was working on issues of forgiveness and letting go of anger and may not have wanted to stir up painful past events. I felt that Marge was in the midst of the cancer crisis in spite of her repeated statements that "it was over," that she was "on the other side."

In fact, those statements, in contrast with others she made, suggest that she was in the middle of two types of illness narratives that had not yet been reconciled. The first story Marge told was similar to what Arthur Frank calls "a restitution narrative," which often dominates the stories of the recently ill.[2] The disease is not a gift, and the entire goal is to become cured and get to "the other side," to where you were in your body and in your life before diagnosis.

The second story, beginning with the words "Cancer saved my life," spiraled deeper. This seemed like a "quest narrative," in which the illness leads to new insights, new purpose, and sometimes even a new identity.[3] To heal from depression and cancer, Marge believed she needed to soften around what she can't change, to forgive herself, and to care for herself. These insights, along with the acknowledged gifts of illness, were part of a narrative that had not yet fully formed.

As Frank explains, different narrative types coexist and interrupt each other. Somewhere between the two, Marge was struggling with night terrors and questions about how she could find balance for herself while passing on a legacy to both her son and her students.

Weeks after we finished the recording, Marge was back in the center of her web, with the same passions and themes as before. But with a difference. She now had a vision of strength driven neither by anger nor action. Instead of falling into a thousand pieces, she was holding a thousand tiny celebrations. And cancer was the catalyst.

Five: "You Can Go Through Anything"
Lorraine McKinley

"A LOT OF PEOPLE tell me that I am like my mother. I can even look in the mirror now and say, 'Oooh, I'm looking more like Mommy, and my ways are easygoing.' My mom was *somebody*. She never smoked, she never drank, she never cursed, nothing. She was always close to the Lord, and I am, too. Whatever people needed her to do, she would always do it or try her best to do it. I miss her a lot."

I've never met Lorraine McKinley's mother, but I see at a glance that her daughter, too, is *somebody*. A dignified black woman of forty-five and mother of three children, ages two, four, and eighteen, Lorraine greets me at our volunteer listener training with a strong handshake and a smile. Her hair is pulled back into a tight chignon, and her attire is Sunday best and carefully tailored, but Lorraine's face is open. She has offered to share her experience of mothering with cancer with our first group of volunteers. Like the mother she describes, she is eager to help.

This is our first meeting. Two years earlier, Dr. Deborrah Bremond, a project advisor, had helped pilot our methods by recording Lorraine's story. From reading the transcripts, I learned that Lorraine had struggled to overcome a speech impediment. My admiration for her increased when she agreed to speak to our group.

Before we begin, I notice Lorraine exchanging hugs, chatting, and laughing with the other panel members—all strangers, all white. When it's her turn to speak, she does so with confidence and warmth. I am struck by the same impressions I'd had when reviewing her manuscript. This is a straightforward woman who has learned to handle stressful situations with grace, a mother who went through cancer without having her story seriously disturbed.

In the following weeks, I puzzle over questions I'd had when first reading her history. Before Lorraine, I had assumed that most people experience critical illness as a transformative event or, at least, one that shakes up a personal narrative. Certainly, my own experience with a less serious disability had fit Dr. Jean Shinoda Bolen's description of illness as initiation into a soul journey.[1] Most sick people I had known reinforced this assumption, especially the mothers I was meeting through the project. Life-threatening illness changed them, often in profound ways.

I had also believed that cancer, in particular, causes significant suffering, intensified by the presence of children. That expectation had been shaped by my experience with relatives who had the disease, by books and films on the subject, and, most recently, by the mothers. In fact, it was the suffering of these women as mothers that was most compelling to me. Yet, beyond some initial shock, Lorraine claimed that cancer had not been particularly difficult for her. It hadn't changed her as a mother or a person, and she didn't fear death at all. Talking with Dr. Bremond, a woman of color, reinforced at least one of my impressions. For Lorraine, cancer was a blip on the screen. Her experience appeared to have little to do with race, aside from the fact that religion has traditionally been a source of hope for many black women.

Lorraine was challenging my ideas about life stories, mothering with cancer, and myself as an unbiased listener. I believe it's impossible to engage in "nonjudgmental listening," a term favored in many hospice, meditation, and psychotherapy circles. However, a good listener strives to become aware of her judgments and expectations in order to keep from imposing them on the narrator. In the context of the project, she tries to maintain an open mind and a willingness to reevaluate preconceptions about illness, death and dying, and childrearing.

Had I missed something in the narrative? Is it possible for a devoted mother like Lorraine not to be torn up over the threatened separation from her children? Can one go through a life-threatening illness and remain essentially the same? I decide to review Lorraine's story before and after cancer.

LORRAINE

As a child, I talked a lot but was very shy and afraid to talk in front of people because of one thing: I stuttered. It wasn't a bad stuttering, but I think it was what gave me a complex as a young girl. My father would say, "Well, can't you talk better than that?"

Sometimes when you stutter, you take a little bit longer saying things, and people don't like to wait and listen. "Okay, Lorraine, hurry up, hurry up, say what you're trying to say." So that would make me feel nervous and uncomfortable. There were times I did feel humiliated. Very, very humiliated. My mom never did it. Never. She would just listen. She was always very loving and giving to us. It was my dad—but that was just his way of doing it.

Growing up, communication in our family wasn't good, not good at all. Basically a lot of tension, a lot of violence, anger, fighting. We never had that close communication where you can share with your parents and they give you good advice. Never could we be intimate, share real feelings. My dad was always negative, so you didn't feel comfortable about sharing anything with him. Months later, he'll throw it back up in your face. Daddy was just mad and angry. His way or no way at all.

So that built up insecurity and that complex I had. Even into adulthood, I would be afraid to get in front of people and speak because that would be in the back of my mind: "Oh, no, I'm going to mess up, I'm going to stutter." When I would get very nervous, you could swear I couldn't talk or read.

As I got older, I said, "I'm going to have to do something about this. I can't allow this fear to paralyze me all my life because it's going to stop me from doing things that I want to do." So I prayed about that, asked the Lord to help me to overcome that. I started learning to take my time to speak, and I claimed that Scripture: "I can do all things through Christ because He's my strength."

I started teaching a skincare class because it put me in front of people to talk. Now I can get up, and I may feel a little uncomfortable, but I know that I need to speak slowly, and then I can do it. It all worked out. I don't feel that fear like I used to.

When I went to college, algebra was really hard for me. My mom never got me a tutor because I never talked about it. I would try to work it myself. But I took the class over, whether it was three or four times, until I came out of it with an "A." I just kept at it. So that was a real achievement.

School was enjoyable. I liked learning, but I was never good with the standardized tests. I got a "C" in some class which had to do with my nursing classes, and the counselor said, "You know, you should change your major. You should get into doing something like secretarial work." And, if I allowed her to discourage me, I would have never gone through nursing school.

I graduated from university in nursing and married the same year and took the Boards, but I didn't pass. I was just a little bit short and took it again and still was a little bit short. I was very disappointed when I didn't pass. I cried. Then, when I took it again, I left feeling that I had passed. And I didn't. I was so bottled up in nerves and discouraged, I said, "I don't want to take it and then not pass. I *am* going to take it again, but right now, my focus is someplace else." I started working for an endocrinology practice doing reception work and, when the nurse wasn't there, taking blood pressures, stuff like that. So, when my mom had her stroke, and then a year later she had another stroke, I never went back.

And when my father would ask me if I passed and I said "No," he just looked at me. He looked at me like I was manure on the bottom of a shoe. Another time when I took the test and didn't pass, and he asked me if I passed it, I told him, "Yes" because I didn't want to hear his discouraging remarks nor see his disappointed look.

I'm not working as a nurse or anything now, and my father has told me on several occasions, "Your education has gone down the drain." And I say, "Well, no, it hasn't, Daddy, it really hasn't because I still stay informed, and I had my children and I monitor them when they're sick, and I cared for my mom." I guess he didn't see it then, but I was there every day, taking care of my mom. I used my education with my brother when he was ill. And I could use it even with my cancer diagnosis. I was able to go to the resources and read up and explore more.

But he just says I'm not working as a nurse, and that's it. Now that I'm doing okay, he says, "You know, I think you still should go back to the nursing." I do plan, eventually, on taking the Boards. I mean,

I don't feel comfortable with myself. I have that Bachelor of Science degree, but I need to finish, I need to be licensed. I *will* do it, and I will pass it.

I think my parents really wanted me to succeed in life. For example, my parents put me through nursing school. My mommy had so much faith in us. She always felt that we would do well. She wanted us to continue our education. My father's very work-oriented. You got to be on a job to succeed. I look at success as being able to accomplish my goals. Finishing nursing school is my greatest achievement.

I always wanted to be married, have a husband and children, a marriage that would last until death do us part, with a husband that took care of the family and where I also would help out. That was the picture that I saw in my mom and dad. They were hard workers. My father took care of his family, working two jobs. We never had to worry about where food was coming from, or clothing, or shelter. We grew up in a good home.

The worst thing is my first marriage not working, and I say that because both of us were—both of us *are*—believers, and I felt that our marriage should have and could have worked. But it didn't. The marriage lasted three years, and our son was born, Joshua, when I was twenty-seven. When I was a single parent, I was blessed because I was able to move back home and work and go to school, and I had my parents to keep Joshua if I needed to work nights. I think I struggled more being out on my own than being a single parent. I was at home until I graduated from nursing school, and then I married again.

I feel that my [second] marriage has been successful. I enjoy marriage, but marriage is something you have to work at. I enjoy our family, having the three children and raising them. I'm glad I'm home with the children. I do not regret motherhood, not one bit. I count it very rewarding, at times stressful, but very pleasurable to be able to raise my children in the nurture and admonition of the Lord. I enjoy being able to give them some sound upbringing and values. I enjoy the playtime with my children, seeing them grow up and develop physically and mentally and spiritually. I really enjoy being loved by them as well as me giving them love. They all come to me and say, "I love you, Mommy," and they kiss me and they hug me.

How do you feel you learned to be a parent?

I learned from my parents. I think that they did a real good job, teaching us the way of the Lord, to live a life that is pleasing to Him. And to enjoy family. To be a good parent, I think you should get some instruction. There's a lot that I still need to learn. I am doing things a little differently. Our parents never told us that they loved us. They showed us love by taking good care of us. I was raising Joshua back home, and I would always tell him, "I love you, Joshua." I noticed that my mom one time said, "Joshua, come here," and she told him that she loved him. So I'm thinking maybe she saw me do that all the time.

What have you learned about yourself that you didn't know before having children?

That I can be stern. I can be very firm. I don't tolerate a bunch of nonsense. Life experiences teach you a lot.

The hard thing is the talk-back. They're smart alecky. Then I think of how I was when I was a child. I was too afraid to get in any trouble, afraid of disappointing my parents. But the hardest thing for me has been with Joshua getting in trouble, getting arrested, going to juvenile hall for a couple of days. He's doing a lot better. He's going to technical school. He's eighteen, but I still fuss at him. As he gets older and more mature, I'm going give him advice, and however he decides to take it and order his life, that's entirely up to him. Every parent wants their child to grow up basically free from all the trauma that's going on in the world, but of course we can't shelter them because they are becoming adults. But I really keep him in prayer.

Since you're mentioning prayer, I wonder if you would talk about other important influences in your life, especially religion.

Well, Daddy was someone who goes to church and that's all. A lot of black people, they just go. But, in order for a change to be brought about in your life, you have to get into the Word of God. The way that I define spirituality is the personal relationship that I have with Jesus Christ and not only studying the Word of God, but living in obedience to how He would have me live.

That is the best thing, to build an intimate relationship with my Lord and Savior, Jesus Christ. A lot of the things that I experienced in life I see as Him developing me and refining my character. That's why I think I'm able to deal with a lot, like my diagnosis—I know that He has a hand in it, conforming me to be more like Him every day. So that is *the* greatest thing in my whole life. Another is my husband and my children. And another thing is Mary Kay cosmetics. I wanted to do something while I was at home, and I thought about doing medical transcription, but I didn't want anything that was so highly stressed. So then someone introduced me to Mary Kay Cosmetics, and I really enjoy it. Now, I'm beginning to learn how to accomplish because we go through a lot of good training. They help us to grow and teach us how to be consistent and how to be successful, not only in our Mary Kay careers but in our own personal lives. So this is getting me out of my comfort zone. It's getting me to talk in front of people. It's building the confidence that I can do it, I can do it.

Mary Kay has a phrase: "We fall forward to success." You fall, but success is not giving up. Success is persevering. If I fall, don't stay down but get up and work at it. Persevere.

Lorraine was diagnosed with early stage breast cancer while she was still weaning her youngest child, a girl not yet two. Her sons were four and eighteen. The doctor discovered the mass during a yearly gynecological exam but initially suspected clogged milk ducts. A mammogram was negative. Five months later, Lorraine began to experience pain in her right breast and arm. After expressing blood from the nipple while waiting to see the doctor, she was sent to a surgeon. He believed the problem was caused by a papilloma, a small, wartlike growth in the lining of a mammary duct that can produce clear or bloody discharge from the nipple. When the growth didn't go away in ninety days, she was finally advised to have surgery.

When I had the first surgery, which was a partial mastectomy, the surgeon went in and took all the mass out, and that's where they found the cancer. He told me he needed to go back in and do a total mastectomy although the cancer cells were so, so tiny. My oncologist drew a picture and showed me why they had to go in and do the modified radical mastectomy. They found that the cancer cells were in three different locations—if they just took out that one part, there would still be cancer cells. Also, the tumors were very close to the duct margins or the walls, and they were afraid that some could have seeped out. They took out seventeen lymph nodes, and those came back negative for cancer.

When I was told that I needed to have the surgery, I didn't think twice about it. My surgeon took my case before the tumor board, and all these doctors agreed to do what he had determined to do. I didn't think about getting a second opinion. I felt very comfortable with what he said had to be done. You think about prolonging your life for yourself, for your children, and for your husband.

After my surgeon told us what the diagnosis and prognosis were, my husband and I went home in the car, very quiet. We didn't say too much. And when we got home, we all prayed together as a family. My son Joshua was at work, so he wasn't with us, but the two little ones and my husband and I, we prayed, and I cried.

I've always been in good health, and I've always tried to be very conscious about what I put into my body to promote good health. Of course, there's times you eat your little sweets or your little chips or whatever, but, all in all, I try to focus on good nutrition. And *whammo!* See, I did everything right as can be. Whoa! And I said, "Lord, what went out of kilter here?"

My immediate thought was I may not live long, and I thought about the children and my husband and that I may be leaving them. I think we focus on cancer as "Oh, no, I'm going to die." And then I began to think, well, not all sickness is unto death.

I would get up for my devotion early every morning at five, and I prayed to the Lord and really shared my heart, and I asked Him to heal me. I went through the surgery and the chemo and some alternative care, which I'm going through even now.

Probably the children were too young to fully understand what's really going on—not even two and four. We told them I had to go into the hospital and have surgery. They knew that I was gone for two days. They knew that when I came home, I was bandaged up on my right side, and they saw that I was resting in bed. They knew that I was going to appointments all the time. And that was about it.

You know how children do, they carry on their daily lives. I don't believe it worried them. But then, my little ones, they did notice the bandages. My little girl knows this breast is not here *[Points to her chest]*, but she sees the left one, so when she sees me get out of the shower, she loves to touch that breast. She even tries to suck again a little bit. She was saying, "What happened to your breast?" I said, "Oh, it was diseased so I had to get it cut off." She says, "Oh." And that's basically how it is. I think that everything still carries on for them because

I'm doing well. And I think the way in which we handled it, they didn't really see it as a downer, like something that was really dark.

The part of me with a professional view of child development shudders at Lorraine's message to her child, who may believe that whatever gets diseased will get cut off. We can't assume that children who don't talk about or show symptoms of distress are perfectly fine. At the same time, I wonder if Lorraine's matter-of-fact explanation and ease in the face of illness might give an even more potent message to soothe a young child's anxiety. However, eighteen-year-old Joshua may not be so easily reassured.

I had told Joshua that I was diagnosed with breast cancer, and his first response is, "Mommy, it's not fair. You eat so healthy, and that's not fair that you've done all this to take care of yourself and it means nothing." So that's where he was, I believe, in a state of confusion. He had a hard time understanding to the point that one of the counselors at school called me and said, "Joshua is really scared." I think the first thing he thought is that he is going to lose me, but he never appeared to me like he was running scared. Then, I noticed he said things. When I was doing better and I was up and around doing things, he was saying, "You not sick, you not sick," and I think that's maybe what he wanted to believe, that I was not sick.

The counselor gave me a number to call where they counsel adolescents. So I asked Joshua, and he said, "Yes." Then he had to do a research paper, and he chose breast cancer. I think that by him obtaining that knowledge, it did a lot for him. We never did see the counselor. He felt more comfortable, and I was doing so well.

I never really felt sick, to be perfectly honest. I had the surgery. I recovered quite well. I would just have little spurts of low energy, and then I would rest and I was fine. The chemo did impact my bone marrow so hard. I didn't know it, but when they took a lab test, there was one time I only had four hundred white blood cells in my body. See, I started out with a low white blood cell count anyhow because I'm considered [as having] benign leukopenia. I was told that's common among black women, and it's nothing. They had to postpone chemo two or three times because my counts were so low, so they'd boost me with Neupogen.

I think the hardest was after I had chemotherapy treatments.

I couldn't move around as fast as I wanted to. That's the time my kids saw me more in bed. If I moved around too fast or did too much around the house, I would begin to feel nauseous. So that was a time that I couldn't really function. I couldn't get up and do a lot with the children. But otherwise, I did fine on chemo. Just a few times, I began to get a little fever. But my temperature never got outrageous.

So, in general, the family routine didn't get very disrupted?

It didn't. My husband went to the treatment center with me. A lot of times, the kids were there, too. It was a family affair. The only person that was not there was Joshua because he was in school, and from school he went to work. The kids were there even to the point where they saw me get chemo. They saw the IV in my hand. Mary would say, "Mommy, what's that?" and I'd say, "Oh, that's Mommy's medicine." My little girl would get up in the bed with me. One time, she fell asleep. And they would watch TV. One time, one of the nurses brought them the videotape of *Toy Story*, so we watched that. It was real normal.

Over this whole period, have you had any concerns about your kids?

They're just really continuing on. The only concern I have for my little girl is I think she eats a little too much peanut butter, and peanut butter is known to be a contributory factor for breast cancer,[2] and I have to really watch her because of me. Otherwise, everything carries on as usual.

Do you think anything good has come out of this for your children?

I think that by me being a model for them, that would be something that will always stay in their minds. They don't have to collapse under pressure or a bad situation. You can rise above your circumstances. So I hope I have been able to show them that.

My hope for my children is that they grow up to be responsible and be able to deal with difficult situations without falling apart. They still may go through situations where they will collapse. But then they can think back and see how Mommy did it, and they can begin to put that into effect in their own life.

What have you most needed through the experience of having cancer?

What I most needed as a parent with cancer? Understanding. When I was going through my diagnosis, my husband was so wonderful, waited on me, everything. He was there from sunup to sundown. It all worked out nicely that he was home with me all that time, even after I had my chemo, because he was also on disability. Then, after I was getting back to normal, he went back to work. But he's back on disability now because of his knee. So the timing was great. He always tells me that he loves me. Then the kids always tell me that they love me, too, so they gave me back nurture that I needed. I get a lot of love and attention from my children as well as my husband, and it makes me even more a fighter, really motivates me.

People come, they visit. They give their support that way, or they're calling to see how I'm doing. One of my good friends brought all the dinners over to my house. I had people come over and pray, and it helped me to rest in that situation. I don't think I could have asked for any more. Everything went beautifully.

I know that some parents are having a difficult time, and they may not know how to tell their children. Their lives may not have gone as smooth as mine. I'm glad that mine was smooth, that my cancer was caught very early. My children didn't have to see me go through a lot of the horrendous upheaval that some go through. It may have been a different story if the cancer was advanced.

It seems that through cancer, all the parts of Lorraine's life had remained intact, supported by family, community, and her unshakable beliefs. Christianity is a cape Lorraine wears in all seasons, not one to be donned and discarded as the weather changes. Still, I keep looking for a place where some part of the story will unravel, or at least change, as it has for other mothers.

Lorraine addresses the possibility of dying when the children are still young.

There was a time prior to diagnosis when I wondered how I would feel if I was faced with a life-threatening illness. You know what I mean? Would I be afraid, would I be stricken? How would I really respond as far as my spiritual beliefs? Am I afraid to die? Then, when I was diagnosed with cancer, it showed how I can really hold on and stand on the Word of God. I learned to put my trust in the Scriptures, that whatever the Lord says is so. I may not understand it at the time that I'm going through it, but I always ask the Lord to teach me what he would have me learn. I learned I can rest in His Word. I was totally resting in Him. Whether I live or die, I belong to Him.

I don't fear death. It's just leaving the husband and children. I know that they would be very well taken care of, but I'd like to see them get older and married and have children, where I can be a grandmother. My husband is a real good nurturer to them. He's there, and he does everything like I would do. I remember a long time ago, when I was in junior college, we saw a movie about breast cancer. They showed how many women didn't have the support of their husbands. Eventually, their husbands left them because they only had one breast instead of two. But I praise the Lord that that's not what concerns my husband. His whole concern is that I am here with him and the kids.

I think that they would really miss Mommy because when I'm gone away on a trip and I call home, [they say,] "We miss you, Mommy. When are you coming home?" But I think everything would carry on.

We know that if something happens to either of us, the children are going to be taken care of through the other of us. If I go, he'll be there. The only thing that we need to think about is if something happens to both of us—let's say, if we both get killed in a car accident or a plane accident. We need to talk about what then.

I've been blessed. Although I was faced with this life-threatening situation, I was able to trust in Him. It is with the resurrection that He came to life, and it's also a hope to me that I'm going to resurrect, too. My family and I, we talk about that. There's family members like my mother, my brother, that have passed, and the kids deal with that very well. They go to funerals with us. And even my little one, Henry, he says, "Oh, Mommy, Grandmommy, she's gone to be with Jesus. She's going to be with the Lord."

Do you see yourself as the same person that you were prior to the diagnosis?

I think the only change was to be faced with the disease. My attitude wasn't one of anger, wasn't one of fear. Of course, you always think about your children and your husband, you want to be around for them, but I see myself as being the same. My sense of self as a mother really hasn't been affected. It really hasn't. You know, I see myself the same to the point of not letting this difficult time get me down. But then I see myself as a little different because I've never faced anything like this before.

At first, I was a person that would be more quiet if something was bothering me, never really bring out those issues, but now I do. I always try to come forth, and if there's an issue that I need to deal with, I always pray and ask the Lord to help me to say it in a kind, loving way but yet firm if it needs to be said in a firm way. But never try to be ugly with it.

If you were given a choice to start your life over again and shape it in any way that you would like, what would it look like?

You know what? I think I would like it to be the way it is because everything is a learning experience and it's wonderful growth, you know, growing more and more in wisdom. I think that you need those little rough sides in your life to help you evaluate things and mature. See, these are things that I can share with my children—the legacy—so that they know what I've encountered, and then I'm able to help them through the rough spots in life. If they go through anything like this, I would like them to be able to respond in a positive way and not to let their diagnosis tear them apart, but to be able to grasp onto the Lord.

I know that He uses me to minister to others, whether it be sharing the gospel with others and leading them to salvation, a ministry to my children, [or] a ministry to encourage other people. Even being diagnosed with cancer has been a ministry for me to share with others. I've met people at the cancer center, and I've been able to encourage them. When people see me, they always see me joyous and smiling because I know who I believe in, and I know that He's intervening, and whatever His will is for me, His will will be done.

A lot of suffering could build godly character. I don't look at it as a punishment. I look at it as the Lord working in me to conform me to be more like Jesus Christ every day. No one wants to go through pain, but it's part of what we go through in this life. When Job went through his suffering, he talked to the Lord about that, and that's what I can do.

I never looked at life as being really difficult. I learned a lot, and I know through your experiences you grow wiser, so I have to say everything to me has been good. Of course, there's little dips, you know. But even though there was a time my husband was in between jobs and things were tight for us financially, everything still worked out. Although our cupboards weren't bursting with food, our needs were met every single day.

What do you most hope for yourself at this point in life?

I hope that I can be a source of strength and encouragement to other people who are going through the same thing that I have gone through, to let them know they can still carry on. It's not the end until you're gone, but as long as you have the breath within you to breathe, you can always make the best out of a situation.

One thing I would say to other parents is to try to involve themselves in support groups. not to feel that they're the only one going through this situation, not be afraid to talk about it. I think sometimes we don't want people to know we have an illness. But a lot of times, when you can share, that's a way you can get support from others. Participating in the project helped me to deeply and profoundly think about things. It takes somebody to ask the right questions and draw out feelings. I found it enjoyable because certain questions I would never have thought about. It resurfaced thoughts and feelings from my childhood. It gave the benefit of really getting into myself, being able to express my thoughts, tell my feelings.

I feel very good about the manuscript because I can look it over later. I like to read and highlight. Later on, I can do a devotional—a small book for other women who are experiencing breast cancer—with the excerpts about things I've gone through and about raising children. It would encourage others that there is hope, and you can go through anything.

Lorraine saw everything in her life, including cancer and recording her story, as an occasion for personal growth and for turning that growth into a spiritual gift. But her story shows that illness is not always a transformative, nor even a shattering, event in the life of a mother. Similarly, being a mother does not always dramatically influence the illness experience.

Lorraine was the first mother to teach me to be vigilant about the assumptions we bring to each new encounter. To protect our own narratives from being disturbed, we want others to conform. I had judged Lorraine as being in denial because of my unexamined attraction to complexity and the shadow side and my discomfort with orthodox religion.

Since meeting her, I have known other mothers who, in the absence of ironclad religious beliefs, go through cancer with ease and minimal change. Years later, Arthur Frank's work has helped me understand that "not every illness story has to be a self-story; even among the seriously ill, many people do not have their sense of coherence disrupted. Little is perceived as having been taken away, so what is there to reclaim?"[3] Lorraine's restitution story illustrates what Frank calls "a passive heroism."[4] Although she was actively involved in treatment, she seemed to surrender her body to her medical team just as she surrendered her soul to her Lord, a coping method that served her.

When reviewing a year or a life, we can list all the terrible things that happened to overshadow the positive and conclude that it was, overall, pretty bad. Or, we can look at all the good that was there, diminishing the import of the negative. It's a matter of perspective. Lorraine was able to look at it all and say, "It is good," and, for her, that made all the difference.

Six: In Limbo:
The Post-Cancer Experience

I AM IN A COFFEE HOUSE waiting for Carla, who has an eleven-year-old daughter, a loving husband, and a busy life. She also has had breast cancer and is four years out from the end of treatment—so far, so good. Carla had offered to do some data management for the project, working from home. Things started off well enough, but over the weeks, she became increasingly unreliable. I guessed that something serious was up and invited her to meet me.

Fifteen minutes late, Carla pushes the door open and rushes over. "I'm sorry, I'm sorry," she starts as we hug and sit down. Hair disheveled, skin gray and pasty, eyes reddened. She starts to cry. I put a hand on hers. "What's going on?"

"Well, I didn't tell you because I just couldn't. I haven't told anyone. But I found out I was pregnant about eight weeks ago, and I've been going through this hellish conflict. I want the baby. I really want another child. We all want more of a family. But I'm afraid. I'm so afraid that if I go ahead with it, the cancer will come back. The doctors tell me there's no clear indication of increased risk in my case, but Fred feels that if something happened to me, he could only cope with our one child. If there were more children and I had a recurrence . . ."

Carla lowers her head and whispers, "I've decided to have an abortion. This weekend, Fred will take Vicky camping, and I'll have it done. I've almost gone crazy trying to decide. I still may back out. But, you see, I can't forgive myself. . . ."

She weeps, blows her nose, and dabs at her eyes with a tissue before continuing. "I've realized I can't sit in front of another child and tell her I have cancer. I can't do it. I can't shatter another child's world for the rest of her life. At the same time, I can't bear to tell Vicky that I'm never going to give her a baby sister or brother. I can't bear that either. I don't know what I'm going to do."

"It seems that what you can't bear is disappointing your child in any way."

"Yes, that's true. That's true." She pauses for a moment, eyes widening. "Cancer is really big, isn't it? What's made it harder is I have a friend, also a mom, who just died from breast cancer. She had to tell her son she was dying, and he said to her, 'Do you get scared sometimes, Mom?' And I thought of my own child and imagined asking her, 'Do you get scared too, baby?' and I thought my heart would blow out of my chest. I just can't tell another child, 'You don't know if your mama is going to be there to see you grow up.' It's a no-win for me. Cancer has won."

I'm uncertain how to reply. I know women who risked pregnancy after cancer and are doing fine years later. I know others who chose not to take the chance and still others who did and had cancer return with a vengeance. Studies have shown that pregnancy following a diagnosis of breast cancer is not detrimental to long-term survival.[1] Some even suggest that pregnancy may afford a protective effect in terms of the risk of recurrence.[2] But many studies have limitations, and the issues remain complex, controversial, and highly individual for women. How ironic that chemotherapy can result in premature menopause or infertility while Carla is pregnant with a wanted child she feels she shouldn't have.[3] I also think about the double standard that might be adding to Carla's pain. Men (Saul Bellow at age eighty-four, Larry King at sixty-five after angioplasty) are applauded or ignored when they have children in spite of shortened life expectancies, while women with similar risks due to disease are often censured or labeled "selfish."[4]

But I don't want to undermine Carla's experience. For her, right now, cancer has won. I give her space to recover her composure. "Why don't I get us some hot tea?" She nods in agreement.

Waiting in line, I recall the day fifteen years ago when my then-husband and I told our seven-year-old daughter about our impending divorce, changing her world forever. I held her and said, "It's going to be okay, it's going to be okay," knowing it was not—not in any way she would want. I grab a paper napkin to wipe my eyes before Carla notices. What can I say to her? I slowly place the cups, spoons, and napkins on a tray and return to the table.

Dipping my tea bag into the steaming water, I feel Carla waiting for me to deliver wise words. I tell her, "You're going to have to make a decision you can live with. Most mothers with cancer feel this anguish, if not for directly causing their children's pain then for somehow not properly protecting them from it. It's inescapable. But things happen to us and to our kids, and we can only do what we can do. You're going to have to choose what's right for you now. If the risks of having another child feel intolerable, then that's the way it is."

I watch Carla closely as she takes in my words, nodding slowly, rubbing her forehead. She puts her hand down and exhales loudly. Her facial muscles smooth out a little. She shifts in her seat and apologizes for letting me down. "Linda, I really want to support the project. I really do. I want to help other people living with cancer." Her eyes well up again.

Without hesitation, I say, "Carla, it seems as if cancer is taking up too much space in your life right now. If you want to give something back to the community, there are lots of ways to do it. You don't have to have the disease front and center all the time. You have a right to respect your limits and take care of yourself. Ultimately, that will be better for Vicky, too." Released for the moment, we both lean back and agree that she will not return to work with the project.

I leave Carla with a heavy heart. In months to come, I frequently remember her haunted face and wonder about cancer's long shadow. It didn't matter that she was four years out from treatment, that her scans were clear and blood work normal, that she still had a chance to live a long and healthy life. It didn't matter that she had made great strides in rebuilding a narrative for herself and her daughter.

Cancer is big, and even in the absence of recurrence, its reverberations can continue long after treatment is over. Carla was beginning to put cancer behind her when her friend's death and an unexpected pregnancy retraumatized her, revealing how much raw grief and fear she was still living with. Cancer the disease had not vanquished her body, but cancer the illness, which involves the total experience of living with the disease, once again claimed dominion over her mind.[5] The wound can reopen without warning.

As I continued to listen to mothers with cancer, I often heard them echo Carla's pain about disappointing children. I heard similar echoes within myself for very different reasons. Carla's suffering had uncovered memories I had assumed were safely buried. I realized that being with these women was going to expose injuries in my own experience of mothering that had not completely healed and to touch places where I had not yet forgiven myself.

Most people do not grasp the long-term aftermath of trauma. Recovery involves going through a number of predictable phases: shock, disbelief, and numbness; deep grief, anger, and despair; the urgent need for information, support, and action; the search for meaning and connection; attempts to gain mastery; and emotional and spiritual resolution.[6] However, each person travels the road to recovery in a different way and on a different timetable.

For mothers with cancer, the extent of upheaval is not necessarily proportionate to the size of the tumor, the type or seriousness of the treatment, or the prognosis. And the post-treatment repercussions can be particularly complex, whether they concern childbearing decisions, work decisions, fear of recurrence, children's risk factors, or the ongoing dilemma of talking with children about cancer or disappointing them.

Mothers need confidence and a healthy illusion about themselves in order to mother. The first stories mothers tell themselves and the first yardstick by which they gauge success as parents concern keeping children safe from harm. "A parent measures herself by her capacity to offer this lifelong protection to a child," says psychologist Louise Kaplan.[7] A mother's impulse to protect children may have some basis in maternal biology, desire, and empathy, but it is culturally reinforced every step of the way and so ingrained as to be assumed.[8] Kaplan may write "parent," but most of us read "mother." No matter how involved in childrearing fathers have become, mothers are still the ones held to the responsibility for protecting their young.

One story mothers tell themselves and their children implicitly and explicitly is that they will be there to protect the vulnerable bodies and psyches of their young and raise them to maturity. The inability to do so can be shattering. Serious illness delivers many blows, but the ones that land with the hardest impact on Carla and the mothers I've met usually involve feelings of impotence, failure, and guilt when the ability to protect their children from pain is compromised.

One mother who had adopted a baby girl only a few years before her diagnosis said: "I've thought about what it means to be a mother whose child may be raised by other people. When I was diagnosed, I had to get through the shock of it, the guilt that she might be losing her mother again. I lost the sense of rightness about adopting her, felt that I had done her a disservice. I got the sense of rightness back eventually. Having cancer changed my conception of what being a mother means. I had always thought that a mother was forever."

While recording her story a year after the original focus group, Irene spoke to this issue. In spite of a good prognosis for early stage breast cancer, she struggled with the challenge of making promises during the post-cancer years to her now four-year-old daughter, Mia.

"There was a point where she was upset and seemed very insecure and clingy. I remember saying, 'What's going on? What are you afraid of?' And she said, 'I'm afraid that you're going to die.' And that was the first time that I was confronted with this notion. Every mom wants to be able to say, 'I'm always going to be here for you.' And I realized that I didn't want to say something that later would feel untrue. I mean, anything could happen. So what I focused on was, 'I'm here for you now, and you're always going to be taken care of no matter what, and I love you, and I'm taking care of myself, and probably everything is going to be okay with me.' I really wanted to say, 'I promise I'm never going to leave you.' The words were right behind my lips. Before cancer, I might have said that. But there's just no way I could. It's always hard to think that I will die when she's young. It's not as tangible now, but it's always poignant."

Empathy attunes a mother to her young, but with it comes heartache—an awareness of a child's pain and the need to alleviate it. A mother can also identify as the child. Children's emotions reawaken a mother's early experience, for better and for worse. Her offspring's suffering can remind her of similar states she suffered when young, complicating her reactions.

Illness intensifies feelings of regression, dependency, and longing for mothering. When a sick mother must disappoint her children, the pain reverberates on many levels. She aches both as a child and for her children, while feeling inadequate to protect either from danger or pain.

Additionally, ill mothers can hurt and feel guilty when they witness their children's suffering at not "fitting in" or being excluded because their families have been labeled "different," "not normal," or "socially unacceptable." The stigma of disease and the questions it raises do not disappear quickly. Is it better for the children to receive too much or too little from teachers and other adults? Is indulging children support-ive or weakening? Is such indulgence more to diminish mothers' guilt than to relieve the children's pain?

After cancer, many mothers feel betrayed by their bodies, by life, by God.[9] When they, in turn, have to break promises of safety, fairness, and belonging, it hurts. It is understandable that Carla would feel dev-astated by having to disappoint her child because the shadow of a more serious loss still loomed. It is also understandable that many moth-ers want to "put cancer behind them," to say to their children, "It's really over."

Children reinforce the mother's desire and the culture's preference to live in a cancer-free story, to return to normal. Susan Sontag writes, "Everyone who is born holds dual citizenship, in the kingdom of the well and in the kingdom of the sick."[10] The country no one wants to visit is characterized by dependency, withdrawal, inactivity, weakness, and preoccupation—exactly the opposite of what children want from a mother. Ill mothers who hold themselves to idealized standards of both motherhood and health before cancer, and whose children have come to expect mothers who personify those ideals, feel more pressured to tell a story of recovery.

Sociologist Kathy Charmaz has explored the subjective aspects of chronic illnesses in her book, *Good Days, Bad Days: The Self in Chronic Illness and Time*. Primary breast cancer, like Carla's and the other women's in Part One of this book, causes an interruption of life that may be short-lived: "Temporary crisis. Life-saving treatments. Full recovery."[11] However, the cancer journey for mothers and their fami-lies does not usually end with completing treatment, passing a five-year marker, or even hearing the longed-for word, "remission," a partial decrease or complete disappearance of the cancer for a period of time.

Although some cancers can be cured, most survivors continue to live in limbo. They dwell in what Arthur Frank calls the "remission society," whose inhabitants, like himself and others with chronic illnesses and disabilities, are "effectively well" but cannot ever "be considered cured." Living invisibly and often anxiously in the "kingdom of the well," "they are on permanent visa status, that visa requiring periodic renewal."[12]

In the aftermath of primary cancer, the challenges of living and parenting are magnified. Making it worse is the anxiety that the trauma is not over, the betrayal will never end. Perhaps Carla felt that cancer had won because of all it had already taken from her and her family—the sense of security, the illusion of control, the hope of another child—and all it might still take. She knew that the fear of recurrence would continue to haunt her.

Anxiety about recurrence is realistic with breast cancer, although the likelihood of recurrence is highest in the first two years following treatment and declines over time. Based on National Cancer Institute long-term incidence and survival statistics, Musa Mayer reports: "More than half of women diagnosed with breast cancer in 1974 eventually experienced a recurrence. . . Some occur as late as twenty years or even more following initial diagnosis."[13]

Almost every mother I have met, irrespective of the type of cancer she has, dreads recurrence. Four years out, Diana was left with "a dull wondering" and the realization that her older daughter still anxiously associated vomiting with dying. Marge had night terrors for herself, concerns about future risk for her son and about how to keep talking with him as he entered adolescence. Even Lorraine, who seemed least changed by cancer, recognized that being diagnosed with a recurrence or more virulent disease would be far more difficult for herself and her family.

Fear suffuses the after-cancer narrative. Mothers treat fear in highly individual ways—talking to a therapist or friend, meditation, information-gathering, suppression, distraction, action—but they try not to infect their children. They also try to revise stories to hold the threat. The story a mother creates after cancer depends on the interaction of many factors. Some carry their psychic and physical scars with pride, some with shame; some as a gift, some as a curse.

For Carla, in spite of a good prognosis, her friend's death

combined with her own pregnancy had raised the fear of recurrence to temporarily unmanageable levels. Her confidence was shaken to the core. Making the decisions, however reluctantly, to have the abortion and stop working in the cancer world helped her reassert some control over her situation. I sensed that her decisions were also efforts to reshape a narrative she could live with for herself and for her child. If she couldn't give her daughter a sibling, she would at least maximize the odds of staying alive. Six months after our meeting, Carla was at peace with her choices and working at a satisfying job on behalf of homeless families.

If some women's medicine is to isolate the cancer, staying as far away as possible from reminders of the disease, others, like Irene, do the opposite. Remaining intimately involved with cancer-related issues becomes a central part of their healing.

Like Carla, Irene decided not to risk another pregnancy, which broke her heart and that of daughter Mia. "It was the hardest part of my grief." Although she didn't express Carla's feeling of defeat, Irene was aware of cancer's traumatic effect in her life and how it separated her from others more fortunate: "Someone once said to me, 'Anything could happen. Either of us could get hit by a bus tomorrow.' And my comment was, 'I've already been hit by the bus. I'm hoping it's not going to back up over me. I'm in the road here.' It brings the whole idea of mortality very close up and personal."

Irene decided to stay in the road in spite of the fact that her diagnosis would have allowed her to sit on the curb (Stage I, no cancer in the lymph nodes, lumpectomy the only treatment). She remained involved with her support group and became a hospice volunteer and breast cancer educator. She insisted on talking about cancer even when her intimate circle urged her to stop: "People had different levels of denial. 'It's all over with, and you're all better now.' Everybody wanted it to be done. My sister says to me, 'Why do we have to talk about this? It's over.' It's never over for me, and not in a way that's negative or that I dwell on. You know, there are times that I still can't believe I have cancer. I think someone made some big mistake. I never felt sick. But it's *always there*. Nobody can understand what it's like to live with this unless you live with this. I don't think I had a great amount of compassion around cancer before I was diagnosed.

"It's become primary in my life. I have lots of friends now with breast cancer. I am involved with organizations. Every month, somebody has a recurrence and is facing the idea that they're not going to live very long. A lot of these people have little kids. It's scary to think about, but I'm glad that we think about it with each other. It doesn't get any easier. It is wrenching every time."

"So why do you think you're compelled to have cancer in your life?"

"There's some way that it's very life-*giving*. It's *very* real. Some people say, 'Isn't that depressing?' And it's not at all. When I have the opportunity to be with people I know who are in later stages of their life, really thinking about their death, I feel like it's a great blessing. And maybe it's been my way to master the losses in my own life. Somebody said to me that my life has been one long lesson in impermanence. That is what I'm learning in this life. Things change.

"You know, in Buddhism, they say pain is part of life but suffering is optional. Suffering is what we do with it. Maybe I could alleviate some of the suffering and some of the sense of isolation. I want to be close to people. It's really important for me to go to funerals. It seems important to not be robbed of that opportunity to grieve. I feel the pain, and it doesn't stop my life. It's just part of it. In my mind, there is nowhere else to go. This is life."

"Staying close to cancer is obviously good for you, but I wonder about the impact on Mia. I remember that after your diagnosis, your first thought was: 'I don't want this to affect my child'—especially with Mia having already had several surgeries for a birth defect."

"Mia hears the words 'breast cancer' every other day around here. I have tried to protect her from this notion that people die from cancer. I don't think that needs to be in her face. She knows that I work with people who have cancer, so, in some ways, it's very everyday for us in a not very heated way. One day, she said, 'Some people have two breasts, some people have one breast, and some people have no breasts.' She doesn't think that's odd. It's been there for half of her life now.

"You know, sometimes I say I want to have a normal life, but I realize, for me, there is no going back. In a way, I feel like I don't have any choice. Cancer is like having a chronic disease—it's always there. I don't ever want to forget that I have breast cancer. I have a debate with other moms who say, 'Don't you want to say you *had* breast cancer?' And I don't. That doesn't feel true for me. For other people, that's really important to say. But when I get too far from going to my group or thinking about it, I find that I'm not living the way that I want to live. I'm too busy, I'm too hectic. It's very grounding, in a way, to remember. The one most important lesson that I've learned in my life is about being present in the moment, making a conscious choice to be how you want to be. The thing I said after I got diagnosed was that I wanted to learn how to be a human *being* instead of a human *doing*. To be able to be quiet. I'm still working on that.

"I think cancer has given me new purpose. Even before being diagnosed, I had been interested in working with people who are dying. It's another idea to work with people who are living with disease, which I think is very different. It's this middle ground, this limbo you live in for a long time. And that's new."

Two mothers. Similar diseases and prognoses. Both with a desire to work in the cancer world, to have more children, to spare their children suffering. Both struggling to accept limitations and discover capacities, to make conscious choices that are true to themselves in the moment.

During a crisis, the human tendency is to revert to a survival mentality and, if we're parents, to protect our children. But raising children is not only about protection. It is also about growth for both parent and child.

All parents will let down their children because of human frailty, the unpredictable nature of life, and the limits of what they can control. But parents also take an active part in encouraging realism in children through a gradual presentation of the world. Fostering children's growth sometimes involves telling hard truths, setting limits, and holding the line. Some developmental experts go so far as to say that parents must disillusion children in order to initiate them into the human condition. For children to be real, parents must first be real—flawed, imperfect, human.

Real life has always demanded that both parents and children tolerate uncertainty and learn to bear inevitable tensions: between attachment and separation, illusion and disillusion, stability and change, health and sickness. And the human condition demands that parents do it all against the inescapable backdrop of mortality, perceiving the whole of reality while maintaining compassion, optimism, and hope. Rarely, though, do the stories mothers tell themselves about promoting children's development allow for serious disappointment or failure. Rarely do they include sharing painful and premature truths like the ones mothers with cancer must impart.

A common, unrealistic parental expectation is wanting life for our children to be simple and smooth when the human condition and the core of mothering are characterized by contradiction, ambivalence, and paradox. Perhaps mothers can find comfort in knowing that perfect security and perfect mothering are neither attainable nor desirable. Children have always suffered. Mothers have never been forever.

part TWO
LIFE ON THE EDGE: LIVING WITH RECURRING ILLNESS

SEVEN: WHEN FEAR BECOMES REALITY

ATTACHMENT AND SEPARATION, lifelong themes in our lives, are central in the world of cancer. As I went deeper into that world, I became increasingly aware of the language used to describe or create degrees of separation. Irene distinguished between those who were safely off the road and those already hit by the bus, but there is another demarcation. An invisible line separates those who have been hit once but have potentially long lives and those who have been struck repeatedly or were hit particularly hard the first time. Living with the dread of recurrence is different from having cancer return or never leave. Living with recurring or advanced illness is also different from being in the process of dying. These distinctions, I began to understand, are not only physical but also deeply psychological and social.

Although Yvonne, a newly diagnosed mother, had been forewarned that she would meet women with metastatic disease in the project's Mothering through Cancer support group, she was upset after trying one session: "I felt guilty when I told the other mothers that I felt great. I have my days when I cry, but then I get on with it and make the best of each situation. I don't want to focus on the negative all the time. They didn't seem to accept that. I am not in denial. I fear that I may die, but I believe that I am going to beat this."

Yvonne, who decided instead to attend a prayer group in her church, did not stay long enough to learn that the tens of thousands of women living with metastatic cancer also "get on with it and make the best of each situation." They don't always focus on the negative, and many believe they are going to beat the disease in spite of the odds. Those with breast cancer know that once it has metastasized, it is "no longer considered a curable disease but a chronic condition that will sooner or later result in death for all but two or three percent."[1] This grim statement still holds possibilities that mothers hang onto. "Two or three percent will beat it—why not me?" is one response. The phrase "sooner or later" suggests that there may be enough years remaining to get the children to a better age, and who knows? A cure may be found by then. In the meantime, there is life to be lived. Twenty-six percent of invasive breast cancer patients diagnosed with metastatic disease live five years or more.[2] Ten percent live ten years or more.[3]

Taking in the stories of others can threaten our own narratives. All of us—especially those who are ill—should be allowed to keep hope alive and to protect ourselves as we see fit. One mother who was six years into metastatic breast cancer explained why she chooses to avoid women with primary cancer: "Initially, I went to several support groups, just shopping. My problem was that my diagnosis was so much more serious than many of the other women who had *in situ* or Stage I. Their mortality was certainly coming up in front of them, but nothing like it was for me, with a small child and a bad diagnosis. So I felt different then—a bit isolated. Now, I'm just not interested in a primary diagnosis support group, even if it were about parenting. Because it hurts. It hurts because I would love to be in that position again."

Support groups are often dedicated either to primary diagnosis or metastatic disease. However, when a woman with a diagnosis of primary cancer has a recurrence, most groups are reluctant to ask her to leave. Rather, members struggle with their anxieties while supporting and trying to learn from the more seriously sick individual.

Fewer services exist to serve those with more advanced disease. The more it spreads and the mother's needs for assistance and comfort grow, the less likely she is to find support, not only from friends and family but also from her cancer peers—unless she's lucky enough to find one of the rare groups for metastatic patients.[4] The degree of fear is much higher, and with it comes greater levels of ignorance and silence. Many highly informed people who understand that cancer is not a death sentence assume that "metastatic" means "terminal" and treat these individuals as practically dead. I frequently have to explain that metastatic cancer patients can live for many years and some will become disease-free in ways that are not medically understood. Even oncologists can become emotionally distanced as disease progresses, equating recurrence or death with failure.[5]

Until Musa Mayer published *Holding Tight, Letting Go: Living with Metastatic Breast Cancer* in 1997, little existed on the subject for patients.[6] What holds true for breast cancer is also true for other advanced cancers and critical illnesses. Her book broke the silence and lessened the isolation and invisibility of many men and women whose lives are permanently changed by metastatic disease.

I knew that the stories of mothers living with recurring cancer would differ from those in the after-cancer limbo of primary disease. As Kathy Charmaz explains, the crisis of primary cancer is acute and temporary, and the possibility of full recovery is real. For the progressive stages of chronic illnesses, like metastatic cancer, there is not one interruption of life but many, followed by increasing intrusions upon daily activities, and, finally, total immersion in disease symptoms or treatments.[7]

Everything that is difficult for mothers with a first-time diagnosis is more difficult with recurring disease: the anguish of disappointing and hurting children, the guilt, the silence, the shame. Fear is ratcheted up and more chronic; losses are more frequent. The choice to pursue increasingly extreme, experimental, risky, and intrusive treatments becomes more complicated because of the potential impact on the children. A mother neither wants to keep frightening children nor turn them into caregivers, but how does she make them feel safe and positive about the future when her health is repeatedly imperiled, when the person they closely identify with and depend on is often too sick to join them in their world?

All the contradictions of ordinary motherhood intensify. The more ill a woman becomes, the greater the conflict between self and other, between holding on and letting go, between the desire to protect and the need to be honest without frightening the child. The balancing act between illusion and disillusion becomes more delicate and difficult. How does a mother hold onto illusions when reality keeps impinging in the form of new symptoms, new tests and diagnoses, new surgeries and treatments? How does she hang onto a sense of self that is healthy and intact as cancer spreads beyond "clean margins," seeping increasingly into family life and demanding more time, energy, and awareness? And how does she continue to talk to her children about what is happening when they are living increasingly separate lives in the kingdom of the well?

I had already learned that ill parents must bring fear down to manageable proportions and then begin the process of revision. As I began to work with mothers whose cancer had recurred or spread, I knew that my emotional challenges as a listener would be greater. But I expected that these women, more than any others, could show us what it is like to live life at the edge. It's a useful story, but not always a true one, that once we've managed to recover from one trauma or major loss, it will never happen again. Like it or not, life keeps challenging us, as it will our children, if not through illness then through something else.

And yet, these mothers, too, need stories to live by. What kind of story can a mother tell herself when recovery seems unlikely and when the disease keeps taking away her ability to project a future? Can she create an illness narrative that, as Frank explains, restores the order that the interruption fragmented, but also tells the truth that interruptions will continue?[8]

The stories of five women living with metastatic cancer follow. Some have had a recent recurrence; others have been living with chronic disease for more than five years. All are juggling two full-time jobs— childrearing and coping with illness and treatments. Several are holding down salaried jobs as well. Each is discovering her way of living with the continuing shocks of recurring illness.

EIGHT: "I WANT TO BE A WARRIOR"
SARA MARKOWITZ

"I WANT TO READ about other moms. To read about other moms honestly. Some of these books are very glossed over and romanticized. I'd like to hear the struggles that the moms had, the issues around their kids."

I am sitting at Sara's kitchen table. With one hand I'm taking notes, and with the other I'm pushing out of reach a plate of chocolate-chip cookies she has just baked. Sara wants to be interviewed—"I have a lot to say"—but in the three years I have known her, she has not been able to create the space to record her life story. A year earlier, she met once with an assigned volunteer listener, but there were crises and cancellations. "My life reads like a Grade B movie. You wouldn't believe it if you saw it." Our plan is to spend two hours together talking about mothering through illness, and then we'll fill in the rest of her story sometime in the future.

If I wanted to interview a mother whose fear of recurrence had caught up with her, I needn't have looked further than Sara Markowitz. Sara had been a member of the focus group in Chapter One. At that time, she had just finished treatment for primary breast cancer. Her lymph nodes were clear, and her prognosis good. She was married and living with her husband, Jerry, and their two children—Ben, almost four, and Eli, twenty-one-months. Throughout her treatment, she continued to work as a counselor in a family service agency.

After several years in remission, Sara's life completely changed. She and Jerry divorced. Two months later, Jerry died suddenly. Three weeks after that, Sara's cancer recurred just as she was packing up the family home to move to the small apartment she and her sons now live in.

"Maybe a Grade C movie," Sara laughs, running her fingers through short, red curls. In the midst of so many changes, her humor remains a constant.

Sara always tries to take Fridays off to cook, take care of odds and ends, pick up her two sons from school, and prepare for the Jewish Sabbath. On this Friday morning, she has finally managed to squeeze in our meeting between dropping off the kids and leaving for a doctor's appointment.

SARA

My mother was diagnosed with breast cancer when she was thirty-five and died of metastatic breast cancer at fifty, so as early as age thirty, I was having yearly mammograms. After one of them, I was called back for something that appeared to be wrong. There was no lump that anyone could feel. I went in, and they thought it wasn't anything and asked me to return in six months.

I became pregnant and nursed my second child. In the back of my mind, I always knew I had to go back to get that mammogram. I remember very distinctly that when I finished nursing, I had to wait ninety days. I made an appointment as soon as I could. It was scary. I was always afraid to get breast cancer.

Two weeks before the appointment, I started feeling a burning in my other breast—it wasn't in the breast that they had been concerned about—and it kept me up for a couple of nights. It wasn't a major pain. There was no lump. I just had a weird feeling in my breast, like something was wrong. I will never forget that day I went to the breast care center and asked them to give me a mammogram right then.

Now, if you know them, you don't go in there and say you want a mammogram. It's like an act of Congress to get one. I said, "Something is wrong, and I really need to have this mammogram today." It happened to be a long weekend, and I wouldn't be able to come back until Tuesday if I didn't do it that Friday. They said, "Do you have a symptom?" I said, "Yeah, I'm feeling a pain, a burning." They said, "You have to go to your doctor because you're having a symptom." And I said, "No! I really can't do that. My doctor's not here, and the weekend is going to be long. I'd like the mammogram now." So they argued with me. I said—and I will put it on this tape—"I want that fucking mammogram now. You give it to me now. I'm not leaving."

I'll never forget the technician's face. She went into a dripping sweat. They gave me the mammogram, and, sure enough, they started doing magnifications, wanting me to wait. I knew something was wrong by then. I had to have an ultrasound of that area, and they did see something, and I'll never forget this either. The technician said, "Oh, look, this looks like a cyst. This is nothing." They shouldn't do that because it did give me some false hope. But the doctor came in and said, "We need to do a biopsy."

I felt complete and total terror. Terror for me, terror for my kids, and at the same time thinking, "This has finally happened." I was waiting for it, honestly. I hate to admit that. I don't think I'm a negative person, but I always felt like this could happen, with genes, you know, and I was scared. A year before diagnosis, I was getting migraine headaches and vomiting and having this feeling of being like my mother was pre-diagnosis. I thought, "This is so horrible. My kids will see me sick." When I was diagnosed, that was the first thing that hit me. My two boys were going to see me sick. So that was the beginning of a journey.

The doctors did the biopsy and found a malignancy, and Sara had a lumpectomy in the breast with the burning, not the one about which there were prior suspicions. There weren't clean margins, so Sara had to go back again for a lymph node dissection. She had thirty-one negative nodes—the good news—but ended up with lymphedema, a potentially chronic post-surgical condition that affects hundreds of thousands of breast cancer patients. The arm near the surgical site swells up painfully with lymph fluid, making it hard to use, and the treatment can sometimes be equally hard.

That really affected me in terms of being a parent. The lymphedema treatment consisted of being wrapped in tight bandages. You couldn't move your hand. I 'm trying to change diapers. I'm a lefty; it was in my dominant hand.

I was having claustrophobic feelings in the middle of the night, wearing the bandages. One physical therapist said to me that I was being noncompliant by taking it off in the middle of the night. I didn't feel like they had a clue. I tried to say to them, "How can I wrap my hand? Can you move it to give me a little more mobility so I can change diapers?" I said, "Why don't you work with me?" It was a guilt trip because my personality is "I want to be a good girl," and I could not.

It was so hard. It was being a parent that was so grueling, doing chemotherapy at the same time. I remember people talking about the chemo part of it: "Oh, you know, you can go to work; do it on Friday, and then you can rest on the weekend." I absolutely could not do it that way. I had to ask them to do it on a Wednesday so that I could be better on the weekend and be with my kids. Another reason was I needed to be able to go to the kids' Shabbats that are on Friday at 12:30. I don't miss that. I go. I always tried my best to make the schedule around what felt important to me in terms of my family.

There was always explaining to be done, but it worked out. I didn't have a lot of problems with the chemotherapy. I tried to rest a lot when the kids were at school. Ben was in preschool, and Eli was in a family daycare. Both places were very, very understanding. So, I felt supported. I was doing counseling at the agency, but I didn't work the one day before the chemo and then the rest of that week. Every three weeks, I would do that. Mostly, I got donated sick days. My co-workers and boss were very good to me. Aside from the insurance that I needed, it was a real anchor at that point to go to work. I needed my identity in that job to remain solid. I was really blessed to have it.

I'll never forget that day of diagnosis. The thing that goes through my mind is how everybody else reacted. How my grandma and my siblings were hysterical, and my husband, too. Jerry was with me, and he said, "This is cancer!" Also, I remember how much I felt that I needed to protect my kids. Three years later, I heard about that movie *Life Is Beautiful* and how the father protects his son from the Holocaust. That's what it felt like. I haven't seen this movie yet, but I really felt it was my responsibility to be honest but not to scare them.

I vividly recall Roberto Benigni's Academy Award winning film, about a father who keeps his young son with him in the concentration camps and protects him by creating an elaborate story that their entrapment is some kind of game. It's ironic that Sara, who is committed to being honest with her sons, has latched onto a movie in which the parent

tries to "protect" a child through lies. I doubt that she knew the specifics
of the plot. I ask her when her own Grade C movie started in earnest.

I was diagnosed four years after we married, and, after I was diagnosed, there were problems in my marriage. Jerry and I decided to divorce. At this point, I had been disease-free for about three years. I had started seeing the oncologist every four months as opposed to three—which is a good sign that things are better. Then, my husband passed away suddenly of a brain aneurysm. It was a very scary, awful time for me and for my boys. They were five and three. Again, I felt a great responsibility to be there for them, to protect them, to let them know that all the emotions they were feeling were okay and that people loved them. The night that Jerry died, Ben said to me, "What if you die? Who's going to take care of us?" Of course, that's always been my greatest fear. I counted on Jerry to be here if I wasn't. I never imagined that Jerry would die before I would. I never imagined that Jerry would *die.* That sounds very silly, but it was such a great shock. I did immediately think of the cancer—"Oh, dear, what control do I possibly have about what will happen to *me?*"—little realizing that at that very time, I did have a recurrence.

I didn't know that until weeks later, when I was diagnosed with metastatic breast cancer that had gone to my lungs. Then, I was confronted with needing to tell the kids again, and when and what and how much was very much in my mind. I was careful. I did talk to people. I have a therapist—I took the kids to a child therapist for about eight weeks when Jerry died. I have spoken to an excellent consultant to the kids' schools. I have called the parent stress hotline many times through the divorce and through this. They've given me resources I try to use. I talk to other moms all the time.

I think that my mind has shifted into saying, "I can control only what I can." I'm going to take care of myself. I'm going to let my children know how much I love them and how many people love them, and assure them that they'll be taken care of. Because now, when Ben says to me, "If you die, who's going to take care of us?" and "Mom, you can't die until I can take care of myself," a lot of parents might say, "I'm not going to die." I don't think I'm going to die, but I can't say that anymore, and I'm not going to lie to him. I think it's okay for me to say, "You know, if I was to die, there are so many people that love you, and I promise you that you are going to be taken care of."

Ben's a very deep thinker, very intuitive. When I was diagnosed the first time, he was three and had a lot of questions about why he couldn't jump on me like he had. Eli was just one, so I didn't communicate a lot with him about it. I wrote Ben the little book, *Ben's Mom and the Bad Guys,* and he liked that book a lot. I wrote down that Mom is fighting these bad guys. I did not name it "cancer" at that time. I said that there's going to be some times when Mom is tired, she has to go to the doctor, go to the mommies' groups, talk on the phone. I don't remember him being extremely upset about it, but he absolutely questioned where I was going. He wanted to know, and I wanted to tell him.

So, when I recurred, what I said to him was, "Benji, the bad guys are back, and I want to tell you now it is called 'cancer.'" And he said, "Is it in your boobies again?" They know my breast is still very sensitive, and my arm, and they know not to wrestle with me because we do a lot of roughhousing, and they think I'm a gymnastics mat *[Laughs],* but they keep the left side off-limits. And I said, "No, it's inside my lungs. I'm going to take some medicine, we're going to fight these guys, and I hope that maybe you can help me. Could you make me a picture? I want to be a warrior." Because we used to always say, "*Ungawa!* Mama's got the powa!"

So, I was trying to use the *Life Is Beautiful* thing again, trying to say, "Let's fight this." I have never said anything to them about I might die or how long because I don't know. They don't need to know that, I don't think, but they do need to know that I get tired, and they do need to know that the next physical thing that is going to happen is I'm going to lose my hair. I said, "Now we're going to try a medicine," and he wanted to know how they put that medicine in, and I explained an IV to him. "They put a needle in, it doesn't usually hurt, and then this medicine goes in and is killing the bad guys. Now, sometimes it has to kill some of the good guys, and one of the places is right in your hair. I'm going to have my hair cut shorter, and then I'm going to take the medicine, and I might look like a little chicken."

He's scared about it for sure. I think it's just a physical thing—Mommy looking different. Every woman, not just every mom,

I've spoken to, the hair ends up being a big deal even though the doctor will say, "Well, it's just your hair." It really speaks a lot about who you are. I'm trying to be philosophical about it. It's only my hair, not my life. I'm going to go to Ben's class. I know all these kids. I need them to know what's going on. I've talked to a few of the parents because I don't want their kids to get scared, either. But I do want to say, "There are some bad cells in my body that we're using some medicine for and—guess what?—it's going to make my hair go, too." I've talked to the teacher, and she thought that was a good idea.

Eli acts differently about everything because he's a little bit younger. He's so used to Tylenol or ear-infection medicine, he wants medicine, he thinks *this is fun, tastes sweet.* I said, "I'm taking this medicine, it wouldn't taste good, and there are these bad guys in there and we want to get them." He's into the Power Rangers, so I kind of use, "Let's fight 'em," and he thinks that is cool.

Where are you right now with medical treatment?

I'll have a few more tests to see how the radiation worked, and then it may be that I have to have a little more radiation. We don't know because the bronchial tube may still be bleeding. I never told them about the blood, ever. I felt like that would scare them, so I didn't say those words. I will begin the chemo in mid-April, and we'll do at least a couple of cycles of that, and then we have to see if I respond. What I learned was: It doesn't matter how you responded last time, this is a whole different ball game. So, one of the choices will be the stem-cell rescue [sometimes called a bone marrow transplant]. Other choice will be some other heavy-duty chemotherapy.

With the bone marrow transplant, the struggle has been very much because of the kids. The social worker said to me one day, "You know, if you do the stem-cell rescue here, you probably won't be able to see your kids for three weeks, or you could see them through the glass." I couldn't sleep for a week because of that. Because, like, who's going to take care of my kids? What am I going to do? What am I going to tell Ben and Eli—that for three weeks I'm not going to see them? What's that going to do to them in the midst of all the stuff they went through? I didn't get to the point where I said, "Well, if I can't see them, I'm not doing it," but I was having a hard time getting to the place I could feel comfortable about doing it.

I met a woman who had two small children, and she had had the stem-cell rescue two weeks ago. I said, "Can you tell me, did you see your kids?" She said, "Oh, yeah, I was able to see them all the time." She explained that sometimes it was hard on them to see her that way, and sometimes it wasn't a good visit, but mostly she felt it was important that they were able to see her. So, I asked my oncologist about it, and he said, "You can see them every day if you want to. We'll gown them, they'll wash their hands, and you can have them come in there." I said, "But do you actually have power to make this decision?" He said, "Yeah, I do." I slept that night. At least now it is an option for me.

Are there other treatment decisions you've struggled with because of the kids?

I can honestly tell you that the first time around—I never told anybody this—I did not want that Adriamycin because I didn't want to lose my hair because of what it would do to Ben. That is really the truth. This time, we're saving my life, and I think that Ben and Eli both can understand. They're developmentally different, too.

But what *do* you do with your kids about your hair loss? How do you deal with that? One woman in my group—I'll never forget this— she and her daughter put [temporary] tattoos on her head. We're going to do that. I've already told Ben and Eli, "Maybe we can do these tattoos—that would be really fun." I'm going to take them to the bookstore and let them pick. Ben has latched onto that. He goes, "Mom's going to lose her hair, and we're going to put tattoos on it." It's like *Life Is Beautiful.* I'm trying to make it that it doesn't have to be horrible. I want to protect my kids. I want it truthful but compassionate for them and sensitive to their feelings and their fears.

This is the third time that you have mentioned Life Is Beautiful *and protecting your kids. It's obviously the most basic need of a parent to protect a child from too much reality, and it's clearly one of the most shattering things to have cancer when reality rushes in and you can't. How do you deal with that?*

Well, a lot of people ask me that. It's a big question. I think some part of it is your natural instinct as a parent. Forget the cancer part for a minute: When things are rough, things at work or whatever, I think that there is a natural instinct to try to protect your child. I'm sure some people do it better than others, and people do it some times better than other times. That's true with me. When it gets to be something big like this—my own little holocaust, as I feel it is—I don't know.

Sara offers me another cookie, gets up to warm the tea, and paces in her tiny kitchen. I keep thinking about the unseen movie that has taken on such metaphoric power in her life. Sara sits down again and continues.

When Jerry died I was confronted with the responsibility that how I acted and how I said things was going to be so important to how they lived in the world. Their life was going to change forever. The night Jerry died, that very night, that was in my head. *What am I going to do to do the best I can?*

Remarkably, I feel good about how I've handled that whole thing. In a weird way, that's a unique experience for me. Because I had to tell them about this major loss, and then I had to gear up again so soon after for the recurrence, and they already are grieving. How I have done it is I try to keep it honest and simple and say, "You know, I need you to know." The reason I had to say something was that there were so many people coming here. This is not the normal experience for them to have. *[Long pause]* Life can't be easy for me, it seems.

Sara's energy appears to flag for the first time, and she looks down at her hands, which have stopped gesturing. Her body seems to slump. But, within a minute, her blue eyes once again peer intensely into mine.

I feel so blessed to have those kids. And I feel sorry for them that they have to live like this. I have a lot of feelings about that from my own experience—to have a sick parent is the scariest thing. Besides that, the parent dies, which is horrid and forever with you. To watch it is a really awful thing. If there was any way that I could have spared them, I would have. So there are moments of weakness where I felt like this isn't fair to them, maybe I should have never had kids! But then, of course, I love them so much. They're like the most important thing I've ever done. It's a hard thing. It's a mixed thing. I wish that I could do something to make it easier for them, and I feel like I'm doing my best to make it easy.

The pain I feel for them is . . . *[Throws her hands up]* It's like the most major paradox because, okay, do I wish I didn't have them? Oh, my God, I can't imagine my life without them, but why did I have to do this to them? I know that sounds weird, but it has made it very hard. All these things . . . The moving is not about me. The moving is about, "What's the best school? What's the best support network for us?" It's all about the kids. If I didn't have the kids, I would go to New Zealand tomorrow and take this big trip, but I could never do that because I can't be away from my kids now. Yeah, I think it absolutely changes everything you do and think. I love my kids so much, but I found parenting *without* the cancer to be really hard.

The other thing—it might not be your exact question—but something that Ben said was that he never got to say goodbye to his dad. I do know that he's going to be able to say goodbye to me. As sad as that feels, as awful, and I don't say this lightly, I'm glad that they can do that. That I can say goodbye to them how I want to. I have to find a place, and sometimes I can, where I know they're going to be okay because this is what is destined to happen for them. People say you choose your parents. I find it hard to believe that I would have chosen the life that happened with my parents, that my kids would have chosen to lose their parents. . . . I was sixteen when my dad died, twenty-six when my mother died, but my mother had been sick my whole life pretty much, for fifteen years. I'm having a parallel experience, and I can't help but feel really bad.

There is an inclination to buy everything for them and indulge them and lose all boundaries that you've spent this really hard work creating. Jerry and I were good parents together. Otherwise, no, but we are the kind of people that the kids have a routine at bedtime. You do your bath, brush your teeth, get your book, and go to bed. The kids have bedtimes. Kids in Ben's class stay up until eleven at night. He says, "Like, why can't I do that?" It's hard—the world is right there.

So, I have had a hard time reminding myself that it is okay that I maintain the discipline. Yesterday, the kids would not get up for school. They would not get dressed. They would not eat breakfast. They would not brush their teeth. They would not get in the car. I don't think it was about me. Maybe they were out of sorts. Who knows? Today, we had a perfectly fabulous day. In the morning yesterday, I was screaming. But that is such a hard thing, them saying "I hate you," and all I want to say is, "I'm not going to be here that long! I want you two to love each other and know you have each other and know how much I love you." When you're parenting day-to-day, life doesn't work like that. I'm dealing with this potentially temporary life with these guys, and I want to make it good. I've got to stick with the program, but it's hard.

That's quite an insight. It's hard for most parents to stick with the program even when they don't have cancer.

Yeah. I've always struggled with that. I've talked to my friends about what they do, you know, just parenting, and I've talked to other women that have had cancer and kids, and they agree that it's really hard. Everyone is bringing my kids a present to indulge these guys, and I always wonder, *When they're getting all this stuff, what is the message to them?* That's not the way I wanted the values to be. I say, "You know, we can't have everything." But, hey, go in their room. It's Legoland!

What are your greatest concerns for your kids now?

That I'm going to die. That about covers it. *[Pauses again]* It's more that I'm going to leave these children behind, that these kids would have to lose their *parents*. You know, I can be angry about it, and I have been, and I can cry about it, and I have. What I'm just trying to do is find a place to be peaceful about it—so *they* can be.

So many moms say they can find peace about dying, but finding peace about leaving the kids is something else. How do you think you can do that?

I'm going to start doing some Buddhist things. There's a lot of good lessons in Buddhism. I think that's more for *me*. For the kids, it's to leave something. I have journals that I've been keeping for my kids their whole life. There's two full journals at least for each of them that I hope to continue. The other thing is that my family and I are going to do videotapes, starting this weekend. All the siblings are going to be together, and we're going to talk about things, funny things about Mom, stories about when I was young, upbeat things. My grandma is going to do a tape about me from her perspective. I was hoping to do—besides what you and I are doing—my own videotapes for the kids, kind of using your questions, and your direction, your ideas.

And then the other *big* thing is if I can know where these kids are going to be, I'll feel a lot better. But it's complicated. Jerry and I talked about this not that long ago. We never wrote a will, we never had a legal guardian. We couldn't do it. We *didn't* do it.

Like almost everyone.

Yeah. Like almost everyone. Now, the ante is upped. We went through all the siblings, but there's downsides to all of them. So there's kind of an auditioning going on. It's very awkward for me, and I have to make a decision.

Sara ticks off the factors concerning potential guardians that she is mentally juggling to arrive at a decision that might bring her some peace. They include: religion, geography, health and mental health, economic stability, lifestyle, values, experience with children, education, the presence of other children, and, of course, love. I ask Sara how she thinks she will decide.

I'm working with my therapist. I make pros and cons lists. What I have to get beyond is: I die, their father has died, they have just moved, and who knows when this is going to be? Is this in two years, five years, seven years, ten years?

Relationships are obviously central to you and your children's well being. Do you want to talk more about how having cancer has affected your most important relationships?

Boy, it's almost hard to know where to begin. I've been both overwhelmed by the help and surprised by some of the people that I thought would be there. Maybe not totally surprised because I saw my mom being sick for fifteen years raising three kids by herself.

But I will say something about Jerry. I think it was very difficult for Jerry to see me being not well. I don't think the cancer did anything more than show me his emotional inability to be there because he really couldn't be. And I did forgive him. When he was alive, he knew that. But it was a fact that he was not there for me—with cancer, I knew absolutely.

In the beginning, he was very supportive. It got harder for him to be so later on. I said in my support groups that if I ever did have a recurrence, I didn't want to be married to Jerry. I knew because of the great amount of support I received from everyone else. It was so painful. I could stub my toe, and there would be flowers and cards and people. I'd walk into my own home and feel—it wasn't nasty, I don't want you to think it was—it just wasn't there.

In terms of other relationships, oh, man, I have been so blessed. I could get into this whole psychological thing. I've always felt insecure.

Everyone always says, "Sara, I never knew anyone who had so many friends. You're this great person." I'm not bragging. I never took that in very well. I've always known that I was a good friend myself, but it was more in the receiving end of things that the wall was. And that wall is Berlin now. It's breaking down. I'm letting a lot of people into my life now.

I have found that you find out who your friends are. My dearest, oldest friends are incredible people. I see how devastated they are. It's connected us more, and I feel lucky about that. And people you did not expect are actually the people you can count on. For example, when Jerry died, a woman called me and said, "I want to help you. I've always wanted to be your friend." She rallied the whole school and raised thousands of dollars for us. I'm sad because I want to be her friend for a long time, and I don't want to be her friend because it's a cancer friend. Man, why do we have to become friends *now*?

How does cancer change relationships? I would say me and my sister have lots of conflicts. I can't look at her without *her* crying. I've kicked her out of here—which is not my usual mode of operation—at least twice since this new diagnosis. I've actually said, "You can't stay here any more."

She's a total burden to me. She's sitting watching MTV, the kids are running around, and I'm pissed off at her because she's sitting there with tears in her eye. And God, she'll say, "I just can't be in this world without you. I can't imagine it." She's like a puddle. She's hysterical, and I'm not.

My brother and my dad fought when he was fifteen, and my dad died of a heart attack. Right then. Right in front of him. And he's never had therapy, if you can imagine that. So, we have, like, major loss in our family and major issues. I've always been the more evolved one. They think I'm Woody Allen, and they are the ones that have been locked into all this pain, where I've gotten all this personal growth out of it—*and* a lot of hard times. So, they are now in a crisis. It's scary for them. I think it's really important to say, "We are all we have—each other." We had a family meeting, and I said to them, "You do not only owe it to yourselves but you owe it to me to get some help to deal with this." For me, I'm trying to find a way to set my boundaries and to be with them and to love them.

Are there things you'd like family members or friends to know about what you've been through or what you're going through now that you haven't been able to tell them?

I've told them a lot. The hand has been forced. But I would reiterate anyway: Please try to understand that as long as I can, *I want my life how it is. I want control of my life.* People are coming in my house, changing it around, thinking that they know the better way for things to look. Comments about my files—"These are so old, get rid of them." I have a lot of stuff. I have my grandma's letters [in] a Grammy file. Why did I keep those? Because when my grandma dies, I want to have all those letters to look at. I've had them for twenty years. I think it's important. Now, when I die, there's going to be a massive bonfire over here, and I've got to let go of that, too, because I can't imagine anyone wanting to keep all this shit.

They mean well—you have to understand, this is all meant well. But people are washing your underwear, in your kitchen, in your face, and, yeah, I get mad sometimes. My sister pushes: "Who are you going to have help during the treatments?" Well, I don't know yet, but I have lots of support, and I have someone picking up my kids every day. "But you've got to have someone there. You're going to get really sick. You're in denial." I'm not. I'm okay right now. I don't want someone living in my house. But people are very worried, and it makes it worse.

This is the thing: Let me be the person that decides what I need, and if I don't know right then, deal with that. I've had a big battle being able to be true to myself, [to] ask for what I need as far as resting. Even to say to my kids, "I'm not feeling great," was hard 'cause I wanted to be Mom and be with them and do things. I've always been considered a superwoman, lots of energy. I'm really hard on myself as a parent. That's why I look forward to your book. How did it work for these moms when they were not feeling well? How did they coordinate the hundreds of phone calls saying, "I will help you"? What did that feel like? It would sure be nice to see how other people felt, in terms of how to deal with all the people who want to help you. It's a huge issue, and it's a hard issue. You end up offending people, with people turning away from you. You end up feeling guilty. You feel blessed, at the same time, terrorized. Because all of a sudden, you *are* cancer. Nothing else.

Do you think that there are ways in which being a parent has helped you to cope better with the illness?

I think so. My first thought that comes to mind is the concept of just living in the present moment. You have to do that so much with kids because they force that on you. And with something like a chronic illness, whatever we want to call it—a terminal illness—I don't know what word I want to use. . . .

"Chronic" until it's "terminal."

Until it's terminal, there you go.

Which could be lots of years from now.

From your lips to God's ears. *[We both laugh]* I do feel that parenting with cancer helps you to be more present, more aware, more grateful. To see what you have. This is how it's been for me. It encourages me to focus on the now and the good because I do have a lot of that. Wow, I have these beautiful kids. I have this support. We have these friends. Sometimes, in your regular life, you don't let yourself see that.

There is no way to know for sure, but do you think that raising children while ill could have any effect on the course of your illness?

That's an interesting question. Being focused and being a parent and knowing that you have that responsibility keeps things calmer on a certain level because you have to keep with the program. A lot of women I talk to say, "I don't have time for cancer. I have to go to the soccer game." So, on some level, maybe it helps.

Having kids is stressful, so I could look at it the other way, too, in terms of the immune system and the stress of it. But my mind tends to go with the first. Knowing that you are responsible for other people keeps you sane. That has truly been my experience. I think there is something about kids that might be good.

Too many women I know have kids and then die, so how much it helps I don't know. It's not like they have kids, and they love them so much, and this cancer dissolved. We *can't* know. People think that Jerry died, and all this exacerbated [my cancer]—people are surmising lots of things about me. There is no answer, and I don't want to take a lot of emotional time to say, "Well, if, if, if." I know that whatever happened was supposed to happen. I know it sounds weird. What my part of it was, they still don't know. I worry about what I ate when I was a teenager. I worry about the stress I had in my life. But I can't spend a lot of energy on it.

Sara looks at her watch and bolts from the table.

Oh, my God, I've got to get going. My friend is going to be here any minute to take me to the doctor.

I pack up the tape recorder as Sara rushes to grab her coat and tries to give me a few more cookies "for your trip home," all of fifteen minutes. Waiting with her on the street, I sneak in one more question: You said you've had a lot of support, but is there anything that you would want that you haven't had?

Regular sexual intercourse. *[Bursts out laughing]* No other commitments, by the way. Just that. Here's my personals ad: "Sex wanted. Short-term commitment or no commitment at all. Come for awhile, laugh, leave." You can erase that if you want.

No, no way, that's an original.

Thank you. Funny that that should come out, but that's what I'm thinking right now. I would like to be freer to go away on a weekend. I have people who could help me, but it's not all that simple, ever. Also, I get emotional leaving the kids, even for a weekend. They'd be fine, but . . .

You can't do all those things. You want to go to acupuncture, you want a massage, you want all your herbs and vitamin supplements, you want to go to these cancer retreats. It's a lot of money to have cancer! There's support groups that are free, and I feel fortunate. The main thing I'd like you to know is that I feel lucky that I have these resources, but I have to speak for all these other people. Where do people who really need some help get it? It's a combination of finding resources and being able to pay and then to feel emotionally okay about that. Wow, how do they do it?

Oh! There's my ride! Talk to you soon! Bye!

Sara blows me kisses and steps into the car.

I stayed in touch with Sara, at first to ask her how she felt about her words and possibly her identity going public. As usual, she made me laugh out loud. "Sure, you can use my name. Use anything. I am a public-service announcement!"

Almost a year after our meeting, when I learned Sara was not do-ing well, I wrote to see if I could come for a visit even if she wasn't yet up to recording her life story. She replied:

Linda, thanks for your sweet note. Hmm, where to begin? This mom is tired! Eli, my five-year-old, broke his leg the first day of kindergarten! He is getting around on a walker quite well now, but what a mess! At least we know this is temporary! My tumor marker is way up these days, breathing affected. Not an easy time. Linda, how I wish this all was just a bad dream! I am not very social these days. The visit will happen. I hope in not too long! I'm doing a video with family and friends that I'm going to give to the cancer center to educate them! I am pleased that you continue to think of me.

Love, Sara

Sara had told me that my questions made her think; her answers opened up new questions and insights. Emotional honesty, anger trans-formed into action, humor, and intimate connection were among Sara's strongest resources. And a talent for fantasy. Over the months, I pon-dered Sara's references to her bad dream, "my own little holocaust," and to the movie that had captured her imagination. Knowing a little about Life Is Beautiful *seemed to have given Sara a way to frame her own experience—to make meaning about it.*

The movie's plot is straightforward: One day, life is simple and beautiful, and the next, it is not. Suddenly, parents are no longer in charge of reality as they once knew it. The Gestapo is in charge, strip-ping away roles, rights, finances, homes, clothing, dignity, identity. Taken to a concentration camp, separated from his wife, a father hides their little boy and holds onto the one shred of control left to him: his capacity to create a story. The child's questions about the abrupt changes are answered with an extraordinary web of fabrications, al-lowing the father to believe that he has done everything in his power to save his son's life and illusions.

If we ask, "How could a movie that strains credulity beyond the breaking point be taken so seriously by so many?" we need only to look to its reassuring message, which speaks to the child within each of us: Ordinary parents in extraordinary circumstances will do anything to protect their children, including sacrificing their own lives. Additionally, many parents identify with the father's quest to make an unbearable situation tolerable for his son. Some ill mothers I've met lie about the seriousness, and sometimes the very existence, of their disease in a desperate attempt to protect their children from suffering.

What kinds of stories can a parent with recurring illness tell herself to maintain strength and optimism when the future appears so uncertain? Sara, who was just beginning her journey with metastatic cancer when I interviewed her, gave me a glimpse into one possibility: her own internal narrative line, inspired in part by Benigni's. Handily grasping the elements at hand—shaved heads and tattoos, bad guys and Power Rangers, fantasy and reality, humor, loving connections, and just plain chutzpah—Sara was crafting a story of herself as a wounded warrior. It was a story that would create meaning out of chaos, return a modicum of control to her, and offer a model of resilience for her children.

The gift of imagination was allowing Sara to make reality more palatable for herself and her children while sustaining their threatened connection. And she was finding a much healthier way to balance fantasy and reality than the impossible example presented in the movie. Sara remained definitely, passionately engaged in real life. In spite of her desire to protect her children, she communicated the truth tailored to their developmental stages—which is what most professionals recommend.[1]

As for myself as listener, witnessing the pain of Sara's existence was mitigated by experiencing her extraordinary life force and generosity of spirit. Ungawa! Mama's got the powa!

NINE: "MY VALUE AS A MOTHER IS JUST BEING HERE"
TINA SALOMON

TINA SALOMON OPENS the door with a flourish and a hug and leads me into the cozy family room where we will hold our sessions. She wears a brown velour pants suit, which flatters her pale complexion and cropped auburn hair. Light makeup is perfectly applied. Tina offers me the rocking chair and sits across from me on a crushed-velvet love seat. When she runs out to get us tea, I scan the precancer wedding and family pictures covering the walls, taking in Tina's long, wavy hair and the men in her life: her husband, Jack, and their sons, Mark, almost nine, and Nathan, three and a half. Their daughter, Rena, died at birth. "I still feel she's my child, so I always say I have three children."

Tina was diagnosed at the age of thirty-six with Stage IV breast cancer that had already metastasized to the liver.[1] She'd had a double mastectomy. In remission for the past year, she was left with a range of physical problems, including heart damage and hearing loss, from twenty months of aggressive chemotherapy and other treatments. "There was no chance at anything that would even remotely resemble a cure."

Tina had written to me, expressing her enthusiasm for the project. She had a great interest in family history, was already "drawing up a will and putting things in Ziploc bags marked 'Grandpa Boris's thimble,' 'Grandpa Norman's wedding ring.'" She had planned to write her memoirs and ethical will for the children but couldn't seem to get to it.

In the envelope along with her letter, I found resources that Tina had enclosed for other ill parents, including a copy of a letter she had written to friends, soliciting their help. This was the first of many generous offers to help further our work. "I've always been a doer." Also enclosed was a copy of a speech she had delivered at a community cancer event about living with metastatic cancer: "Breast cancer is not just a life-threatening illness, it is a *life-encompassing* illness. . . . With my metastatic cancer diagnosis, all of our plans, hopes, and dreams were exterminated, with no real hope of resurrection. While today I sit before you, blessed to be alive, let alone in remission, almost every small and large aspect of our family life is affected. . . . My husband and I live from test to test, holding our breath and fearing the other shoe might drop . . . all the while trying to maintain the smiley-faced, positive attitude that everyone tells us is so important to cancer survival."

Tina returns, goes to the closet, and hauls out photo albums, maps, and mementos that she has compiled to assist her memory in recording the family stories. She wants to relate all the stories from her childhood, the sad and the sappy. "What can I say?" she laughs. "Control is important to me." As if to prove the point, Tina then interviews me about my knowledge of child and adolescent development. "I'm not a psychotherapist," I say, "but I know quite a bit, and I'll be glad to listen. I trust that through the process of listening to herself tell her story, a mother will usually find her own answers."

Tina nods and then begins to talk about what is going on with the kids and her illness. "My older one, Mark, came home yesterday really upset, saying his life was a complete mess. Then he started listing the reasons. I was so relieved that there was a list, starting with school cafeteria lunches. My cancer only got tucked into the middle. Then Nathan started screaming, "I hate you, I hope you die," and I had to call the parental stress warm line. I can't tell the difference between what's developmentally normal for a three-year-old and what's due to my illness. Of course, the experts don't know, either."

Tina smiles wryly. Sighs. Her mouth quavers. Her voice lowers.

"Well, I just got bad news. The cancer's back. Another recurrence in the liver."

The other shoe had dropped, a little under three years.

"But I still want to do some fundraising for you."

Her lips set in a determined line. Tina lets me talk her out of hosting an event in her home but won't hear of backing out altogether.

She plans on writing a solicitation letter once she knows what's happening with the treatment. I make her promise not to overdo. "Yeah, okay. *[Long pause]* I used to be like city water. I could run all day and there was always more to draw on. Now I am like water drawn from a well. I have to be careful not to draw too much at any one time, lest the well run dry."

When I return the next week to tape her family history, Tina greets me, again looking as if she has a social engagement, rather than a nap, to rush to afterward. "I'm going to have to leave the phone plugged in. The doctor may call. I'm going crazy trying to get another opinion about the liver biopsy."

Tina explains why these stories are important to preserve: "I knew my great grandparents, and it was always important for me to know about my family and my history. It's been tremendously valuable to look back and understand how people get to be the way they are because it brings an understanding of yourself. I want to be able to share that with my children—and their children as well. Also, my husband and I have different recollections of what happened in our marriage. My kids can get my version of the story and then his."

She speaks about her late-in-life discovery of Judaism as a worthwhile "frame of reference" in which to raise children and as a guide to her values. "Teaching your children the values in the tradition, handing something down, is important." Tina tells the stories behind the objects and photographs, starting with her great grandparents and grandparents. "Chemo brain" or no, her memory is superb. We both forget about the phone and the time until the tape recorder clicks off. Two hours have passed.

"Oh, my God, there's never going to be enough time to cover it all!"

"Never enough time" becomes a recurring theme. Tina thinks it has as much to do with her temperament as the cancer pressure. But she grudgingly accepts the disappointment that she won't be able to include every story, mumbling, "I can't control anything."

The next time we meet, Tina looks like she has just rolled out of bed, hardly the fashion plate I have come to expect. "I think I'll let you ask me questions today. I couldn't get any preparation together for what I was going to cover." Her voice is weary, her skin pigeon gray.

I expect more medical news, but Tina dives in. As she tells the stories of her early years, she sheds light on her sense of responsibility and need for control.

Her father was "a very difficult man," "abusive," and "extremely unpredictable." Tina concluded early on that "that was what fathers did. Mothers were nice, and fathers were mean." When her siblings were born, she became a "miniature adult. My sister and brother were always called 'the kids.' I was *not* one of the kids—I never remember being carefree."

Tina survived by staying out of her father's way, trying to please him with top grades, and planning her escape: "One of the ways that I survived my childhood was that I knew that my childhood was temporary. Sixteen is when I ended up graduating from high school, and then I was on my own." But she was left with a "sense of perfectionism." "He held me to very high standards, which I still hold myself to now, and that's good and bad."

After working her way through college, she moved to Washington, D.C., where she entered the world of technology and finance and soon became a department manager. Tina then met Jack, who was starting a business in the same field. They married, built a business together, saved money, bought a house. Their single-minded rise to success changed dramatically when she became pregnant.

After the session, Tina shares two pieces of information. She is throwing Jack a surprise fiftieth birthday party with seventy-five guests, and she is going to her third tumor board to check out her next treatment options, including a stem-cell rescue—both within the next few days. "This one doctor, who I really like, said, 'Well, I have kids, too. If it were me and I was pushed, I would probably do a bone marrow transplant.' Then he said, 'You're so strong and assertive.' I just looked at him and said, 'I'm a *mother*.'"

Tina is ready to tell the story of becoming a mother, which, she says, will quickly get into being a mother with metastatic cancer.

TINA

Work has no importance to me any more. It was important to me then in the context of the times, during the eighties. The whole economy was, at least for the middle and upper-middle class, expanding so we were achieving tremendous financial success. I loved my work, but once Mark was born, I didn't want to work as much as I had to.

The more important thing was to be able to be home with the kids, so that led to a lot of problems for me. I ended up having to go back to work four weeks after he was born. I really resented it. It taught me a lot about the value of being there as a mom—I mean *physically* as well as emotionally. I don't know that I wanted to stay home full-time, but I really miss that thing I never had—neighbors chatting over the fence, hanging laundry or doing our weeding, sitting at each other's houses and drinking coffee and going to K-Mart or whatever before the kids come home from school. That sort of thing. That's what I was raised to be! My mother was a stay-at-home mom, and I didn't see anything wrong with that. I hit junior high school, and all of a sudden, the world changed. No one asked me. *[Laughs]* I really miss that thing that I never had. For all the gains that "women's lib" has made for women, I don't think that anybody could foresee what kinds of changes it was going to bring. What's gotten lost is what it takes to maintain a household and raise children. *Somebody's* got to be there. I think it's a mess right now. I wanted balance and I didn't have any balance. I don't really think there can be balance, to be honest with you.

In my social circle, which is mostly socioeconomically advantaged, a lot of women have gone to law school and business school and have nannies and are stopping work and realizing that *this is not working out.* So I felt incredibly trapped in the situation I was in and was really pissed off that I hadn't married a man that could support me financially so that I could stay home and have my babies.

Is there anything you'd like your kids to eventually understand about your marriage or the way you and Jack have parented together?

There's a lot. When Jack and I got married, I think that we made the decision that this was going to be it for us. We're very good friends. We've always been on the same level. I don't think it ever occurred to him that he was giving me equal footing or somehow granting me anything. Jack is a really, really good man, and he's a really, really good husband, and that's been very comforting. But fatherhood has become the focus of his life, so it's changed our relationship.

Tina fights to hold back tears; I pause the recorder until she's ready to continue.

It's painful to think that the kids would have to come to know our relationship through a story told like this, that I won't be able to share it with them myself. *[Long pause]*

Jack has always been the dreamer and the creative visionary in the relationship, and I've been the person who's done the thing. Which doesn't mean that Jack walks away from things when he's finished envisioning them, but the bulk of the responsibility for making something happen had always been mine. When Mark was born, this came out even more. He absolutely fell in love with Mark, and he was totally involved with his care from day one. He's a wonderful, natural, absolutely fantastic father. But the down side was in terms of the day-to-day operations of the business—I was better at it than he was. So, when Mark got sick and had to stay home, Jack was the one who would stay home with him. When there was late work to do and somebody had to leave to go home to get Mark, Jack would be the one to do it.

Mark's first year, we landed the biggest contract we've ever had, and I was the person who was running the whole project, literally working seven days a week, eighteen to twenty hours a day. I would come home at two in the morning and have to get back up at five. It was unbelievable. My first Mother's Day, I remember Jack had gone to Safeway and got me a balloon and a card, and he brought Mark into the office for a few hours and kept me company while I was working, and I was consumed with anger. I was angry at Jack, I was angry at life, I was angry at myself, at the situation, everything. It was really, really stressful.

I had a bad problem with my back. When I was twenty-two, I hurt my back moving books from my mother's apartment in a grocery wagon. My back was never the same after that. When you're young, you always think that you're invincible. *There's* a lesson I want to teach my children! *[Leans forward toward the microphone]* "Don't take your bodies for granted, and don't think that because you're young you have this bubble around you—even then, you can do damage."

Toward the end of my pregnancy with Mark, I had a lot of problems with my back, but they went away after the pregnancy. When I was pregnant with Rena, I didn't have back problems until the end.

I must have ruptured a disk during the emergency delivery. I was out of work on disability for about six to nine months after that. We both wanted to have a child right away. In that loss of Rena, there was hopefulness, also. After we lost her, we lost another baby through a miscarriage, and even then it was like, pick up the pieces and go on and have Nathan. I went to a lot of doctors, but they would not recommend surgery and then getting pregnant right away. I had to make a choice, so I decided to have the baby instead.

And then, when Nathan was about nine months old, I got to the point where I said, "I can't live like this any more," the pain was so . . . well, I don't need to tell you, I'm sure you know. *[Points to the back support I carry with me]* Living in constant pain is incredibly debilitating, and people look at you, and you look completely normal. It's sort of like cancer. Everybody says, "Oh, you look so good," and I say, "Yeah, but by the time I get to the point where I don't look good, I'll be dead very soon. Looking good doesn't mean I'm not sick." But it was horrible, just horrible, and I think, if any of those things contributed to the cancer, that contributed to it, living in pain for such a long amount of time.

I ended up having a microdiscectomy to remove some of the ruptured material, and in the process got a staph infection. I was really sick. But I was back at work, acting like I was normal. Finally, it came down to selling the business, which was arduous. We had the business sold, we had a letter of intent signed, and we were dotting the i's and crossing the t's on the contract the week I was diagnosed with cancer.

Everything was so pressure-filled, and it had been for such a long time. Right before I was pregnant with Rena, we had finished building this house. So, from when Mark was born, we've been on seven years of a lot of stress. I remember getting to the point after Nathan was born where I would drive home some nights, and I would think to myself, "How can I get into a car accident that would be serious enough that I could get out of having to work, but it really wouldn't hurt me that badly, wouldn't destroy my life completely?" That's the space I was in when I was diagnosed. The stress and eating on the run and having a drink after work and never having any time to exercise, that all becomes the things that "cause" your cancer.

I imagine you know that that's somewhat dangerous thinking.

Oh, I know, but that doesn't change the fact that I still think that way. This is a perspective that I want to share with my children. There's a level to which I blame myself for the cancer. I'm a very intuitive person, and I wish I had paid more attention to the intuitive part of me. I allowed myself to be trapped in a work situation in which I was *extremely* unhappy; it was keeping me from mothering and constantly making me choose other things over my children.

Normally, as a listener, I would not disagree or suggest alternative interpretations. However, I am disturbed by the way cancer patients, especially mothers, blame themselves for their illness. I can't help questioning Tina's need to find someone—especially herself or the work, or, by implication, her husband—to blame. I ask why she feels the need to come up with an explanation when there are so many complicating factors, perhaps environmental or genetic ones, beyond her control.

I think partially, if I were able to understand why it happened, I might be able to undo it.

That's a trap, you know. It seems you've already made many of the changes you wanted to make in your life, and that's valuable, irrespective of the cancer.

Then why is it back? *[Laughing and crying]* When Rena died, there was a structural explanation for what had happened to her. She was choked by the umbilical cord. I got the statistics of how many times that happens and why it can't be prevented. There was anger and frustration and disappointment and loss, but I know what happened. It happened. Her death is a lot easier for me to understand and accept than my illness. You get into these rationalizations of, "Am I a good person or am I a bad person, am I being punished, am I being taught a lesson, is this somebody else's lesson?" I go through a lot of stuff about evaluating my sins, so to speak, against other people.

One of the more profound things my husband said to me was when we were talking about losing Rena in the context of cancer, and about karma, and that somehow losing Rena had to do with the balance of something: "Well, how do you know that it's your karma that's being played out? Maybe it's mine." There's an incredible amount of unfairness about this, an incredible amount of rage, and there is a tremendous need to make some sense out of it.

It's pretty hard with this recurrence. Living with cancer takes away a large part of one's frame of reference, especially right now, being in this limbo of not knowing whether this treatment is working or not. My husband and I have lost the ability to make plans—short-term, long-term, whatever. All I have is the present. That's all any of us have.

I guess the rest of us have the illusion that our plans actually control what will happen to us in the future.

Right. Well, I want the illusion back! *[Laughs]*

Tina excuses herself to call a doctor, leaving me to my thoughts. I realize that she cannot create a recovery story in which cancer will only be a temporary interruption. Recurring critical illness like hers makes it impossible to hold onto a narrative line that is intelligible and predictable or to project a future. Without a story to fall back upon, and in the absence of an explanation for cancer, chaos threatens. Perhaps Tina's determination to preserve the past is also an attempt to restore the continuity of her narrative.

Tina and Jack do make plans, but they are limited and tentative. Because of the loss of Tina's income and her "low chances of long-term survival," Jack cannot do anything to risk the family's financial security—making a career change, which he would like to do. Nor is the family able to move because of being geographically bound by Tina's health insurance.

Cancer granted Tina's wish to be home with the children. But being sick creates a whole new set of stresses and preoccupations, not the least of which is dealing with the medical system. With a little time left in our session, I ask whether her healthcare providers have helped or hindered her need for relief from stress.

You've hit a raw nerve for me. I think that this is a much bigger deal than healthcare providers realize. They minimize and trivialize the physical and psychological toll that the diagnosis and the treatment take. As a result, I don't think that women are prepared for the absolutely incredible physical debilitation that's not obvious.

"Tired" means "sleepy" to people. It's not sleepy—it's that there is nothing to draw on, there is no well, no reserve. And how do you get dinner on the table, how do you look at the kid's picture and go, "Ohhh, what a beautiful house you drew there"? *[Pretends a child's voice]* "It's not a house, Mommy, it's a dog."

And yet, the medical professionals are telling you, "If you schedule your chemo on Friday, you should be able to go to work on Monday or Tuesday. Maybe you could cut your hours back to thirty a week and somebody can take your kids until dinnertime." Dinnertime's the time you want to collapse and go to sleep! "You know, there's wonderful anti-nausea drugs." Well, nausea's not the only problem. It's everything else. It's the fact that you can't have a bowel movement without feeling like you're going to rip yourself open, and everything burns and hurts, and then your husband wants to have sex, and the kids wake up in the middle of the night, and the alarm goes off in the morning. . .

We would have these horrendous Monday mornings. I was totally flipped out because I knew I was going for chemo. But there's this total lack of acknowledgment from the medical community that anything bad or debilitating is happening. Then, that snowballs because it affects whether you have disability insurance. If affects how your employer's going to accommodate your job. It affects your own ability to accept help. People are saying, "Can I bring meals? Do you want me to take your kid tonight? Do you want this or that?" Well, you don't want to impose on people because you're being told that this is not a big deal.

So, what do you want from the medical community?

Not only do I want acknowledgment, I want doctors' orders. I want the doctor to be telling me, to be telling my husband, to be telling my employer, to be telling disability or social security or whatever, "This person cannot work, this person has to go home and go to bed, this person is neutrapenic—meaning your immune system is impaired—this person is at risk for infection."

I want to feel . . . I want to feel fragile. I want to feel like I have a right to go into bed and pull the covers over my head and put my Bernie Siegel tape or whatever on and cocoon.[2] My therapist talked to me about treating the time that you're going through chemo, treating that first year—she said *year*—as a sabbatical. "Take a sabbatical, and your job is to take care of yourself." It really angers me that there's not this support. They can be optimistic and positive, and they can say to me, "Let me know what ails you, and I will do something to help you," *but acknowledge the fact that I'm going to have ailments.* Say, "This is heavy-duty stuff we're giving you."

Did any of your medical practitioners actually ask you about your children?

No. *No!* And you want to know something? I felt as if I played the mother card. I brought my older son with me when I had blood tests because I wanted people in that doctor's office to see me with a child so that they would put more value on my life and on treating me well because they knew that I was a mother. I brought pictures of my children to chemo because I wanted my doctor to see these faces, *[Crying]* and I wanted his heart to break so he would do something to save my life.

Do you think it made a difference?

I don't think so. With doctors, you're just dealing with people. My little one was still in diapers. He had no concept. There was nothing in the chart.

When I had surgery, the anesthesiologist knew the names and ages of my children. I didn't tell her. Somewhere in my chart, she knew there was a Mark and a Nathan, and she knew how old they were. She took the time. She talked to me about where they went to school. I know it was all to allay my fears, but I felt very differently about being in her care than I felt about being in the care of somebody who did not acknowledge my children.

Tina is right in saying that doctors are people, but they are also part of a powerful culture with its own specialized language and narrative demands: Cure is the only acceptable story. She was trying to interject her voice and truth into the medical narrative.

A week later, Tina is distraught. She has decided to have an oophorectomy—the removal of her ovaries—in order to suppress hormone production that might spur cancer's growth. Her hormone levels have been off, and the doctors are concerned. "Also, I have a lump on my side, and the doctors don't seem to be responding quickly enough. I'm afraid the cancer is growing wildly." She wants to start with the topic of motherhood and cancer, letting the talk go where it will.

We wanted to have more kids after Nathan, and that's been taken away from us. I'm waiting for myself to get past the panic of the cancer aspect of it so that I can get hit with the realization of what all the underlying issues of losing my ovaries are. Right now, I'm rationalizing to myself that they're superfluous appendages at this point. It's like, when you think about having parts hacked away from you, where is the person? I mean, I know I am not my ovaries or my breasts.

It makes you think about the essence of being human?

Yes. There's nothing about having the mastectomy that I ever cared about anybody knowing. I had huge breasts, and I'm actually happier with the mastectomy than I ever was with my breasts, if you can separate it from the cancer. But last night, when I heard Jack talking to somebody on the phone, telling him that I was going to have the oophorectomy, I was like, *Who is he telling this to? The world doesn't need to know.* Sometimes I'm just an observer to my reactions.

What else would you like to say about mothering and raising children while ill?

I think, first of all, of the overwhelming sense of responsibility. Talk about being responsible! My reaction to the illness was always oriented toward my reaction as a mother. One of the most important things that I thought of at first was, *What do I tell Mark? How do I tell Mark?* Mark was barely eight. Nathan was sixteen months; there wasn't anything to tell Nathan that I had to be concerned about.

We had this whole network that had come to us around Rena's death. Somebody said, "Basically, approach it the way you approach talking about sex. Give a little information and stop, and let him ask questions, and just answer the questions that he asks. No more."

That really worked for me. I also found that I had to be very truthful with him—for two reasons. One is that Mark and I have always shared a very intuitive sense between us, so it's impossible to keep a secret from him. The other part was that the psychiatrist Mark had seen focused on the issue of trust. The difference between answering questions and lying is tremendous. It was very important that Mark—and Nathan, as he got older—could trust us to be truthful but not give more than he could handle.

We said that I had gone for a check-up and the doctor had found a lump in my breast, and they weren't sure what it was, and I was going to go for tests and find out, and it was possible that it was going to be cancer, and did he know what cancer was? My mother-in-law was sick with cancer at the time, and we had differentiated her situation from mine and said that there were a lot of different kinds of cancer.

I tried to be, not nonchalant, but matter-of-fact. I didn't act like it was nothing, but I didn't fall apart, either. It was really important that he feel secure, that his world wasn't going to come crumbling down around him. I have a clear memory of having this very practical conversation with him, talking about the cancer, how chemo works, and different ways they treat it. He was concerned about Nathan because I had breastfed Nathan. Was Nathan going to get cancer because he was drinking the cancer? He wanted to know why they can't cut it out, so I talked about the idea of cancer throughout the body.

He had zillions of questions, but the questions would come up piece by piece at very odd times, sometimes out of the blue. The thing that really blew my mind was, after we had been through all of this with him and I had had surgery and was going to start my chemotherapy, as he was getting out of the shower and I was wrapping him in his towel, something I said triggered him to look at me with utter shock and amazement. I will never forget his eyes, open as wide as can be, and he said to me, "You mean you have *cancer?*" I just stood there, and I thought to myself, "Huh?" You kind of visualize this level of sinking in, you know, *literally sinking in.* Somehow, through all of that, he never got that I had cancer. Never assume, never assume.

He was devastated. He was crying and sad and had a lot of questions. I guess he was stuck back in that part where we didn't know for sure and never really got the part that, yes, now we know, and now I'm going to go for treatment and have the mastectomy and all of this other stuff. Somehow, in his mind, the chemo was something that you would do *in case* you really did have the cancer.

This week, Mark has sunk into feeling horribly sorry for himself. I got irritated and started telling him about all the people who had much worse things happen to them in their lives, and he stomped off and went upstairs, and I suddenly realized, *What am I saying to him?* That's a terrible thing to say. I mean, would I ever want anybody to compare what I'm going through to the horrors that other people suffer? There is no comparison.

So I went and apologized and told him how incredibly wrong I was and how bad I would feel if somebody had done that to me. I didn't know what the connection was, but he said, "Oh, and then every single day, when I see my teacher in school, he asks me, 'How's your mother?' I don't want to hear that question all the time. I want to go to school and forget about things."

Well, his teacher called last night about something. I was telling him this story, and he said, "Well, it's funny because the other day,

I was asking another little girl how her mother was doing. Mark came over and said to him in a very irritated way, 'How come you don't ask me about *my* mother?'"

So last night, Mark had come into our room, and I said to him, "So, what's going on with Ellen's mother?" I never discussed it with him before, so that question was innocuous. He could have answered anything. He was flipping through a magazine and said something like, "She's fine, but Ellen's got a lot to learn about life." I said, "What do you mean?" and he said, "She thinks her mother's going to be cured of cancer."

Well, cancer's not a generic thing, especially not breast cancer. There's all different forms and levels of it. In some ways, the level that they found in me was one of the worst. I said, "Sometimes it's practically curable. You never know, it might never be a problem for Ellen's mother again."

He flipped another page of the magazine and didn't say anything, and the vibes were very clear that the conversation was closed. You cannot imagine the different issues that come up. If you're not listening and paying attention, a lot of harm can be done.

What about Nathan's reactions?

I think I'm a good mother, but in a lot of ways, I feel like I'm not there for them now, especially Nathan. I went from not being around because I was working to not being around because I was sick. He always thinks I'm going to meetings. What he needs from me that he doesn't get is more patience. I am very worn out, and I have been since he was born. I had my back surgery when he was nine months, and since then, it's gone from bad to worse. There were a lot of problems for Nathan around the concept that I was sick and my door was closed and he couldn't go in. I mean, literally. I had a bad time with healing, and so I went through multiple surgeries and was constantly needing to be physically protected from being hurt. I had a lot of nurses coming into the house, I had a PICC[3] line in, and I was having infusions and constant problems with dressings and drainage.

He's always hearing, "Mommy's sick, Mommy's tired," and then he starts being sick and tired. Sometimes I have noticed that Nathan closely identifies with any kind of an illness that I have. He tells me he has the flu a lot. He has to lie in bed with me. I feel so bad for him. But what he needs from me that he *does* get is a lot of acknowledgment and validation. He's such a *being* in our family. That's something important I want him always to know.

The thing that's so weird about cancer is that cancer generally is the kind of disease where you are well until you are diagnosed, and then, when they treat you, they make you sick. I always felt like I had to be very careful about how that was presented to the kids because I didn't want them to feel that doctors or medicine would make them sick or hurt them. Each little piece had to be handled in its own way.

Like Nathan questioning me about why I didn't have breasts. Recently, he asked me something about why my bra was so heavy, and I said to him, "Because I have different booby pads in them right now, and they are very heavy." He said, "Why do you have the booby pads in your bra?" He knows I have cancer now, so I said to him, "Because I have cancer." He interrupted me and said, "Oh, so you wear your booby pads so you look more like a regular person in your clothes." And I said, "Yeah, that's right." I stopped there. There wasn't anything more to say.

He just turned four, and pretty close to that time, we were looking at old videotapes. We got into the concept that Grandma was dead and how did Grandma die. . . . Well, Grandma died from cancer. He asked me about some other relatives, and, as it turned out, all the relatives he was asking about died from cancer. I said to him, "Not everybody dies from cancer." I told him about some people who have cancer that aren't dead. He asked me if kids can have cancer. I said, "Some kids can have cancer, but not many children get cancer. It's something that mostly happens when people are grownups."

I said something really terrible to Nathan the other day, and I was horrified when I said it, but, you know, I'm not perfect. He acts out a lot with kicking and punching and things like that, and this was right after I had come home from my surgery, and he was very focused on the fact that he could hit me and hurt me. So he decided that he needed to do that. I'm being sarcastic, but he does this all the time. I was putting on his shoes, and he started to kick me, and I kept telling him, "Don't do that, you can hurt Mommy. This is not a hitting family. This is not a kicking family," whatever. Then he did it again, and I got very upset and said, "Don't do that! You could hurt Mommy very badly. You could kill me if you kicked me like that after I've had an operation!" I thought, "Oh, God, now I've done it. Now if I die, it's going to be on his conscience that he killed me." Sometimes kids think that they can wish for things and that they really can happen.

Are there other parts of mothering that are difficult for you?

Recognizing that they are complete, separate human beings that have their own will. You can underline and capitalize that! *[Laughing]* And that I can't make them do what I want, and I can't make them understand me, and sometimes it just drives me crazy. But I think mothering provides a nice distraction to having cancer. *[Laughs]* The intensity of mothering—all the tasks involved, keeping track of their schedules and washing the clothes and making breakfast and remembering who likes avocado this week and who doesn't—that's very consuming. Dealing with their emotional issues outside of cancer is very absorbing and can give me large blocks of time when I don't think of myself as anything other than a "normal person."

So what do you think mothers need in order to be "good enough" mothers, especially when they're ill?

First and foremost, mothers need to be happy with themselves, and then they need breaks from their children. And help. I definitely subscribe to the theory that the healthiest thing for my children is for me to be happy and healthy. I spend a lot of time taking care of myself, which is not, on the surface, doing anything for them, but it is. With cancer, I don't feel like anybody is taking care of me, with the exception of some physical ministrations from my mother. The rest has been me taking care of me while other people take care of everything else. I try to be in touch with what I need and want and follow that—going to Beverly, my therapist, going to my group, going to acupuncture, going to the body worker, doing this project with you, volunteering at the kids' school when I want to and not doing it when I don't want to.

That's the thing that's transformed for me a lot since the cancer, which I did not have before: a sense of valuing myself as a person and realizing that preserving myself physically and mentally was a service to other people. After I was diagnosed, I wasn't sure who I was or why I was important. I was amazed by how much people seemed to care. I used to think that my importance as a mother was what I *did*, meaning driving or shopping or whatever, and with a lot of help from Jack and Beverly, I've come to realize that my value as a mother is just being me, being here. That's a hard thing to learn, to accept. And with these surgeries, I have to keep questioning, "Which part is *me?*"

I was thinking of the same thing earlier. Your ovaries and your breasts are not what's important to your children.

Right. Or your hair. That's the thing that has been so wonderful. Mark is completely nonchalant about the fact that I have no breasts. He was completely nonchalant about the fact that I had no hair. In fact, he loved it when I was bald.

So what's most important to you now?

I think my purpose is raising my children. But not in a sick or twisted kind of way—the overbearing mother that has no outside life. . . . The source of my greatest joy and inspiration, and the source of my greatest fears and horrors and disappointments, are around being here to mother them. I *am* a mother, and I always wanted to be one, and I can't even remember not being one. *[Crying]* It's my job, it's *me*, you know?

When I was first diagnosed, I told my doctors that my goal was to stay alive for my children and that whatever it took, I would do it. *[Crying]* They always talk about cancer, particularly breast cancer, in terms of five years' survival, and I'm constantly thinking ahead to what's a good age for them to be for me to die. If I can see Nathan through to kindergarten, if I can see Mark's bar mitzvah, if I can make it till Nathan's bar mitzvah or until Mark graduates from high school . . . I'm constantly bargaining with God: "Just let me finish my job." And I've realized that that's sort of like falling into a trap of, well, what happens if I live until they're that age? Does that mean then I get to die? *[Laughs, reading a smile that I can't suppress]*

I don't think it quite works that way because entire generations of mothers would have croaked one day after high school graduation.

Right. There's this other part of me that thinks that I know what they need and I'm instinctually tied to them and committed. But then I think, *So were a lot of mothers who died young from cancer.* That's not going to be my salvation. Then what if I do die soon and they're left on their own? What's going to happen to them? Will I have ruined them or failed them by dying? Is this illness and the potential for my early demise the thing that's going to make them into stronger, better people? I don't know.

I've heard frequently that children need to feel as if their parents did everything that they could to not die and will blame the parent for dying. Like, if you'd only gone for the bone marrow transplant or if you'd taken your vitamins . . . It influences me a lot. I'm also guarding myself very carefully against doing anything that might leave them with any feeling of guilt or responsibility.

You probably know you're not going to be able to control all of that.

But it doesn't stop me from trying. *[Laughs]* I could never believe when people would tell me something can't be done. I remember stopping for directions once, and this man thought and thought and finally said to me, "You can't get there from here." I guess the theme of my life is that *of course you can.* When people tell me I have metastatic cancer and there's nothing you can do, I'm like, "Wait a minute. There is a way to solve *any* problem, let's look into this."

The most important thing for me is to be alive, and the approach that I'm taking to managing my illness is to keep stretching it out as long as possible. The fact that I have to go through these "difficulties," I guess would be a word for it, *[Laughs]* I just do it. It's what I have to do. About the only part we can change is how we feel about it. I like a combination of "fight like hell" and "go with the flow." Like that "Serenity Prayer": Change what you can, and accept what you can't, and be smart enough to know the difference.

You said earlier that you were amazed that people cared. How have the people in your life responded, whether helpfully or harmfully?

A lot of people want to help, but they don't know what to do. Certain people feel like they shouldn't ask or call or write because somehow they might be making me feel worse by reminding me of my troubles. Well, like, "No, you're not reminding us of something; it really helps to know that people care. Cards and notes and people telling me that they were thinking about me and knowing that I was included in people's prayers helped me. The fact that they were praying has value, but that value is magnified tremendously by telling me. It helped Mark to know that so-and-so from his school was sending a note or that his teacher called. Several of Mark's teachers actually brought meals over, and I think that was very special to him or to hear the messages on the tape.

As Tina said earlier, metastatic cancer is life encompassing, influencing most relationships. She has been estranged from her brother for a number of years and, although he tried to reconcile after she was diagnosed, Tina decided to avoid the emotional turmoil of communicating with him. With her sister, there's a different issue: "She had her baby when I had my tumor. I don't begrudge her; it just makes things awkward sometimes." And then there's her mother.

One thing that's been very troubling to me has been my relationship with my mother. The response from my mother was the same as when Rena died, which is that it became *her* problem, and I needed to support *her*. I felt very strongly that I was the one who needed mothering. Through my therapy, I've realized that this is a theme that goes all the way back to my childhood.

In the groups I've encountered, I've been surprised at the frequency with which women have found that their mothers have not been able to support them in a way that they've needed because their mothers feel so much pain. This cancer is infinitely easier for me than if something were to happen to one of my children. It sickens me to think about it and makes me scared to talk about it. So I try to have compassion for my mother. I try, and I can't find it in me. *[Crying]* I want her to take care of me.

One thing that disturbed me came up when I was having a conversation with Jack and Mark. It had to do with my going for the bone marrow transplant. Mark said to me, "One thing about you, Mom, you're a rock." And the way that I heard it was that he was seeing me as very strong and able to survive *anything*. I took it in a very bad way, not outwardly to him but to myself, which was that my child sees me as being hard and cold, rigid—the negative, unemotional connotations of a rock—not as soft and warm and nurturing, somebody that feels pain and joy. It still sticks with me now. It's like, here come the tears. . . .

Why do you think you heard it that way?

[Crying] Because I think that that's always been my role. That is what Tina is about. The outside of me is the person who can have her ovaries out on Monday and be picking the kids up at school on Tuesday. One of the most horrible things somebody said to me when I was first diagnosed was, "Well, I know if anybody can beat this, it's you. You're the strongest person I know." And I thought, *Well, if there was ever a set-up for failure, if there was ever a set-up to disappoint . . .*

This was a big issue with my recurrence. I really felt like I let everybody down. I was supposed to be the strong one that beat everything.

People say variations on, "Oh, I can't believe how well you're handling this. You're so brave." A nurse once said it to me when I was lying on the operating table. I said, "I can't figure out a way in which handling it badly would improve the situation." *[Laughs, then sobers]* I think it's possible to be strong and capable and optimistic and also to be fearful and feel pain and not have all the answers. I don't think of it in terms of anything other than: *This is what I do.*

Part of the problem is that people don't understand what breast cancer—probably most cancer—is all about. People ask stupid questions like, "Are you cured?" They don't seem to understand the life-threatening aspect and the fact that there isn't a magic bullet. They don't understand what it means to have survival statistics read to you. How their mother's or their cousin's experience with it last year or thirty years ago is of no relevance. I've been amazed at how many times in the past I had been insensitive, now that I've been enlightened, so to speak.

Tina recognizes how her strength and stated determination to "beat everything" often seem to contradict her equally powerful need to be nurtured. Her story opens up a critical question that has plagued me for years: How does a mother keep nurturing when her own well is close to dry? And there are new questions: What's a life worth? What's a long-enough life? A good-enough life? What is the essence of being human? After losing hair, breasts, ovaries, how do you recognize yourself as a woman and an individual?

These issues become heightened as Tina faces another medical crisis. When we meet again, the day after the oophorectomy, she hugs me more gingerly than usual, the only physical sign that she has just been through major surgery. But her close encounter with death and loss is on her mind.

So often, I think about what a horrible thing this is to have happened to *them.* I don't think about that it's a horrible thing that's happened to me. It happened. And I'm not afraid of dying. Everybody in the world that's ever lived before me has died, and obviously it's deal-with-able. You know it's going to happen. It'll be part of the journey like everything else. The issue for me is the timing of the death and the nature of the death and how that pain will play out for the children.

This comes out of my desire to protect my children. One of the biggest fears is that I'm going to go through a long, lingering, degenerative type of death as I have seen so many people with cancer go through, where they waste away and lose a tremendous amount of their dignity and create an enormous emotional burden on the people around them. The idea of my kids coming home from school day after day and going upstairs and seeing me in my bed getting frailer and frailer and sicker and sicker and becoming incontinent and having tubes coming out of my body and perhaps losing my mental faculties and getting to the point where I have been with relatives with cancer, of wishing they would die already because it's just too much . . . and feeling so frustrated and angry and pained . . . I really, really, really don't want to see them go through that, and I'm so frightened that that's going to be the reality for them. Not only am I not going to be able to protect them from that, but it's something *I am going to cause.* [*Crying*]

I don't feel that doing anything proactive to hasten my death is within my rights as a human being—any more than I am allowed to take someone else's life. So, *que sera sera.* [*Wistful*] I would want them to know how sorry I am and how much I would want to be able to spare them that. [*Crying*] What did these two absolutely beautiful angels do to deserve this kind of fate? It tears me apart. I might not be able to comfort them. I might not be able to. . . .

Look, this morning was Purim at Nathan's school, and everybody was going to wear a costume. I've mentioned this to Jack a dozen times. When Nathan came down in his Power Ranger costume, Jack was like, "What's this?" *[Shakes her head]* What if I wasn't here and Nathan was the only kid who came to the school without a costume because Daddy didn't remember? That's *my* job, and that's something they're going to lose. Life does go on, but it is very painful to me.

Jack and I had a horrible incident before I went into the surgery. I thought to myself, *You know, why am I doing this? Why am I fighting, stringing this thing out? I'm prolonging the agony for everyone. Why don't I die and get it over with and let them move on? Let Jack find a new wife, let Nathan form an attachment to a new mother. Mark will be young enough to make some sort of a transition instead of constantly going through this trauma of Mommy's next illness, Mommy's next operation, Mommy's next depression.* I even felt that way after I was first diagnosed. I didn't see the possibilities that I could have something other than an ever-downward spiral.

Let me give you a brief version of what happened on Friday, [the day of the surgery]. I made this decision to have my ovaries out very clear-headedly, very pragmatically, very aggressively. That didn't mean it wasn't fraught with other issues. I was sitting there in the gown, waiting for them to come and get me, and I said to Jack, "I'd like to share my feelings with you," and I told him how upset I was about the idea of losing my ovaries. Everybody in the medical professions was being so practical and nonchalant, sort of like, "Oh, it can be in-and-out surgery, you can go home the same day," that kind of thing. I had given the doctor the example of, "What if somebody said to you, 'You can have your balls cut off and it's no big deal, just in and out, you know, we'll cut them off, a couple of stitches, send you home.' Like it's nothing." If they would say, "You are going to be in a lot of pain" . . . They don't ever use the word "pain"—you're in "discomfort." I think that it's a combination of them trying to protect themselves from what they're doing to other people and also maybe a way of allaying your fears and not making too big a deal out of it. I said to Jack that I was really feeling bad about the fact that no one was acknowledging the other side of the coin, the loss and the pain and the downside to all of this.

He got angry. "You know, this was your decision, you're the one who wanted to have the surgery, you're the one who made the arrangements for it, you're the one who was in the big rush to do it, and I don't understand." And I said, "Yeah, well, that's the whole problem—you don't understand. You don't want to talk about it, you don't want to go into counseling." And at that moment, the guy came to take me to the operating room.

I was sitting there in tears in what they call the "staging area," and I got up and said, "You have to get my husband. I need to talk to him." I said to Jack, "What's the point? Why don't I just go home? Why don't I let myself die and move on with this?" He started in with, "Do you think that that's what I want?" "Well, I don't know what you want because you don't discuss your feelings."

We did ultimately have a chance to get it straightened out. This is not a bad man that I'm talking to you about, *[Crying]* not an unfeeling man, not an uncaring man. He never has learned that aspect of communication. I don't know how to share my experience without it sounding like a criticism. It's not hard for me to show my vulnerability. It's hard for me to not have it perceived. I think he needs me to be the rock. I need somebody to be the rock for me. *[Laughs]* Basically, it's a stalemate.

Tina and Jack did go for counseling shortly after this, which relieved the terrible pressures and grief both of them were experiencing. Meanwhile, my questions multiplied. Before knowing Tina, I had assumed that a mother who is gravely ill but carries an unbearable burden of responsibility might need permission to lay the burden down, to let go. Now I think the converse might also be true, that a seriously sick mother might just as well need permission and encouragement to keep fighting, even if her life poses a burden to the family. I ask Tina whether she really believes her family would prefer for her to die.

I don't think Nathan has any kind of frame of reference to know. I don't even know if he would remember me when he grew up. Mark, no, probably that's not what he wants, but he can't have what he wants, anyway. Jack, I don't know. No, I don't think that's what he wants. . . .

The uncertainty hangs in the air. Once again, Tina is trying to get her reality validated. I see how an ill person's narrative is interwoven with those of others—like physicians and husbands—and how difficult it is to maintain confidence in one's own version. Tina is as assertive in confronting physicians as she is with Jack, but the cost to her is great. Understanding that the men in her life are human beings with their own stories does not diminish her pain when she feels that her emotional truth—especially her experience of vulnerability and loss—is unacknowledged or misunderstood. Tina looks exhausted and indicates that she is done with the topic for now. I ask her if she has found anything of value in living with cancer.

I've always been hesitant to look at secondary gifts with this illness because I don't want to candy-coat it, but if I could have the option of not dying young, I'd rather have had the cancer than not. Parenting with cancer made me a stronger, more motivated, more clearly directed person. I think a tremendous amount of growth and transformational experience have come out of it.

I don't know whether there's a purpose to life. But I believe that within people, there's a tremendous power to advance beyond a very superficial realm. That's a realm that I was living in until I was diagnosed with cancer. I was always running and doing and never really thinking about things.

I feel that I'm on the cusp of understanding myself in a very different framework than before. I've been able to get in touch with a spiritual and creative aspect of myself that constantly surprises me. I guess if I have one negative mantra about myself, it's that I'm not very creative. I have found that I have more creativity than I realized. I'd love to learn more. I'd love to read more. From the point of view of being more charitable, I would like to be able to do more. I would love to take in a foster child. I feel there's lots more for me to do, lots and lots and lots.

I have a lot more to offer my children. I think they will handle adversity better than people in general do. I don't want to say that they'd be stronger, better people for it, but they won't be destroyed by it, either.

When I lost my father—I was twenty-six—I was very afraid of moving out of my intense grief because I was afraid I was going to forget how much I loved and missed him and how angry I was. I was afraid that it would be like he never existed. It doesn't work that way. When they say, "Time heals all wounds," it doesn't say, "Time *erases* all wounds." It heals them. You still have the scar. I think that's very important that they understand.

Would you like to say something to your children about this story you've recorded?

I almost feel like I want to give an apology. If I were to die before I had the opportunity to chronicle for the children all the details of my growing up beyond what I've done so far, I guess I want them to know—I don't want to say that I did the best I could, I just did what I did. It would be nice if there were more, but there is what there is. My mother-in-law used to bug me to put dates on pictures, and I used to think to myself, "Why isn't she just happy that I'm sending her pictures?" Now, I go back to pictures, and it's like, "God, when was this? Was he two? Was he three?" I guess I could say, "There are the pictures. I'm sorry we don't have dates on them. There are these scanty journals. I wrote what I could."

Probably a lot more than most people do.

I know. *[Laughing]* That's what my accountant says to me every year when I apologize. "Oh, God, most people bring me a paper bag full of stuff. You're apologizing." I cross-reference with post-its. It wasn't as much as I wanted to do, let me put it that way.

After Tina and I completed the taping, I gave her the manuscript for editing. We talked about not creating a monster for herself, and, in fact, she decided to drop her elaborate plan of separating the story into packages deliverable at different ages. Because of her complicated life, she held onto the unfinished manuscript for two years but knew that it was "good enough," even if "imperfect."

As Tina eased her tight grip on control and made living her priority, I began to see both the pattern of our sessions and her coping style more clearly. Before and after each interview came action: Throwing a party. Planning a PTA event. Scheduling medical appointments. Organizing meals. Tina the "rock": responsible, in charge, and almost always looking her best.

And during the interview? She seemed to use our sessions as she used psychotherapy, as "time out" for herself, a place to unload and be validated for who she was. She told an uncensored story, gave in to overwhelming grief, and even allowed chaos to enter when admitting that metastatic cancer may be the one problem she cannot solve. In the face of radical uncertainty, Tina sometimes blamed herself, but at least she spoke her truth in order to wrest her narrative back from the forces that threatened to overtake her. Then, marshaling her will, she would move back into action.

Ravaged and "enlightened" by cancer, Tina was learning to value herself just for being. Insights would bubble up, giving a sense of the new story she was creating: "All I have is the present." "Fight like hell, and go with the flow." "There's lots more for me to do." I finally saw her attention to fashion, to preserving heirlooms, and to entertaining guests as having little to do with vanity or perfectionism. She was insisting on her own individual style of meeting illness, taming chaos through the creation of beauty and order.[4] She was being the creative person she had always wanted to be.

TEN: "YOU GET WHAT YOU GET"
JULIE RENAUD

JULIE RENAUD'S PLAN was to put a copy of the story she was recording for her seven-year-old daughter, Erica, in a safety deposit box. "My hope is that she will know me better even if she can't remember very much about me. I think it's a process for myself as well, part of the journey toward death *and* toward life that is valuable.

"Yesterday I turned thirty-nine. Since my recurrence of metastatic breast cancer six weeks ago, I have been trying to think of ways I can leave my daughter documentation of my life. This is extremely important to me. I have had difficulty organizing my thoughts and priorities. My hope would be a feeling of peace. I could check off this important priority on my 'things to do before I die' list."

It was only after Julie told me that Erica had been born during the year she and her husband Greg sailed around the world that I realized how much their house feels like a ship. The hardwood floors are mainly uncovered, as are the walls, with the exception of a few black-and-white photographs of ocean liners on the high seas. Light streams through the large, open windows. A floral scarf is tied tightly around Julie's head. She could be a young sailor.

In the kitchen, rose petals are drying on the stove, vegetable soup simmers on one burner, and green tea steeps on another. A breakfast nook overlooks her flourishing garden. Julie clasps her teacup with both hands, looks lovingly at the plants and flowers, and then nods to me to press "record."

JULIE

I grew up surrounded by brothers. I was *the* tomboy. I asked my mother about myself as a young baby, and she said, "Julie, you were really on your own." I never felt as though being a woman would impede my goals. I didn't have career choices all lined up. I wanted to experience as much as possible for the sake of learning bigger pictures and different ways of life. Travel wasn't just a phase; it stayed important.

I graduated college majoring in landscape design and worked for a couple of years as a gardener and designer. I loved it. As soon as I quit, I used the money to go on a trip to the Southwest by myself in my 510 Datsun stick shift. My "Freedom Car" I call it because it took me *everywhere!* I met Greg the week before I was leaving. Then I drove off and had a fantastic time by myself.

With Greg, I found someone to be with whose life brought me a lot of travel. We went sailing for a year on the ocean. A lot of women told me I was out of my mind. Fear alone would keep them from doing it. But I felt Greg knew what he was doing, and the boat was well equipped. You cannot control the uncontrollable, so you gotta let go and go for it. And that's where Erica came from—somewhere off the coast of Hawaii. Unplanned but, needless to say, glorious. There was a very short-term panic about it. It wasn't a negative shock—it was just "Wow! Okay, now we have to go from here."

When I found out I was pregnant, I had some glimmer of the devoted mother that I would be. I think that's what gave me pause. I never expected to have children so young. I had questions, but deep down inside, I knew that this was it. I was now pregnant, my path was completely altered, we would adjust to that path.

We went to a doctor, who advised me that I should not sail to Canada. We read and thought about it and decided to do it anyway. I was quite active, quite healthy. But it was still a scary thing to do. Sailing can be lonely. It's a soul searching, very introspective time, and that appeals to my nature. Pregnancy is more of a community, social, women's thing. I was missing that and yet having a wonderful time.

There were some middle-of-the-night 2:00 A.M. winds whipping from the south, and the waves are coming from the north . . . we were just slamming. The boat would go up and *slam* down, and go up and *slam* down, hour after hour. You couldn't do electric steering; it all had to be manually done. And I'm standing out there five months pregnant. I can't even zip up my foul weather gear anymore, and I'm getting *slammed,* and then the sail is knocked down. . . . *Okay. Enough! I shouldn't be here! I don't think this is a good idea! [Laughs]* But there's something to endurance, and there's something to getting through, and then there's something to the rainbow when the sun comes out, and it's utterly spectacular.

My mother was there for the birth. It was a significant emotional experience for me to have a new baby and to be with [my mother] at the same time. I remember dreading her leaving, and I couldn't say why. I remember crying at the airport, waiting for her flight. I've hardly done that around my mother. We are not a tell-it-how-it-is family.

This was beyond a hormonal roller coaster. The next generation had come, I was now in the middle, our whole positions had shifted, and I was so afraid of her dying. Not that she was in any imminent danger, but I realized she was the grandmother, and now she would be the first to leave, and then I would shift into that position. I could only do one shift at a time, and I suppose I was afraid for her. I really *needed* her to be there, and I couldn't say any of those things, especially not at the airport five minutes before her flight. But I was very aware that the universe had shifted and I was the mother. *[Thoughtful pause]* It's ironic how things are working out.

And yet, the way things worked out was for the absolute best. As things went with cancer, we barely got Erica under the wire. There *is* a reason for things, and there's a reason she chose to come when she did, and for that I'll be forever grateful. Because without her, the meaning of my life would be so very different. And in some respects, it gives my death more meaning, as well.

I was thirty-two and Erica was a year old. She had just taken her first steps. I was nursing. I felt a lump in my breast, had a mammogram, and the doctor called and said, "It's cancer. You have to have a mastectomy next Tuesday." So I nursed Erica in the mammogram waiting room, and that was the last time. I was told to stop nursing right away and began to go to a series of doctors. We went through two or three weeks of very painful weaning before they could do anything. So it gave us a little time to see doctors. I really wanted them to focus on my case.

A young mother, breast cancer, let's try to save her, please! *[Laughs]* I felt more unique because of my age than my parental status. I'm sure that they saw in me a "desperate-ism" to survive.

It became clear that the cancer was rather diffusely spread through the breast so a mastectomy was the only option offered. I was in treatment from when Erica was about thirteen to twenty months. After surgery, it was understood that it was Stage III-A, which is serious—I was told that it had most likely become systemic, although there was no evidence of that. I began chemotherapy, and then I did a stem-cell transplant. So that was three weeks in the hospital. Erica spent her time between Greg and my mother, who now lives nearby. Then there was radiation and a long recovery from the stem-cell transplant.

Four months later, I began the long road of adjusting to living with a potentially terminal disease, but at the same time feeling as though I had made my choices in large part based on Erica. It was important to me to be able to say to her that I had done everything I could to stay with her. My case certainly warranted it; it wasn't a question of over-treatment. But I didn't want to think, "Oh, if only I had done such and such." That was part of my motivation for doing the stem-cell transplant and signing up for pretty much everything that came along.

It's been an evolution of six years now. Every year was a different adjustment. There were the first two or three years, very worrisome that it would come back because often if it does, it comes back in those first years. Life became extremely precious *with* her. Having cancer cleared out a lot of things I was doing. Sometimes when people have terminal illness or are told they may die, you think, *Oh, I'm going to travel and do all these things before I die.* But my reaction was more to go within, to circle the wagons. So, my world got smaller in some ways. Richer but smaller. I didn't have the strength to work, I didn't have the interest, I just wanted to be with Erica.

I am intrigued by the ways mothers differ in relation to work outside the home after cancer but even more taken by what each mother chooses to focus on as priorities change. Listening to Julie reminded me of a conversation with a colleague that had troubled me for some time. A psychotherapist who works with cancer patients, she had shared her distress about a very sick young mother who wanted to be with her child rather than invest most of her time and energy attending support groups or pursuing alternative and complementary healing practices that might extend her life. "This mother needs to focus on herself and commit all her energy to fighting this disease," she told me.

For some women, limits on money and time prohibit taking advantage of various treatments. For others, like Julie, being with their children may be the most crucial part of their healing, engaging the will to live.

When I was first diagnosed, naturally, my first thought was, "Who will be her mother?" *[Begins weeping]* I was so preoccupied with her experience of losing a mother that losing my own life was secondary. I'm sure she was aware that there was sadness and that Mommy didn't feel like getting up right now, but I really didn't feel as though there was a lot of worry or fear.

Erica was speech- and language-delayed. She didn't speak until she was about three-and-a-half, so I became her interpreter. We became extremely close because of that, *extra* close. I knew what she was trying to express, and I would alleviate a lot of her frustration by letting people know or helping her along. I do believe that I was reacting to her needs, not creating her problem.

As far as the first few years after treatment, I never felt confidently cured. I certainly *hoped* for it, and as the years went on, the likelihood seemed greater and greater. But I was always a little more tenuous than some people that I know in the same situation, declaring that they're "done" with cancer. I was never done with cancer. At the same time, as the years went on, I felt it is time for me to have work of my own. [I thought], *Gosh, if I am going to survive, I need to move on! [Laughs]*

Then the fifth year came. That was more of a milestone than I expected. That was a letting-go a little bit, a beginning-to-hope. A beginning-to-think, *Okay, now Erica is in school. Time to organize and find something for myself.*

Within that year, I think I was having a recurrence, but it was really at the six-year mark that I had scans that showed extensive recurrence. So all of that momentum of finally crawling out of the futureless state of mind went *whoooooosh*—went away. That was just a few months ago, and that's been a big loss because it was a long road to get there. I do realize that I was lucky that I got six years.

Julie pauses and once again looks toward her garden, her face relaxing as she does.

After the bone marrow transplant, I knew that I wanted to move off the boat. We were living on a sailboat for many years, and when Erica was born, we were still there. After the bone marrow transplant, we bought this house, and I worked in the garden and used that as sort of healing, day to day, here and now. It was time to get my fingers in the dirt. I've always had a botanical touch. I get extraordinary joy that I can't describe out of nurturing plants. When I'm with plants, I'm in awe. It's complete, everything else is gone, fingers in the dirt, can't wear gloves. If you're talking about pure let-go pleasure, it's with Erica or in nature. Nature really sustains me.

I like to see new things and grow new things. With plants and nature, everything is momentary, and then it changes. It goes with my nature, accepting change and actually *inviting* it. I get such satisfaction out of seeing something blossom that I thought had died.

Now Erica's having that same childhood connection to certain smells and rocks and plants. If you take a child out in nature enough when they're very young and they see things grow, they see green grass in the spring, they see brown grass in the fall, they see the dead mole on the path, they see the hawks circling—why is the hawk circling?—they see death, life, death, life, they get a sense of the cycles of life. As I see it, that is the spirituality that one needs to convey to one's child. It's something I've tried to do with Erica, simply the child being in nature enough to come upon these things in the natural way. My mother did that for us unwittingly. I think it is helping me come to terms with an early death. I should tell her how much I appreciate that.

Because Erica couldn't speak during all that time, she had no words during my treatment. When she was about four, she wanted a baby brother or baby sister very badly. I told her that when she was a baby, I had had to take some very strong medicine because I had cancer. It was supposed to make the cancer go away, but it also meant I couldn't have any more babies. And then I would say how *happy* I was that at least I got her! I had to tell her over and over again.

Then, when I recurred three months ago, that first night we needed to tell her what was going on. She asked if I was going to die. Greg said, "Well, possibly. But we don't know." I told her that the cancer had come back, and that I would have to take some strong medicine again, and that it would be hard, and she would have to understand. There was that first month of shock and coming to terms with things. She had lots of questions. She would ask often if I was going to die.

With a recurrence, I had to go straight in for surgery, and I was gone for five days, and then I started chemo right after that, and I was *very, very* debilitated. With all this trauma going on and me being in the hospital, a couple of weeks after that, she said, "Oh, I'm so glad Mom didn't die." So to her, it was *that* time that I was going to die. Her first grade teacher had had cervical cancer and was tutoring her and would drive her home. Often, Erica would bring something up, and the teacher would tell me. In protecting me, she was opening up to her.

At the moment, we are saying, "We don't know." I've told her that chemo is our friend and the doctors are working hard. She has asked if I'm going to have cancer the rest of my life. I said, "Yes." I wanted to know why she was asking that. It came out that she was checking because she wanted to know if we were going to wrestle again. Often, I find there are very concrete reasons for her questions! *[Laughs]* So I try to get behind her questions.

I don't like the limbo that saying "Nobody knows for sure" leaves. I don't think that's good for a child. But she's seven, so she's very *now*. If you said, "Well, yes, Mommy is going to die of this eventually, maybe not for a year or two," she would expect me to die next week. So we've not done that. As I step onto the assembly line of chemos and metastatic breast cancer, I let her in on it incrementally, let her get the feeling that this is progressing, without just saying, "Yes, Mommy is going to die." And you *don't* know. Let's pretend, let's go on for five years. I mean, that's a lifetime to her. It's pretty serious, so unfortunately I think it's not going to be a huge amount of time.

I try to bring it up when I have a specific thing to say. She knew I had a doctor's appointment today—so I try to give her a little piece of information: "I went to the doctor today, and the chemo is still work-ing, but it's not as strong as it was so we might switch to a different one." I don't like her thinking I went to the doctor and I'm not telling her something. Then I said, "But the cancer is still there, too." And she said, "Well, I have a lot of hope." It's difficult because if she hopes and hopes and hopes and then it doesn't work out the way she was hoping,

I don't want her to turn away from hope. To walk that tightrope of tempering the hope but keeping it going is what I find the biggest challenge with her.

I felt cruel at the time, saying, "Look, Erica, some things are just not fair." She got an early dose of the fact that life is not fair, and I don't know how that will turn out. The death of a mother: What's less fair than that? On one hand, I felt obligated to teach her fairness—that one has to treat people fairly and one should expect a certain amount of fairness in return—and on the other, that life is *not* fair. Things happen, like losing your mother and me losing my life.

And what about you? Are you walking that same tightrope in terms of hope?

Oh, yes. I'm a little more realistic, a little bit less hopeful. But still I have a place of hope. I am generally a realist: one who likes information, gathers information and distills it, and tries to know as much as anyone can know where I stand.

After my surgery, I remember Greg saying to the doctor, "You know, everything has been bad news. When is the bad news going to stop?" And the doctor said, "Well, I think it stopped now." I learned later that that surgeon had had a hard time and couldn't tell me how bad things were. He just said he wanted me to keep up my hope. He told my therapist this! He went to my therapist for consolation because he found it so difficult to tell me these things. I think I reminded him of his daughter. I was livid when I heard that I wasn't getting all the information!

Having parented almost entirely with cancer, that first year before cancer seems like another world. It was a blissful world. I didn't know it *then*. But, oh, everything was out in front—a new family. It's wonderful now to think of it.

There have been wonderful things in the last six years, as well. But cancer came from nowhere. I was a very healthy person all of my life, very physical, and to go from extraordinarily physically fit to cancer and chemo and the physical transition was huge. I went through treatment when she was one, and I went into menopause when I was thirty-two, and I couldn't have any more children.

The early years were difficult because in her preschool there were many pregnant women, many women with two or three kids, certainly not in menopause! I felt separate, and my issues were different. I think when people learned of my story, they tended not to share as much about their own happiness, their pregnancies, whatever. I tried to put them at ease and let them know that I wanted to be part of their experiences, but there was a distance. While going through all the joys of young motherhood, there was a cast of shadow.

Also, intellectually and spiritually, maybe, I was wanting a little more depth than the usual diaper conversation, potty-training. Even though I reveled in every aspect of those simple conversations, often I felt like, *Yes*, and then, *But* . . . Often I felt women were taking their lives for granted—"just another baby," that sort of thing, and a lot of complaining about what a struggle it was, which it is. I wanted so much to be a part of that and complain about one's husband, and I did, but I was always separate from it. There was a barrier. There was a little bit of what mortality does for you. It pulls you out from the inane, and I resented that a bit. As much as it has deepened my life and made for a lot of contemplation, I really wanted that bliss, that ignorance.

Listening to Julie, I wonder whether a very young person facing mortality would have a sense of fullness in a brief life. Had Julie developed some philosophy from this experience? I ask her how she thinks about accomplishments.

Because I've had a varied life, accomplishments are in the moment, and then there's another moment. I see accomplishments as something *within* more than something that shows. My goal has been to have a varied life, and I've accomplished that. I've had an amazing number of experiences. A lot of women have told me they could *never* live not knowing where they were going to be or what was going to be happening or what their bank account would look like. For some reason, I *have*. It's not something I set out to accomplish. I did set out to go with my nature. And now I feel, should my life span be forty-some years, I have done more than some eighty-year-old people have done.

Through it all, I have considered myself a good friend, and that's a sort of accomplishment. It takes work, it really does. I feel as though I have supported people, listened to people, and given myself to people in a way that helped them. But, again, I go with my nature, and now that I am needier than most in the friendship department it's coming back. So there was a reason. There is an order. People have been so forthcoming, and I feel I need to keep it coming from me as well, and that's become a little bit difficult because time is . . . I'm so frantic. And I still give.

Of course, the crowning achievement is Erica. Erica has been my passion for seven years—watching her grow up and accepting who she is and imagining how these characteristics may develop over time. She's been probably the greatest challenge yet about the only experience of unconditional love that I've ever had. I think that having survived this long has made a huge difference in Erica's life as far as her emotional expression and self-confidence. That is a huge accomplishment because I set myself that goal.

Being human, I have a pull in both directions and at times have wished I had something of my own. Sometimes I wish I had stuck to a subject enough to be more advanced in a field. I was working on that, trying to find what that would be, right before recurrence. My goal now is not in the future. It's now. And it's the past—trying to organize the past and impact the present.

Another thing I feel good about—again, it's not an accomplishment, it is part of my nature—is a confidence. Whatever I do, I can do. I don't hold myself back because I'm a woman. Part of that is a natural thing, maybe denial, *[Laughs]* that it will work out. If it all goes away tomorrow, I can adapt, and I'll do whatever I have to do. I'll go get my minimum-wage job and get by, and I'm perfectly confident about that, so I don't feel dependent. I *can* take care of myself.

I certainly have other areas where I have held myself back for self-esteem or shame issues. But danger was not something that kept me back. I had a confidence of being able to physically get through and also a way of letting go of control when I really *had* no control—stormy seas, horrendous nights, whatever it was. And now cancer.

Julie grows quiet. She has expressed intense feelings and described turbulence, but there is an unusual sense of calm in the room. With little prompting, the stories, thoughts, and ideas flow onto the tape.

After I was diagnosed with breast cancer the first time, I was trying to understand if there was a connection between my emotional, psychological state and my diagnosis. I resolved that fairly quickly in my mind—that my emotional state had *not* caused my cancer. And I feel that still today. I'm not responsible for it.

When shame is built up in a person, it flows into other directions in your life. I think shame creates silence, and shame moves you inside. Being diagnosed with cancer can do that. With a recurrence, it's even more demanding that I let that stuff go. So, I have tried to bring Erica out and *not* be silent, and I try myself not to be silent.

There's only so much you can control, and you can drive yourself nuts thinking there's some way around that. I don't think I would have learned that lesson without cancer. I would be a more controlling person. I consider that an accomplishment.

But, as far as Erica goes, I feel that I need to make some plans and hold onto the control as long as I can. That's why I tried to talk to as many people as possible about my wishes. So it would be witnessed. And I talked to Greg about it.

Something Greg said early on after my cancer diagnosis stuck with me. When Erica was about two or three, and I was obsessing about dying and leaving her at such a young age—How would she ever possibly survive? I still have those feelings—Greg said, "You know, she is her own person." It struck me at that moment that she *is* her own person and that she must know that she is *not* responsible for my cancer or my death or in any way for me.

There's a lot of things I *want* to control about my own death, for goodness sake. And, yet, if you're going to live in the moment which, if you don't have a future, is all you have—then control is a greater illusion. I have managed to let go of a lot of control and let be, and I know in my heart that no matter what happens, Erica is her own person, and she *will* be okay, and she *will* grow up, and she *will* learn to control her own life without me. But some of the difficulty of living with cancer for as long as I have is that understanding of how little we control but still living in a world where most people believe we can, and feeling that isolation.

I have been living with cancer for a long time. It's so much now a part of *life*. Why did I make it six years? I will never know. I've thought about that quite a lot. I have my own feelings about how much control one has over one's cancer, one's body, and one's immune system. I feel relatively out of control in that respect. But if having to get up in the morning and go on helps your system, or if having a reason to live has an impact on your longevity or your quality of life, then, yes, parenting would be it!

I've been very down in the last three or four days. I think I'm going through a secondary coming-to-terms with recurrence. Erica's in school half a day, and I can think and grieve, but, boy, when one o'clock comes, I'm down there. "Okay, get your stuff. Now we gotta go. Let's go home, and we'll do something fun." I *have* to hold it together, I *have* to go on, and I *have* to hold up. Being a parent requires me to put myself aside a bit and continue on. That is not a bad thing.

How I would be reacting to this if I wasn't a parent, I have no idea. I imagine one could become quite morose. I'm not a morose person, so I don't know if that would happen. Still, one would have to work so much harder at finding something else to live for. I really, really, really want to get as much time as I can with Erica. That could affect one's longevity. I *so badly* want to be with her. . . . *[Begins to cry]*

I think cancer has made me a far more patient parent, far more sympathetic. Just slow it down, listen, hear what's really being said. I suppose one doesn't want to be too mean because one doesn't want to be remembered as a mean person. That sort of clearing out of priorities and letting go of a lot of things of my own is something that every mother does, especially in the early years. But, for me, it *stayed* cleared out. Motherhood wasn't a phase, something I was going to do in the young years and then get on with things.

But leaving the earth is far more difficult. *[Weeping]* If I didn't have a child, I would be grieving my own death, I would be grieving leaving so young, and it would seem so sad. But with a child, especially a young one, it's utterly tragic. I sort of understand why religious organizations don't allow people of their order to have children. It is *so* grounding—it just attaches you to the earth in a way that nothing else really can. I don't want to spcak for thc spirituality of other people, but it puts your feet in the dirt and makes it a lot harder to leave. At the same time, it enriches the life that you do get.

But I am concerned—because Greg and Erica are *not* as close, just by pure time—that losing me may be even more of a vacuum. Greg has to travel a lot for work for economic reasons; it's just her and me all week long. It makes the transition to *not* having me seem even greater. When we lived on the boat, Erica was with me every single minute. She never knew where she was when she woke up. The places changed, the beds changed, the climate changed, the airplane rides—everything changed, but Mom was the same. I was the continuous thing in her life, so we are probably closer for that somehow. I have been that center pole for her, which is great for me to have experienced and given her, but it makes it more difficult now with the thought of dying and leaving. I'm not sure how much you can replace a center pole. I think you can support from the outside, but I'm not sure if that pole can be found again. *[Continues crying]* Well, I'd like to talk to Erica.

Julie turns to the tape recorder and begins to speak directly to her daughter. After describing aspects of Erica's personality that she appreciates and her difficulty with speech, Julie records an ethical will for her child to receive sometime after her death.[1] She includes her own philosophy and values as well as messages to children recommended by the project. Excerpts from Julie's ethical will are included at the end of the chapter.

I met with Julie a few weeks after the tapes were completed. During our first conversation, she had said that she hoped to find more peace. I asked her what she hoped for now.

Sustained remission. Prolonged. I would never ask, "How much time do I have?" and I would never ask for a certain amount of more time because it's never going to be enough. But medically, I hope for a long enough remission to emotionally come to some kind of peace. I think I've come a long way in the peace department in the last six years because I've had that time. But on the issue of separating from Erica, I have a certain amount of panic: Do I have enough time to make that best possible transition for her *and* for me? Because I'll *never* be ready to go. So I'm not sure that that's really an attainable goal at all. I'm never going to be at peace with leaving Erica, and maybe because I say it that way I never will.

I'm not one to advise, but I think it's critical to keep communication open. Talking to people is something that I've really needed to do. Especially lately. It does get the mind to calm down, and it gets it out—otherwise it goes around and around. The greatest emotional support is accepting my version of reality and listening and not trying to make it go away or denying it.

My family has been pretty good about that. My mother doesn't ask questions, but she listens. I do my best to say it so she knows what's going on, step by step. She'll call after I've had a doctor's appointment and ask me. My father has a bit of a positive attitude, so that's been a little struggle lately. Friends, as well. The ones who can't walk on both the bright side and the dark side tend to disappear. It's very, very limiting and draining to me to not walk on the dark side. People who feel you can make or break your own health, or defeat the cancer with your attitude, nutrition, or any one component, have fallen by the wayside. I mean, really quickly!

But I would speak for most mothers, all mothers who are dying and leaving a child. *[Weeping]* One of the biggest fears is fading in the child's life. What Greg remembers of his mother is shockingly little, even at eleven. Erica is only seven. I can ask now: Please try to keep me alive in Erica's mind and in her life. Her experience of me over time will change because of her age. Each phase has to be addressed and re-addressed and then re-addressed. One of my fears is that I will become Mom-back-then, the persona a long time ago, and not re-addressed and held forefront. It's a natural, selfish feeling. Lives go on. It's inevitable. But I want my friends and family to continue to be vigilant—talk to her about me, tell stories, *tell the same stories*, whatever it is.

I imagine that, eventually, I will become so weak that letting go will be a relief for everybody. And that will be right at that time. Hopefully, there will be some peace there. In the meanwhile, I have all of these day-to-day things to accomplish with Erica, and I have longer-term organizing of my life, making it presentable in a way that can be kept for her. I don't feel as though I am progressing along that path fast enough, according to how this disease progresses. So it's causing me some anxiety. Then I step back and say, "You do what you can, and then you let go." I'm constantly going back and forth between those two things.

But I want that balance between trying to organize and preparing to die and living and hoping to live. There are four components at least there! I have been focusing on the living and the trying to prolong time—those two things. I certainly have emotionally been thinking about dying a lot, but not in the physical preparing and anticipating. So, on the one hand, I tell myself I'm doing the balance that's right for me. On the other hand, I have to be aware of what's not done.

What sustains me? Just the moment, really. Erica *in* the moment. I feel like there's so much to do in so many areas, between making a dentist appointment for Erica and trying to write down my wishes for her in the future! *[Laughs]* That whole spectrum sustains me. I have to keep going. I really have no control over what sustains me or what will eventually kill me, you know? I just continue to *be*.

Sitting with Julie in her breakfast nook felt completely comfortable. In spite of her waves of emotion, I never felt either of us might be overwhelmed. The outside world became smaller, but mental horizons expanded, and each moment became deeper, richer. Just as she described.

I found Julie's story and her advice to her daughter in the ethical will that follows so useful that I have turned to them in helping my daughter navigate her own path into adulthood. Her wisdom about parenting was connected to two words that, in her original transcript, slipped into her sentences sixty-seven times: "nature" and "natural." Unable to project a future story for herself, Julie used her understanding of nature to create a narrative of flowing with the cycles of life and living increasingly in the moment. Her attachment to the earth and her grief at leaving it did not diminish. But she modeled an ease in being present, here, and okay, just by being.

From Julie Renaud's Ethical Will and Messages For Her Daughter

After I was diagnosed with cancer, when you were one, every day has been special. The special moments are so numerous that it's difficult to choose one because I have been so "here and now" with you—the future being so uncertain—and so aware of special times that seem ordinary to most people.

Not very long ago, I walked out into the backyard in the afternoon, and the sun was coming in from the west and shooting through the yard. There was a magical light in the whole yard. The yard was glowing, and this beam of light was hitting the steps that go down into the lower lot, and I called you because the pine tree up above was full of these small birds on every branch. I called you, and you came out, and we sat in the sun in that ray of light, and you sat on my lap, and we watched the birds, and they were chirping. It was as if time did not move. It was a glowing moment where we sat there together, and you probably touched the moles on my neck and watched these birds. And then they flew off the tree in five or six groups, and we wouldn't know when the next one was going to fly. You were uncommonly still and quiet, and you just watched these birds. You understood that this was a moment, and so did I.

Over the course of a half an hour, we sat there, and then, as soon as the last birds flew, the sunray stopped, and the yard was back to its usual feeling. I haven't any explanation for it. It was a moment I'll always remember because you were there with me. It was a message of some kind, I'm not sure what. But I was extremely grateful to be there with you. Those are the kinds of experiences that make leaving you so difficult, for all those moments that were yet to come and that won't be. You may not remember that moment, but it will be inside of you somewhere, and it's inside of me. So as much as I wish I could stay and be with you and have more of those moments, we do have a lot together, and I think that that connection will continue even after I'm gone.

I'll go on to some of the wishes that I have for you, right now, at seven years old. I wish that you will experiment, learn a variety of skills, but then *know* yourself. Know what gives you utter confidence, know what really makes you feel good, know what is easy and you do anyway, and then take that to a depth of skill. It might be woodworking, it might be theater—there will be a variety of things that you're good at. Find the path that feels at ease, but I would support your choice regardless of what it was. I really regret that I may not be there to watch you develop those skills.

I really, really wish that after I die, you can continue to grow emotionally. That you won't shut down. I think somewhere in your heart you will know that I loved you, and you'll know that I know you loved me, and that I would be there with you if I could be. I am not leaving voluntarily. I tried everything within my belief system to be there as long as I could. I've blended Western medicine with Chinese medicine, relaxation, and visualization, and then, most importantly, being there with you. You've taught me more about being in the moment than any religious path could ever teach me.

I think you have a deep understanding, a security inside of you. I hope that from this safe place, you can reach out and find support and love and friendships. Know that there's nothing you have to feel guilty about. There's nothing that you've said or done that has made life difficult for me. I've never questioned your love, and, in time, hopefully you will come to understand how much I loved you. I really am grateful for the years I did have with you because I can see now, even at seven, you have a formed character and that you will be okay.

You know your dad, Greg, lost his mother when he was twelve, and it was a huge turning point for him. He was very angry at his mother for leaving him. If you do feel angry at me for not being there, that's okay. Sometimes it's hard for Greg to let love in, and I hope that'll be different for you, that you will be able to allow love in, as well as to give love to the people that you care about. Also, I wish that you eventually find someone to be with who can walk down a variety of paths with you and to depths of contemplation and emotion. I hope that my death will not make it difficult for you to trust people and to form lifetime friendships and loves.

Erica, I would like to continue speaking directly to you because that feels good. I have been struggling with bringing a new life into the world and at the same time contemplating leaving the world, and that, I'm sure, has changed your life. It certainly has changed mine. But cancer just happens, and there isn't a lot of explanation for why. I hope that it doesn't become too much of a quest for you to know why. I have stopped asking "Why me?" and tried to focus on living with cancer for the past six years, most of your lifetime.

I read you a book lately, *Lifetimes*, by Bryan Mellonie and Robert Ingpen. Every living thing has a lifetime, and this will be mine, however long I live. Hopefully, you will be able to have a long, full, fairly happy life, you can keep my love for you in your memory, and it will eventually become a source of strength for you.

One of my biggest hopes is that I've been with you long enough to give you a foundation of security and safety and love that you will be able to handle the struggle that comes after my death. I know that I have to let go and allow you and Greg together to go forward and live as best you can. There may be more struggle for you, more loneliness, more sadness than other kids that you grow up with and maybe even the adults you're around when you're older. I think you will know loneliness more than most people. And there will be really tough times when other kids are with their mothers and you're not. I know this partly because Greg has told me how it was for him. Counselors have told me that kids who have to go through struggles when they're young *can* grow up stronger for it. It's a small consolation to me, but I hold onto that right now, that somehow the struggle will benefit you despite the overwhelming tragedy of losing your mother.

I don't know what you will learn from my death and what your feelings about death will be. I don't fear death, but not knowing my own journey, it makes it difficult to know how that process will be for you. Again, though, I'm hoping there will be some benefit for you—to watch the process, to *know* death. I think to understand mortality at such a young age can somehow strengthen your soul and can only be deepening for you, in a different way than having had a mother all of your upbringing would have fortified you. But you will certainly learn self-reliance the way Greg has. And that's not a bad thing, unless it's taken too far. Unfortunately, all the grief and pain must also go along with that deepening of your soul. And I regret that more than anything.

There is no question that looking at mortality at a young age has deepened my life. It's created priorities for which I'm grateful and basically given me more confidence to say what I feel, do what I want, and let people live with it. But I'll never look at it as a gift. I would have preferred ignorant bliss to a deepened soul from cancer. And I would have wished the same thing for you. But those are wishes, and the reality is that you get what you get, which is a favorite expression of yours. "You get what you get," and that's what we got.

Greg will be there for you. He loves you more than anything, although sometimes it's hard for him to show it. I think you can trust him with your feelings, and I think that by doing that, it'll help him tell you his feelings. But my advice is that you open up first, and then Greg will open up, and please cut him some slack. He tries hard, but it's very difficult for him to express himself.

I know that sometimes I've been critical of Greg for small things in front of you, and I *have* tried to change him. But I want you to know how grateful I am to Greg. He has been there in the ways that he could be there, with his full heart and soul, and he has been extremely steady for me going through cancer. I never doubt that he will be there. He will be there for me as long as I'm alive, and then he will be there for you as long as he is alive.

My wish is that he will eventually find someone to be with who loves him and he loves her, and you can have a stepmother. I have often reminded Greg that he must consider how this person will be a mother to you. I know that it's more important that Greg care for her and that she care for Greg first, but my maternal gut instinct screams out that you be considered as a primary focus in choosing a new person to be with. It could be difficult for you, no matter what, because she is not me. But I really wish that you have someone in your life as a step-mother. For all the problems that can come up, the benefits are greater if it's a healthy relationship. So long as she's a *Democrat*.

It's been difficult for me to settle on any particular religious up-bringing for you. I certainly didn't have a particular religious path. Nature worship, I suppose, would be the paramount influence in my spiritual life. When I say "nature," I mean literally being in nature. Be-ing quiet. Listening to the wind. Listening to water. Listening to silence. I see in nature all the living cycles and all the cycles of death. It's com-plete. I am most at peace in nature, and I think spirituality, religion, is a quest for peace. I've tried to expose you to a variety of models. You have to seek out what works for you.

I am much more resigned in my late thirties to the inequity of the world. I was never necessarily interested in saving or changing the world, but I did have that wonderful naiveté as a young person that the world would change for the better. Now, I'm a little more understand-ing of how slowly things change, and sometimes how quickly things change, and how sometimes when things change very quickly, they change in a very unexpected and not always healthy way.

I found myself saying to a friend the other day, "Change is the only thing that stays the same." We paused because it seems like such a con-tradiction, but it isn't. Change has been the only thing that has stayed the same in *my* life—and, I suspect, in the world as well.

I do believe that we're all just separated by our perspectives and it's an illusion to imagine that reality is the same for any two people. I think that often I'm just a little perspective away from another way of thinking about things. Your perspective changes from day to day, from year to year, from decade to decade. If that's the process for you, you have to imagine that that's the process for everyone else. Life to me is not a knowing thing, it's an illusion, a changing perspective—that you choose. That major lesson has made it easier for me to accept other people's perspectives, not judge them, and learn what there is to learn from them. I hope that as you grow older, you can hold your own perspective solid and not rush to judge somebody else's religious path or model that they have chosen to explain the universe or hardships in their life.

Someone called me courageous, so recently I've been thinking about that word, "courage." Courage to me is how you deal with fear, and I think in this culture, courageous people are thought not to have fear. In fact, I think courageous people have as much fear as anybody else—it's just the way in which you channel your fear and face reality.

I think there are different ways of approaching fear, especially with cancer. Some people tend to run away. They want to deny it and have it be gone and not say it out loud because sometimes saying things out loud gives it more credence. Then there are people who fear and explore that fear and get information. That's the type of person that I am. I talk to people and look that fear in the face and say, "How do I dispel that fear?" Most of my fear and anxiety come from not having information, not being able to get it, or that *nobody knows*—it's an expression I hear all the time from my doctors. I'd rather have bad news and know about it than wonder about it and not be told. I don't want to judge other people, but I judge this as a positive thing because I want it for *you*.

One of my biggest focuses has been to encourage your curiosity. I thought I would succeed as a parent if you were a curious person because if I'm not always there to answer your questions, then you can go find out for yourself. You are a very, very inquisitive kid, and I'm hoping that your curiosity can evolve into my way of dealing with fear and the unknown. Put the fear in a place on a shelf where you can live with it, take it out, look at it, see how it's changed over time, see if you need to find out something more about it. It takes too much energy to *deny* fear. This process seems to me a better way to face fear, face *grief*. I know those are two different things, and one is a much longer process than the other. But one of my biggest fears for you is the turning off of your curiosity as a way of trying to turn off your fears and your grief.

So, whenever you read this, I hope that you can think about how you face fear. Whether it's a very tricky driving situation, a break-up of a relationship, a feeling of abandonment, or feeling as though you can't live up to the expectations that somebody has of you—see how you cope with it and how you move on from it. What gives you the most peace? Perhaps a religion will be there for you. Perhaps you'll have it all worked out yourself.

Erica, I want to summarize. But summarizing means ending, and I don't feel as though I'm ready to end this process of talking to you because there's so much more. Hopefully, I have connected with you, that you will know me from within yourself most of all. I don't really expect you to remember me if you are under, I don't know, ten when I die. Even if you can't remember my voice or you can't remember specific things or times with me, it doesn't really matter. I think that I'm in you. I don't want you to feel bad about that. It's a natural thing for kids to not remember what their mother's voice sounded like or what she looked like. You have videotapes of me and yourself when you were different ages, and you'll have this book to read, and you'll have some audiotapes to listen to. And some writing in my own handwriting. I'm saving all of my calendars because I would be curious to see my mother's calendar books. And, of course, you have people who knew me to talk to about me; they will remember me in their own way.

The last thing I'll say is how grateful I feel that I got to have you in my life. Every day, I feel so grateful that you came to us, that I got to experience being with you and watching you develop. It seems the biggest tragedy that I have to leave you. But even that does not overwhelm my gratitude. I hope in time, as you get older, that the tragedy of my leaving will somehow be overcome by the gratitude you feel for being in this world and having had me, even the short while that you did.

I know I speak as if my death is definite, but I do live with a tiny box of hope that something will come along, that I will be an exception, that I will survive longer than expected or perhaps lead an average life span. I hold out for that in a small way, but it's more important in my personality to be realistic, and realistic means the likelihood of my surviving metastatic breast cancer that has spread to my bones, my lungs, and my plural chest wall. It's a pretty extensive metastasis, and it does not often allow much time after recurrence is found. I need to be focused right now on preparing for my death but hoping to live. That's the struggle I live with every day. I wanted to let you know that you gave me a real source of strength to endure the treatments. I did it for myself, but I did all that for you, as well.

I guess my biggest wish for you is that you go through the tragedy of my death—that you can move forward and not withdraw, but stay expressive, find joy, find love, and eventually find some peace. I really wish that you're able to hold onto hopefulness. You have a lot of hope right now that I will get better. You said it to me, and it's so sweet. I hope that my death will not be a giving up of hope for things in your future, that being hopeful now didn't work so you give up on hope. I hope that after my death, in time, you can believe in hope because it's essential to keep a balance in your life between hope and despair. So, even as I face the reality of what could be seen by many as hopeless, you are my continuation of hope. You embody it. You are it. Having you there gives me something to hope for. I don't mean that to be a burden but an explanation of where I draw my sense of hope from. I want you to find and follow your own source of hope.

So, in closing, I'll just tell you I love you, and I know you love me.

ELEVEN: "CHRISTMAS IS EVERY DAY NOW"
JANET JOHNSON

JANET JOHNSON LIVES on a dead-end street in a San Francisco Bay Area neighborhood most people wouldn't want to visit at night. A short, ample, African American woman, Janet has been watching for me from the front window of her small frame house. I enter a living room that is sparsely furnished and neatly arranged. Family photos are the only wall decoration, and they are dominated by the handsome, beaming face of Janet's sixteen-year-old son, Jordan.

The day is warm, and she suggests that we talk in her front garden. She leads me to a concrete patio the size of a carport crowded with a table, three folding chairs, and a scattering of potted plants. During our hour together, the postman and several neighbors go by, each greeting Janet with affection. She explains that this is the neighborhood where she and her six siblings were raised. Her family, except her mother, who died less than a year ago, are all within walking distance. "I never moved out of the neighborhood. I've always lived next door or down the street. I've been really lucky because I always had family around."

Living with family allowed Janet to stay home with Jordan for five years after she became a single mother at the age of twenty-six. Her younger siblings had already had children, as had all her school friends. "I was kind of a late bloomer." Later, having her mother down the street allowed her "to go to work and have somebody there that would take care of my son. So that was really, really good."

At first, Janet responds with reserve and clipped replies. She tells me she is afraid to break down on tape. "See, I'm going to be crying and crying, and then my son is going to listen to a tape with a bunch of crying on it." I reassure her that she can use the pause button while she gathers herself. Soon, Janet's warmth and sly humor begin to emerge. So do the tears.

"I would like to leave my son with something he can remember me by. My mother, we don't even have her voice. There's not a day that goes by that I don't think about her. If I could hear her voice now, it would make me feel pretty good." Janet also says that it would do her good to talk to someone. And that, through this story, she hopes to help other women like herself "to better express themselves because a lot of women, I think especially black women, have a hard time expressing our feelings, such as fear."

Janet has not had a mastectomy. By the time breast cancer was diagnosed two years earlier, when she was thirty-eight and Jordan fourteen, it had spread too far into her lymph nodes for surgery to be beneficial. A year later, cancer metastasized to her bones. Scans, blood tests, and chemotherapy have become a way of life. Still, she is determined to continue her full-time employment as a food-service worker in a local hospital, as much for psychological as economic reasons.

"A lot of people say, 'Why are you still trying to work? Why aren't you on disability?' Well, because that's what I got to do. I don't feel like a disabled person. I've been on disability a couple of times when I felt there was a need but never longer than a month or so. Even with chemo, I've always felt pretty good. I didn't want to make myself feel like I was sick. I felt like, as long as I was able to work and do, then I was okay. It made my son feel better, too, because when I was home, he would kind of worry about me. He used to tell me, 'You know, if you could get up shopping, you can go to work.'"

For Janet, being a mother "is the most important role because you have a person dependent on you to take care of," and employment is a way to be a good mother. "Some people try to make you feel like you should stay home. Well, I couldn't do it. I had to work and take care of him. I just did what I had to do. I didn't neglect him to go to work. I feel like I was there. I still participate in his school. And I think we did very well, and we're still doing okay.

"It's been an experience, I tell you. It's been an experience, trying to raise him, trying to do the right thing, trying to work and take care of him. When you're trying to raise a child by yourself, you don't want to be coming down hard as you're already the mother, you're the father, you're the disciplinarian, the teacher, the nurse, the doctor. You're all these things rolled up in one. It's been kind of hard, but I don't regret it at all. Not at all. I think he's the best thing I ever did.

"I got to finish raising my son. And I'm going to finish raising him. So that's what keeps me motivated and pushing on."

The next meetings are held in a colleague's office a few blocks from Janet's job. Unfortunately, the borrowed keys don't open the front door when volunteer listener Michael Ann Leaver and Janet arrive to tape their first interview. But, with Michael's persistence and Janet's forbearance, the couple "break and enter" through an open window and leave in the same fashion. Later, Janet tells me the story in her own words.

JANET

We really wanted to hold that meeting because when you want to start something, you want to start it. We were there, we were gung ho, we're going to do this, and I'm saying, "I can't believe this! This door is not going to open. I came all the way from work! Oh, my God! This is not fair." *[Laughs]* This is just too much for anybody to have to go through!

I said, "Well, we're burglars now. Oh, my God! Is anybody looking?" I expected somebody to come back: "Somebody just reported two people climbing in a window. Where's the security people?" Yeah, that really broke the ice. *[Laughs]* Yep. Go out the same way we came in. Everybody looking at us. Oh, that was funny.

But it worked out. Some things are meant to be, and that's all there is to it so I'll leave it at that. But find another office!

With this, Janet shifts gears to begin her cancer story.

I've always been a "show me" person. It's not that I didn't believe in God because I do. I know there's some higher force that's keeping us breathing and keeping us with a lot of knowledge. But it's been really hard for me because I've always been a person who wants to see who I'm worshipping. If He's supposed to be real, why can't I *see* Him? I didn't have a lot of faith. The only faith that I had was in myself to do the things that I needed to do to take care of myself and my child.

When I first went to the doctor, I said, "Oh, I got a lump under my arm," and he said, "Well, we'll take a mammogram." I remember being very scared about taking it. But I also remember that people always said if they don't come back and take no more pictures, that pretty much tells you that everything is okay. I believed in that. So when the woman came back, she said, "You can go." And I felt like, "Phew! This is okay." I got a little paper in the mail, said, "No cancer shown."

Anyway, I was having a problem with my shoulder, and I went back to the doctor and happened to mention, "You know, I still got the lump under my arm, but I took a mammogram and it came back okay." Of course, she didn't know anything about it 'cause she wasn't my primary doctor, but she was female, and she was concerned. She said, "Why don't you take another mammogram?" So, here they go again.

I took another mammogram, and they still didn't pick up anything. I was feeling pretty confident that everything was okay. Then, with her being very persistent, she asked me did I mind seeing a surgeon. I said, "I don't mind," but I didn't understand why because this machine just said that I was okay. So I saw a surgeon, and she said, "We can do surgery on it and see what it is. You may have had a low-grade infection at one time, and your lymph glands swell up sometimes when you have infection." I remember being scheduled for surgery. I trusted her and everything. I felt like she did what she could do.

The doctor came in, and she said it was cancer, and I was like, "What is she talking about? What is she talking about? I just came here for them to take a look. They didn't say nothing about no cancer!" They were sure it was breast cancer. I didn't understand how could it be breast cancer when it's not in your breast. So it's a fast course of learning. Breast tissue is not just the breast. It's all the way up to your shoulders and under your arm. Looking at the cells, they could pretty much tell.

I wasn't expecting it because I had put my faith in this machine. I remember hearing her and then not really hearing her at all. It was like my mind was in outer space. It was like, "My God! I don't believe I'm hearing this." One day I was okay, and the next day somebody's told me I have cancer? I just *really* did not believe it.

I was with my sister, Donetta, and I was like, "Is she *crazy*? What is she talking about? I did what I was supposed to do, I had my mammogram, they said it wasn't anything, so what is she talking about?" My sister was crying so hard that she could hardly even see. I don't know how we made it home.

And I can remember my mother coming out and looking at both of us and knowing that something is wrong. She never shed a tear. She just said, "You gonna be all right. You gonna be fine." I remember other family members crying and pretty upset 'cause it's a very scary thing. And, oooh, I remember wanting to go home, people saying, "Oh, don't go home. Don't go home. Just stay here and be with family." *[Begins crying]* I just wanted to go home. I wanted to be by myself.

I remember walking down the street, opening up the door, and falling on my knees and asking God why. "Why? Why? Why me?" And I tell this to people all the time. In the slightest whisper in my ear, something said, "Why *not* you? Who are you to think that you can't go through things like other people?" And when I heard it, I jumped up 'cause it scared me. I didn't know what to think. I was kind of dumbfounded because it was so clear in my ear.

Janet pauses and sits back in her chair. After a few minutes of silence, I ask her why she thinks God gave her this challenge.

Because I tended to be a person that wanted to be in control. So I think He took me, He just say, "Look, I'm in control." I'm not going to say it's been one of my downfalls 'cause I don't think it has been—but I've always wanted to control every aspect of my life, do what I wanted to do. I've always been a responsible person, so I guess that ties in with having some kind of self-control, kind of like keeping your eye on the prize.

I *thought* I had control over my health. I had control over my child. And when you're single and you're trying to raise a child, you're used to doing things on your own. I had a child, and I've taken care of that child. I didn't ever want him to get sick. I would get so frustrated if he got a cold or something. "Oh, he's got a cold! How did he get that cold?" Well, he got a cold because kids get colds.

But you don't know you have somebody higher that's controlling you. The hardest thing with the cancer is taking a back seat and let God do the driving, relinquishing control over something I never had control of. I think He's been in control all the time. I really do. You don't even know what your faith is. He's *giving* you that faith. So He's working with you all the time, but you don't realize it 'cause you're thinking that you're doing this on your own, and that's not true. And this is a challenge. *[Laughs]* This is a challenge, I tell you. So that was the hardest thing. It felt like I was out of control, and I didn't like that feeling.

I think I was more resentful of changes that I would have to go through than anything else. I had to go to the doctor all the time, I would have to take blood tests all the time, and I didn't want to do that! I didn't want to go to no doctor all the time. I didn't want to go sit up in no hospital. I *work* in a hospital. I don't want to sit up in there. This is what I'm saying. Oooh, things can happen in your life that can change from one day to the next. It's funny how one word can change your whole life.

Another really, really hard thing was making decisions, having doctors and people coming into your life. I can remember being so overwhelmed when I was diagnosed. I had good physicians, but these are things that I've never had to deal with. They're talking about bone marrow transplant, they're talking about chemotherapy, they're talking about radiation. You can either do this or do this or this. And I was like, "What are these people talking about? I don't understand! What's going on?" I didn't have any control over anything anymore.

People were telling me what to do, what they would do, what they have done, what they should've done, what they could've done. And all you're thinking about is, "Who's going to raise this child? Oooh, God! Who's going to take care of my child? Who's going to handle that responsibility?" I would've liked for him and his biological father to get more close, where his father could have been there. So that's the worry, that cancer worry, but also the fear, living with the fear.

That was two years ago. What has it been like for you to deal with recurrences and metastases?

When somebody says "cancer," it's always associated with death, with being a life-threatening illness, which it is. And then, with the recurrences, it doesn't help at all. I met a woman that had had cancer nine years ago, and all of a sudden it comes back. So when people say, "After five years, it's not going to come back," I kind of look at them. I mean, this thing's in God's hands.

It certainly is a disappointment when they say, "Your cancer went someplace else." And, unfortunately, you get tired. Go through another test? I have to do this? But if your tumor markers are up, quite naturally, my doctor's going to say, "Well, I want to run some more tests on you," so she can find out if there's a problem. Looking back, I appreciate her being steadfast and trying to find out. If she hadn't, it could be a lot worse.

It's been quite a challenge, I tell you. But it's certainly not worth giving up for. I've had a few setbacks, but we've all had setbacks. I used to wonder, "Oh, God! I have breast cancer. I had a metastasis." And my mind just going way out here about the metastasis. You think, when things happen to you, you're the only one they're happening to. I took it all so personal. And you have to put things in proper perspective and say, "You've had a metastasis. Deal with it the best that you can do. You're not the only one this has ever happened to." When I go over to the cancer center, I see people younger than I am, and we're all going through the same thing. I'm not alone in this fight. I sit back and look around and wonder about that person, "How do you feel? Do you feel like I feel? Do you fear like I fear?"

What are your beliefs about death and dying?

Petrified. Pet-ri-fied. When I was younger, I always thought I would die young for some reason. Listening to my mother, her mother died at a young age. I wasn't exposed to a lot of people dying. I was just always scared of it. I guess the fear of the unknown. That's the biggest thing—not knowing, especially if you're a person like I am and want to know everything. And not being able to know, really. But, see, that's where the faith comes in. It's a faith thing.

I feel like the Lord has been carrying me. He's had to because I don't feel like I could've did it by myself. So I know it had to be somebody, something, and I guess that would have to be Him. I wouldn't say I'm fanatical, but I know that there's a higher being because He's been there for me, walking hand-in-hand with me when I go to the doctors. So I say, let Him be in control. This is something I can't fight alone. When I heard that whisper, I had to kind of back up a bit and say, "Well, Lord," and really start praying and give it to Him.

It's like a little spiritual awakening. It's opened up a whole other door. Of course, me that I am, the human side of me still wants to be in control. It's not that I don't have the faith. I do. But it's like you want to be in there helping. *[Laughs]* It's hard to give up the reins. But it gets easier and easier, and you kind of learn to put your trust in God and to know, whatever outcome, that's the way it was meant to be.

Earlier you mentioned the difficulty of making treatment decisions, and with metastatic cancer, you have constant decisions to make. Has faith played a role in your decision-making process?

You know what? Actually, for me, there is no process. Just take the basic information and kind of go from there. It's not that I'm trying to say ignorance is bliss 'cause it's not. I certainly think that knowledge is power. To be a part of the decision-making in your illness, that's important. I ask questions, listen, and try to get an understanding. But I don't want to know the statistics and gory details. I really don't. You already told me I have breast cancer. I'm already living it. All that other medical mumbo jumbo, keep it to yourself. I think that's what keeps me functioning. If I feel too overwhelmed, then I start getting a lot of fear. People might say that's not a good way to do things, but knowing all that other stuff is not going to prolong your life. Because you're dealing with God here. God gave doctors knowledge to help you. That's how *that's* being done.

I've been very fortunate to have a good oncologist. It's all about being honest and able to have a rapport, and we've got a good rapport. I trust my doctor to know me. I trust that she has my best interest at heart. I trust in her judgment and her knowledge, and I also pray that she be okay, too, so she can continue to take care of me. *[Laughs]* I certainly don't want nothing to happen to her!

Before cancer, control had been important in your parenting, too. When Jordan was fourteen and you were diagnosed, how did you handle breaking the news to him?

He was at summer camp so it kind of gave me a little time to figure out what I was going to tell him and to get myself together. First of all, try not to fall apart yourself. I thought about keeping it a secret, but then I thought about somebody opening up their big mouth and telling him, and he wouldn't appreciate that. Honesty always pays off at the end. So I thought the best thing to do was to tell him myself. When he came back from camp, I told him. *[Sighs]* He already knew that I was going to have a little surgery under my arm, so I told him what it was. Then my mother talked to him. She told him everything was going to be okay, so she kind of reassured us both.

So you used the "C" word?

Yeah. I used the "C" word. *[Chuckles]* But then I downplayed it and told him that the surgeon got all of it. I really didn't know no details myself, so I couldn't give him information that I didn't know. I was as in the dark as everybody else. It's not often that they find breast cancer under the arm.

So how did he react when you told him?

He was quiet. For a few days, he was really quiet. He didn't have much to say. I think it's pretty typical of him. Uh-huh.

Over the past two years, with the recurrences and treatments, have you talked to him differently?

Maybe a little differently. This last recurrence I had, I was very skeptical about telling him. I remember being adamant, telling my friends and family, "I'm not going to tell him." I know I told him out of anger because we were just going back and forth about little things, and he was sounding a bit cocky and selfish to me. Let's face it, kids are like that. They go into that little teenage mold where it's all about me, me, me! And I try to tell him, "You know, it's not all about you all the time."

I think I blurted it out. I didn't want to do it like that, but it happened, and he asked me, "How long have you known?" I told him, "Four or five days." "You wasn't going to tell me?" I said, "Well, no, I wasn't going to tell you." "What else are you hiding?"

Janet lowers her eyes briefly. She seems to be struggling with mixed emotions: frustration and anger about her son's self-absorption, confusion about the best course of action, and remorse about losing her own resolve as well as a bit of her son's trust by withholding the truth.

You know, you want to protect your kids from everything, but you can't protect them. You can't hide things. Keeping secrets from people is very stressful. I've always tried to be as honest and open with him as I could without burdening him down. And we do discuss it at times. In as far as him discussing it with anybody else, I don't know. He's a very private person. I wish that he would've gone to a support group. But you know how kids are. I don't want to push him. So I would hope that he would feel comfortable enough to come to me with questions. Knowing that this is no fault of anybody's. This is just life. Unfortunately, things happen to people, and we don't have any control over it. I certainly wouldn't want him to feel guilty about anything—just know that I love him. *[Crying]*

Do you feel like the two of you have gotten closer through cancer, or has he gotten more distant? How is he managing it, do you think?

Well, he's a typical sixteen-year-old, starting to talk on the phone, that sort of thing. Kids, I tell you. They start transitioning into getting to be a young man, then the girls start calling, and you're looking at him and saying, "This is my baby. What is somebody doing calling for him?" We've reached that point now—God! *[Laughs]* He doesn't want me in, as he says, his business.

It lets me know that he's okay, these are the normal things that are going on in his life, so that makes me feel pretty good. I think he's doing as well as can be expected with it. Sometimes we feel like kids can't take things, but I think that we have to give them a little more credit. As a matter of fact, I don't think I used to give him much credit, but now I see that he can really accomplish a lot.

I know he's a strong person, very strong. Talking to him about this illness, he says, "Oh, you're going to be all right. You're going to be fine." Kids believe everything's going to be okay. *[Thoughtful]* I think he's going to be fine.

The thing that is hard to me is being a *mother*, but then being able to let him go and trust him enough to know the direction he chooses is going to be the right direction. I certainly don't want to smother him. He's sixteen. And you have to let go. That to me is the hardest thing, letting him go. *[Long pause]* Just letting go.

Janet says these words over and over. Sitting quietly with her, I wonder how she sees her son growing into manhood, possibly without her.

I'm not going to be able to protect him from the things that he may have to go through, but I do want him to be self-sufficient. That alone would be enough for me, that he takes care of himself and is self-reliant and responsible and gets the most out of this world while you're here. Like I told him one time, "It's not impossible for you to have the things that you want because as long as you're living and God is breathing life in your body, anything is possible."

That's why I push education so hard with my son. I kind of wish I went further with my education. We all graduated from high school, but being on the job now, I see how hard it is, and I know it's going to be even harder. The only issue that I have with him is that I want him to do a little better in school. He's going to scream, "Mama's talking about education again!" but it's important to me. If that's a message that I want to relay over to him, so be it. *Finish school! [Chuckles]* Because, no matter what, once you've got it in your head, nobody can take your education away from you. Nobody.

So with your kids, you try to give them a little insight, and you try to smooth it out for them. You want them to not have to learn things the hard way. I think that's what parents really want for kids, to learn from mistakes and not keep making them over and over and over again.

But you know what? You can't smooth it out for them 'cause they going to hit those rough spots, and they have to learn things on their own. You do the best that you can do and hope that some of those values that you have instilled in them pay off in the long run.

Is there anything else you'd like to tell your son on this tape about how you're doing, how you're coping, what this experience is like for you?

You know what? This has been one of the toughest things that I've ever had to go through. I try to tell him that we don't have control over every aspect of our lives. I don't know why I was faced with this challenge. I don't think it's a punishment or anything. It's just something that God wants me to go through.

I want him to understand that I'm not angry about it. Because I know people have been through a lot worse. And I would really want him to not be bitter about anything. Because I'm certainly not. You can't look at the why of it. It's just one of those things. That's all a part of life, facing a challenge and overcoming it and facing another challenge. So I feel right now I'm facing another challenge. And I'll get through it. That's what I would really like him to understand.

And to be thankful for every day that you have. I always try to remind him that he's very lucky because people are sick, people are going through things, so thank God you're young, you got your health and your strength and don't take everything for granted. Because tomorrow's not promised to any of us. Anything can happen during the course of a day. That's why, before I leave, we always say we love each other. I try not to let my last words to him be out of anger. I really try not to. Life is too short to walk around holding grudges.

It's very important to me to show affection. If you don't show no affection to kids, some of them are rigid. When you go to hug them, they don't understand why you're hugging them because they haven't been hugged. So we do that hugging, and he kisses me, and a lot of times before I go to work, I'll go in his room and tell him, "I love you. Have a good day."

I ask Janet if she believes the cancer experience has changed her as a person.

Yes, the way that I look at life now and the everyday things that people take for granted, you don't take for granted anymore.

But she also says that she does not think it has changed her mothering style or the way she communicates with her son.

"We've always been really close, we've always communicated, and that hasn't changed. We still do things the same way we normally do."

Janet's messages to Jordan about education are expressed by many parents but are especially important to lower-income parents who recognize the economic necessity of finishing high school. The awareness of mortality adds far more urgency to her messages. Mothers with metastatic or aggressive cancers may find themselves riding their children hard around one issue or another that's important to them. One mother said that for her—and others she knew—it was pushing her kids to grow up fast, to reassure herself that they could survive without her: "I know it puts terrible pressure on the kids, but I can't help myself." I ask Janet whether she wants to share other concerns about parenting Jordan.

Well, it was kind of strange, me and him had a little blowout yesterday. I guess with me being so overwhelmed with everything, I felt like, "God, I'm not getting enough from him." Certainly not wanting him to feel any guilt, but I felt like, God, you know? But, then, you still have to think about him being sixteen and having his own mind and his own faults. So we got into a little respect thing. I respect you, you respect me, *[Laughs]* and had a pretty good little talk.

I was sitting on the porch, and he came and said, "Did you really say you hated me?" I said, "No, I didn't say I hated you, but sometimes I hate some of the things that are going on. That's the way I feel about it, but certainly not hating you. I was really angry. I said some things I shouldn't have said."

I felt pretty good about it afterwards. We have our little spats, but we don't let it escalate. We can always come back together and sit and talk about it, say we're sorry or let's not do this anymore. I like that rapport that we have.

So he's pretty straightforward about what he thinks?

Oh, yeah, very straightforward. Sometimes too straightforward. *[Laughs]* But that comes from me, that's my mouth. I was kind of flip-mouthed. As a child, I had to have the last word. It kept me in trouble with my mother all the time. I said to my father this morning, "This is a payback. Your own kids come back and haunt you." *[Laughs]*

I was talking to my son one day a couple weeks ago. I think I had been for a treatment and had called him from my room, and I didn't expect for him to say anything, but he say, "Did it ever occur to you that I don't want to go with you when you have your treatments?"

I didn't know where it came from. Maybe it was something that he had been thinking about. That lets me know how much he's growing up. What I wanted him to do was come on a day that I didn't have chemo and meet some of the people that have taken care of me—the doctors, the nurses, the social workers, people that have really, really been there for me.

So, it kind of got me to wondering. It's really hard knowing that is your mother having this life-threatening disease. I had to go back and reflect on my mother's illness.

You never think nothing will ever happen to your parents. You don't even want to think about them being sick, let alone being sick enough to leave you. I didn't want to see my mother sick. Even though you're grown, you still have that child mentality—as long as I'm here, she going to be here!

To me, it's selfish to keep people here that are really sick. Even my mother—she had chronic lung disease, and she had a hard time, her little lungs were so small. Sitting there seeing her struggle for breath, I knew she was suffering. But I can see her and touch her and kiss her and do all those things. That was my thing. You want your loved ones there. So I'm not going to snatch that away from him. I had to tell him, "You know, I understand. I understand what you're trying to say."

I am curious about whether Janet has talked to Jordan about what she calls a "spiritual awakening" catalyzed by cancer.

I've talked to him. As a matter of fact, I'm trying to get him to go to church, but, like I say, you can't force them. I let him know that I believe in God, and, no matter what happens, everything works out the way that He wants it to because it's all in the plan. You want to see your parents live forever, but that's not the way it is. Everybody wants to see their kids get grown and have grandkids, but that's not promised to anybody. We're just passing through this life. Some of us go soon, some of us go later, but this is the one thing that everybody's going to have to do.

Once you realize that the people around you are going to keep a watchful eye out, it eases a bit. It's important for me to know that he's going to be okay. I know they're going to be there for him. That's how my family is, you know. *[Softly, long pause]*

We kind of discussed it a little bit, me and my son. I always say, "Go stay with my niece, Benita." She checks on me every day. We've gotten very close. To the point that I say, "Well, if anything happens to me, that's where I want my son to go." She's a young parent, but she's got a good head on her shoulders, she's very well rounded, we have the same values and kind of think along the same lines.

I think the biggest issue is trying to make sure that your child has some place to go, just in case, and this is not just because I have an illness. Things can happen to you in a second, and the next thing you know, you're gone. I really feel comfortable with him going with Benita. But hopefully, he'll be grown, and I'll still be here. That won't be an issue. I do plan on being around a long time. *[Laughs]*

I hear Janet give herself permission to let go when the right time comes; I hear her hope to have a future with her son. I wonder how she is thinking about her future, aside from mothering, and whether her spirituality has had impact in other areas of her life.

As much as I hate this disease, I have met a lot of good people along the way that I wouldn't have met otherwise. I think He put me here to tell many people about different things I went through. It's frightening, but if that's what He put me here to do, then I guess that's what I'm going to be doing, maybe help somebody and be able to talk with them without scaring them.

During the course of this illness, a lot of women at work have asked me about mammograms and when did I think they should have them. People come to me and say, "Oooh, you know, I feel a lump in my breast." I feel pretty good about being able to share a little bit with them. Of course, I'm no expert. I can't tell them no medical mumbo jumbo. I can only speak for my experience. But I tell women, "If you feel like your body's going through changes and you feel something there, then I think you should have a mammogram. I don't think nobody should tell you, 'Oh, no, you're too young to have a mammogram.'"[1]

I didn't think I would be able to do this because I was so bitter about mammography. I felt like it let me down. Then I realize that it's just a machine! It's not foolproof. And I know mammography detects cancer in a lot of people. The most important thing that I would want to tell women is, "Keep going to the doctor, have your mammograms, and get to know your body. You know when things are not right. Don't depend on mammography to detect breast cancer. Check your breasts, and note the changes." That's what I want women to do. And it's good to have some knowledge of family history.

It seems like you're doing a real service because some African American women don't go to doctors in time, and they don't get diagnosed early enough.[2]

No, they don't. They don't. And there's a lot of myths out there about breast cancer.[3] I would say, "You know, I used to wear my bra too tight." And now knowing that those things don't have anything to do with getting cancer. I think people are trying to figure out how did they get this disease, "Did I eat too much fatty foods or what?" I think especially black women need to come to some kind of consensus as to the myths. They're really in the closet with it. And they don't want to lose their hair. You have a lot of women who don't want to discuss what they're going through, but I don't have a problem with it. If I'm able to help a person, that's worth it to me.

I also have this thing about telling people to take advantage of things. Your health might not always be there for you. You know, when I was coming over to record my story, a lot of people were like, "What you doing? Where you going?" The times I did tell somebody, they were like, "Oooh! Why you doing that?" I guess people think that you're rushing your time. And I said, "No. You don't have to be sick to do this here." I always use Princess Di as a good example.[4] I said, "She's a woman that had everything, and she went out one night, and now she's gone." They said, "That's true." So everybody's like, "You know, this a good idea. I'm going to try to do that."

It sounds as if you're finding a new role for yourself, like a community health educator.

Yeah. You know what? I feel like I'm in a good position to help a lot of women going through this thing. I think that would have been a good calling for me. I enjoy talking to people. I really don't think it's too late in the game. I think it's just the right time. Maybe this is what I'm supposed to do. I would like to do some work for the American Cancer Society, to give back to people who have given me so much. 'Cause you have to give something back, you have to give back something.

I have picked Janet up at the hospital where she works for our last session. Earlier, she had spoken about the importance of work to her economic and psychological well being during cancer, but she looks particularly drawn today. When we're settled in my office, I ask how she is faring on the job.

I really like working in food services. Being able to go to work and get out there and be among people and supporting myself and my son, that really keeps you going. So as long as I'm fortunate enough to be able to do it, then I'm going to do it. But I don't like working in cold storage, in a refrigerator. To me, that is very, very hard—cold and your nose running and you don't even know it's running! It compromises your body.

I want to work. I feel like I *can* work. I have a right to work. I've been there eleven years, and I think I've worked pretty good, and I've given it my all. But I don't feel like a job has to physically tear you down in order for you to make a living. I'm very scared that I'm going to injure myself irreparably. That's one of my biggest fears, maybe lifting something up and really messing my back up.

My lower back's already been diagnosed with arthritis and inflammation. I don't want to compromise my body too much, and I don't feel like I should have to. If I want to work, I may have to be accommodated on certain things, but they should do all they can to make sure that I can work. I'm in the process of trying to change the kind of work I'm doing to where it's not as physical. But, for the most part, it's been okay.

Have they made good-faith efforts to help you do that?

No. I haven't really pushed it because I'm still working with this cancer agency to get accommodation under the Americans with Disabilities Act. We're just now getting the ball rolling. I'm not the only one who's going through this. I sympathize with my coworkers because a lot of them have arthritis, a lot of them have had injuries, and a lot of us are older, and we can no longer do the real physical work. So I want them to be accommodated, too. I try to look out for everybody's best interests. I don't think I would be able to do what I do if it hadn't been for some of my coworkers. They take the load off.

"We want as much of our lives as we can have." That's what Sara had said in our first focus group. For Janet, that means continuing to hold a job. The determination about working that she expressed during our first meeting is still evident, but so is her exhaustion. She is sometimes short of breath, and her eyelids droop when we pause. I ask if she would have worked this hard through the illness and treatments had she not had a child.

I don't think I would have. And that's not to say that I would be just giving up, but I don't think I would've fought as hard. When I look back, I think I should have taken a little bit more time for myself, just to relax. It's hard for me to be working and stuff like that.

Me and a coworker talked about this. These kids don't know what we have to do to try to bring food to the table. You're doing manual labor—if you're not lifting nothing, you're pushing something. And sometimes you don't feel like they really appreciate what you're going through. Sometimes you get a little bit angry about it. It's like you're Superwoman. They're all, "You haven't done anything today," and you've pushed carts, you've lifted up milk crates, and oooh, like my back is *really* feeling the effects of it.

I think we kind of get sidetracked when we have children. Sometimes, you lose sight of your needs because you're so busy doing for your kids. I know I'm guilty of it. I'm like my mother in a lot of ways. As long as everybody else is satisfied then that satisfies you, and you sit yourself on the back burner. A lot of times, I neglect myself. I'm buying a pair of pants for him, then I'm looking at this dress I want, and you always say, "I can come back and get that dress later." Well, I don't plan on doing that anymore. If I see something and have the means to get it, just get the dress. I really don't do enough for myself. I want to be more into taking care of me, spiritually and emotionally, on the job, off the job, even in a relationship. That's one of my New Year's resolutions—to be good to myself. To take care of my son like I've always done but think more about myself and what I want. It's one thing to say, "You know, I've got to live for my child." That's fine, that's true, but you got to live for you. You're important, too.

It took me a while to think that. It was, "He's all alone, he's my son, is he going to be okay?" I didn't have time to focus on my own needs. But I think once you realize that the people around you are going to keep a watchful eye out, it kind of eases a bit. Then you tend to focus more on yourself, see.

Now, I *know* my son is going to be fine. I comfort myself knowing that he's still typical. He's not letting this—I'm not going to say bother him, but he's very optimistic. I don't know if I would call that denial, but as long as he's okay, I don't have a problem. That makes me feel a lot better, that feeling in my heart that he is going to be okay, and holding onto that, just holding onto that. That takes a tremendous burden off your shoulders.

Many of Janet's statements could apply to any woman raising a child and especially to those who are single or poor. Black women, in particular, have taken care of others both from necessity and tradition. But how do you care for anyone else if you don't care for yourself? I think of the words of the sage Hillel: "If I am not for myself, who will be for me? If I am only for myself, what am I? If not now, when?" Caring for oneself precedes caring for others.

As a mother living with cancer, Janet is beginning to focus on herself now that her son is sixteen years old, she has guardianship arrangements in place, and she is almost convinced he will be alright without her. But, if she is going to be better to herself, it will require relying more on her relationships with others. I ask her if cancer has changed her relationships and if her family now treats her differently.

Uh, no, not really. They don't tiptoe around me or anything like that. And I really don't want nobody treating me any differently 'cause I'm still the same person. Everybody has their challenges, you know. It's just when it's cancer, to people it's always associated with death.

Are others aware of your needs so they know how to help?

Well, sometimes they don't know that I need it 'cause I tend not to ask. When I do ask, they do come around, but I've always been a very independent person. I think that's really one of my downfalls. I'm not going to let nobody dictate what I'm going to do. I think if I wasn't as persistent as I was, I wouldn't have come as far as I came. So I think it has its advantages and disadvantages.

Are there things that you'd like your family members or friends to know about what you've been through that you haven't been able to tell them?

Some people think that you're a rock. Well, I want them to know I'm not a rock. I'm not a rock. I cry about this. People say, "Oh, you're so strong." "Oh, girl, how do you do it?" I just keep doing what I'm doing. It's not that I'm trying to pull any magic strings. I have horrible days, horrible! I'm not this strong person that people see all the time. No, I'm not strong. I'm not strong.

What would it take for you to let the people close to you know how you feel?

To be braver. *[Laughs, then becomes thoughtful]* Anger, probably. Anger. I've done a lot of anger outbursts. Sometimes even with my son. You know, "Look! I'm just going through it. I'm not this person that ya'll think, 'Oh, she's strong. She's strong.' I'm not. I'm not. I cry at the drop of a hat. I don't want to be strong for nobody."

I have heard this now from several mothers, like Tina, who so clearly disliked being called "a rock" or "courageous." They see these comments as a way for non-ill people to distance themselves. Even those who work with ill or dying people hear similar comments: "I don't know how you do it." These kinds of statements make the wall between us palpable.

At the same time, Janet knows she is caught in a bind partly of her own making. She wants more support but has a hard time asking for it. Like many ill people, she hates dependency and insists on some measure of self-sufficiency but is pained by others' perceptions of her as stronger than she feels she is. And others don't necessarily want to see her vulnerability or need. They are buoyed by her strength—and relieved.

I ask her if she thinks it's time for her to get some nurturance.

Yes, it's overdue. But, you know, you have this thing looming over your head. How do you tell *men?* How do you break the ice to tell somebody that you're going through this without scaring them off? I would like to be in a relationship now. But when you're a woman and you're going through something like this here, you always question, "How do I look?" and your hair and your whole femininity thing, the sexual thing. So I don't know.

You want somebody to take care of you a little bit?

Yeah, uh-huh. Yeah. *[Chuckles]* That would be good. Real good. I was telling a friend today, "God, you know, good friends and family, that's fine, but I believe that I would do a lot better if I had a companion, somebody to let you know they're there for you, they're in your corner, someone that would go to the doctor with you sometimes." That I really do wish I had. I think it makes a big difference.

A lot of people downplay that. People say, "Girl, you don't need nobody. You're alright." That's not true! It kind of angers me when people say, "Well, you got family and friends." That's fine. Nothing wrong with that. But when my mother was sick and my father waited on my mother hand and foot, I say, "Boy, he took his vows very seriously, in sickness and in health." That's what I'm talking about. Somebody that's there for you through the good times and the bad times. I think women that have significant others in their lives do a lot better dealing with this disease and everything else, I really do. Yep.

But, for the most part, it's been okay. For the most part, I've been very functional. But now, this particular treatment I'm taking, this Taxotere, has really, really taken a toll. You know, the muscle aches, the bone aches, and I have to go up there and sit in a refrigerator in the cold.

Today was a hard morning for me, I could really feel the aches and pains, and even my father came down. I told him it was the chemotherapy and the side effects, and ain't too much you can do about the side effects, just got to roll with it. Unless you take some pain pills, which I did, so I did feel a little bit better, and I was able to get up and come here today. I knew this was the last session, and I really wanted to come.

I realize that Janet had not gone in to work at the hospital today. She had nonetheless traveled there by public transportation so I could pick her up for the taping. Had I known, I would have offered to postpone or to meet her at her home. So much of what she has been saying points to her total exhaustion. We are almost at the end of the session, and I offer to stop, but she wants me to complete my questions.

You said you've continued working longer because of your child. I'm wondering if that's also true about your medical treatments?

I was just thinking about that today. *[Long pause]* Yesterday, I was at work, being in this chemo fog, and, you know, no taste buds at all from the chemo, and I love to eat. *[Sighs]* And even though I'm going through this, I really try to stay positive. At the same time, I guess, wondering, what is this all for? And then, you know, you have children. That's what it's for. All the things you have to go through, the drugs, the chemotherapy . . . *[Crying]* It's hard. *[Very softly]*

Hard to keep going?

Yeah. *[Crying]*

What's the hardest part for you?

God, I don't . . . whooo . . . I don't know, I think trying to deal with it. All of it. Treatments . . . It was never like it was a denial thing, but . . . ah, I felt like I was just too young, you know.

You were just thirty-eight. Life is full of surprises, huh?

[Laughs] And they say this is a challenge. Well, this is one of the biggest challenges that I've ever had to go through. God, this has been a challenge. I can remember at work yesterday, I got angry. I got absolutely angry. I said, "You know, I'm so tired of this, so tired of this. I've had the chemotherapy, and I can't taste anything. Nothing tastes right. I am just sick of this!" To the point where you're like, "God! Is it worth it?" And then, of course, you backtrack, and you say, "Yeah. It's worth it." But sometime you get to that point where you could chuck it all away.

We sit in silence as tears roll down Janet's face. I don't try to hide mine. I feel moved by her pain as well as her trust. I am with her as she moves back and forth between despair and hope, the desire to let go and the desire to keep fighting.

So, what keeps you going, Janet?

Well, let's see. My son, for one. And number two, my mother. She was there for me when I was sick, and if she ever had any fear, I never saw it. If she cried about it, I didn't know. But, you know, for her, I stay and fight. She'd say, "Oh, you going to be just fine. You going to be here to raise your son." It's like she had an inside track on what was going on.

And then, when I think about other people going through worse, that kind of set me back on an even keel. Lot of people are not fortunate enough to be able to work, and I am. I guess I'm still treatable because they still treat me, and a lot of people can't be treated. So it's a lot of things to be thankful for, 'cause, as much as I feel sorry for myself, I look at the kids that have cancer, and, God, their little bodies, to even be taking chemo.

So I have to kind of reel myself back in and get away from this pity party that I have every now and then. *[Laughs]* I have to put things in perspective again. Even if I'm not well, I don't complain about the ache or pain because if I didn't feel anything, I wouldn't be here.

So this illness has really been a teacher for you.

Oh, yeah. Oh, yeah. Now I'm in school, and I'm really having to learn. I may have not liked school in the past, but I'm going to a school now, and I'm having to deal with a lot of things, read a lot of things. This is just like a school 'cause I'm faced with it every day.

I thought about Janet's two-year education in the school of cancer. I thought about her crisis of faith and how that whisper that she called "God" opened her eyes and led her from a story of control to one of faith. What she saw—expressed in the old saying, "Man plans, God laughs"—could have been a recipe for cynicism or despair. Instead, in surrendering to her human limits, Janet gained perspective, clarity, and a sense of purpose . . . on some days.

On others, she had to struggle to stay afloat among the contradictions: between surrendering control and doing what she can, protecting her son and knowing that she can't; desiring to give up and needing to go on. Since Janet liked to have the last word, here it is.

I don't ever remember believing in Santa Claus. I knew where my stuff was coming from. *[Chuckles]* But the day before Christmas, me and my son, we went to Toys R Us and did a little shopping. When I got home, I got this phone call. "Janet?" and I say, "Yes." They say, "This is Ramon, Dr. Swartzman's nurse." And I thought he was calling to ask me about how I was doing because they check up on you and see how the treatment was. And he said, "Dr. Swartzman told me to call you and tell you your tumor markers are going down."

I said, "Oh, my goodness!" I said, "What a nice Christmas present." And he said, "Dr. Swartzman said that you would say that."

And I started hollering, and my son, he ran out of his room, and I told him, "My tumor markers are going down!" Well, he didn't really know what tumor markers are. *[Laughs]* So he hugged me, and I spread the good news to my family. They don't quite understand, but they feel like if I'm happy about it, it must be something good. I don't think I could ask for a better Christmas present. I really, really don't. Just being here is Christmas enough for me. Christmas is every day for me now.

And my girlfriend called up, "How long you been up?" I said, "I've been up since, oooh, six." "Girl, how you do that? Why you up?" But, you know, I open up my eyes and know that I'm still here. That's enough for me. That is just enough for me. And I guess that's why, when I go outside now, I look up in the sky, I look at it with a whole different meaning than I used to. And that's kind of strange to me 'cause usually we go outside, look around, and go on back in, but now, when I get up in the morning, I open up my eyes, it's like, "God, another day! This is another day for me!" And that's what I like to share with people, just open up your eyes in the morning.

Twelve: "The Story Has Not Ended Yet"
Carrie Arnold

I.

"I CAN'T CHOOSE," Carrie declares, looking over the menu of options for organizing her story. "I can't choose. I can't even think straight. I'm too anxious."

A small, bald woman peers at me through thick corrective lenses, then continues pacing like a nervous cat as we go through the simple introductory materials given to all project participants. Carrie Arnold's thin face is gray and haunted, perhaps due to a recent stem-cell rescue for metastases in her chest wall.

"I'm just a very anxious person," she says shortly into our first hour together. We're sitting in the apartment where she and her eleven-year-old son, Jaime Mendoza, live, a tidy two-room unit in the working-class flatlands. I jot down the facts. Diagnosed with breast cancer four years earlier. Recurrence and hospitalization within the last ten months. Caucasian, single parent of a biracial son. Member of a metastatic cancer group.

Carrie expresses a long list of concerns. Her worries about confidentiality are only partly allayed by our consent forms. She is unable to complete the biographical information sheet because it brings up too many painful issues. She offers a critique of our first evaluation form and points out some typos. My attempts to think through her story with her are met with a grimace and more resistance: "Our talk is raising all my demons."

Carrie's pacing stops abruptly. She stares into space and speaks with deliberation. "Two sentences come to mind: 'My life has been characterized by struggle and upheaval,' and 'Having Jaime has been a highly transformative and healing process for me.'

"What came to mind was a dream that I had when I was pregnant. When I was pregnant, I was terrified as old as I was, thirty-five, because I was so afraid of doing to Jaime what was done to me—passing on the lousy parenting I got. So, in this dream, one of my brothers bites me on the neck and tells me that I have to do the same thing to Jaime. And I say, 'No! I won't do it.' This dream was very significant because if there's any theme to my parenting, it's been to try to be conscious and to work on my own stuff so that I'm present for him. I don't know how successful I've been."

Carrie has discovered the beginning of her story and decides to start with the "lousy parenting" she had received. Eight days later, we begin taping.

CARRIE

My mother and father did not get along very well, and I was the only girl in a family of three brothers. My father did not respect women. Plus, I got all this sexist stuff from my brothers. My mother would alternate between telling me to keep my mouth shut and sticking up for me. Then, my older brother, Ron, molested me when he was fourteen. I was ten. And that has greatly, greatly affected me.

I remember about four or five times, although I'm not real sure. My brother worked on me and worked on me, told me that his friends were doing it. I wanted his approval and love so badly that I did it. I felt really icky about it, really icky. I knew it was bad.

I have no relationship with my brother. He denied it. He called me a liar, and one of my brothers sided with him, so I have a relationship with only one brother now, Bradley. Jaime has always wanted to know what happened with Ron and me, and I've never been able to tell him because he's too young, but I always intended for him to know someday.

It never occurred to me to talk to my mother because I was sure she would blame me. Not to mention that I was totally ashamed, and the idea of spinning out that shameful scenario to her was unthinkable.

My mom is. . . what is my mother? God, I feel all blocked. Maybe you should stop the tape while I gather my thoughts. *[Pauses]*

My mom gave off a lot of contradictory signals. On the one hand, there was this very self-sacrificing quality to her mothering. On the other hand, she was extremely narcissistic and self-involved, so that was very confusing. . . . Oh, God, I feel like I'm making such a mess of this. . . . It's complicated, and it's hard to just tell the story.

Within five minutes, Carrie has blown the lid off. However painful the telling, this mother is clearly determined that her son eventually understand who she is and why she has cut off part of their family. Narration will be difficult for her, although it might lead to some healing. We pause the recorder repeatedly as Carrie expresses concerns that she is "all over the map." "This is really hard because it dredges up a lot of stuff."

With such an emotionally charged topic and so much anxiety, an indirect approach might be best. I explain that it's sometimes easier to start with family or personal history—perhaps she'd like to begin with her birth.

Okay. I was born in Cleveland on June 10, 1956. There was a problem because the umbilical cord was wrapped around my neck and strangling me as I was being born, and so I wasn't breathing. It really scared my mother a lot. She cried when she looked at me for the first time. A difficult beginning. Living has been so difficult for me a lot of times, I wonder, was there a part of me that didn't want to be born?

Carrie was six, brother Ron ten, when twin brothers were born.

It was a terrible stressor for our family. My father never helped my mother, and my mom was overwhelmed. On top of that, her own mother was sick. Things started getting really difficult in the family. That stress had to go somewhere; I got a disproportionate share. I was the girl. And I was a real sensitive kid, and a sensitive kid is a magnet for that kind of stuff. I cried very easily. I couldn't help it. I didn't feel my mother loved me; she just tolerated this ugly kid. My father would make these alliances with my brothers, and they would tease me, and it was real sadistic sometimes. I hated my brothers deeply. I wished they had never been born. But I never voiced anything I was feeling in a direct way.

God, what a family. All we've got are difficult relationships. But it wasn't all terrible, either. There were some good things about being a kid, too. I remember how everything was so wonder-filled. I remember sitting on a sidewalk watching bugs when I was about four years old, just watching life very close to the ground for what seemed like hours. I enjoyed school a lot. I was a real smart kid, and I knew it, and it was one of the ways I tried to make up for other things I didn't feel good about inside myself. I was reading stuff at the college level when I was ten. I wanted to know about the natural world, the human body, the mind. I liked to draw.

I was a pretty good child, too good. A lot of stuff was boiling inside of me. I was lonely, very lonely, a time bomb. When I was about eleven or twelve years old, I exploded. Overnight, my whole personality changed. Whereas I had never dared to confront my mother, all of a sudden, I couldn't do anything else. It was bitter and terrifying because every time I would fight with her like that, I felt more alone, more scared. So I was a pretty upset, gawky kid.

By the time I got into junior high, everything deteriorated. All these feelings I had about my father and my brother and the injustice of my position in the household erupted. The hormones—being off balance was enough to tip me completely over. It was like being plunged into darkness.

All of a sudden, I had problems making friends. School became a nightmare. I was a lousy student. I would end up in detention for talking and for being uncooperative, and I was very slovenly about my personal hygiene. I felt bad about my body, and ugly, and I carried myself in that manner. It was a dreadful, dreadful period in my life. My mother and I were always screaming at each other, and my father and I were always screaming at each other. I went down the tubes. I went down the tubes.

When I didn't go on to college, that was a big failure, and I felt that failure keenly. My grades were horrible. I continually tried, and I continually failed. I could barely stay alive from one day to the next without going under. Finally, my mother said to me, "You have to go to work. You have to do something." I was living at home, and I would get fired from every job I would get. I didn't have experience, I didn't have skills. I was incompetent and felt totally inadequate, like I couldn't do anything right. I was just such a mess.

I was in and out of one depression after another since my teens, severe clinical depressions where I would wake up at five in the morning unable to sleep, all the somatic stuff where the actual colors change to gray. It's not just a metaphor. And when my parents divorced—I was twenty-five-years old, but my sense of self was tenuously grounded—it was too much for me. I thought a lot about killing myself, even though I never made an attempt. I was paralyzed. I had no life of my own. It was hard for me to keep friendships because I was so needy.

Oh, man. When I talk about my life, it's incredible to me. I know I had fun, too. I don't feel like I'm giving the whole story here. It wasn't unremittingly grim, though that's what it sounds like. *[Pauses]*

Well, I was thirty years old, and I did not know how to get out of this circle I was caught in and start moving in a line. I always felt like Sisyphus rolling up the stone, and the stone would come down again. So I thought, "I have to do something really drastic. I have to start creating a life for myself, or I'm just going to die." That's when I decided to move to the Bay Area. It was a do-or-die thing.

I took a major leap. I moved here and found a job at a health clinic and stayed for three years as a receptionist. It took me a couple of years of floundering around, but I think that moving here has been a very, very important thing for me, and I made it work out of sheer desperation. This job I have now at another health clinic and this apartment I'm still living in today are the first real stability I've ever had in my life, a kind of low-functioning stability.

I was living with Jaime's dad, Herman Mendoza, and we'd been together about a year. I wasn't using birth control, and I knew what would happen. I wanted a child. I wanted more than one child, but my life didn't turn out that way. We had talked about having kids and getting married, but actually, having the kid was the main thing for me. I got pregnant.

By the third taped session, Carrie is having new symptoms and diagnostic tests. She brings her anxieties but has learned to relax a little and trust the process. She is ready to talk about the beginning of motherhood and her earlier statement: "Having Jaime has been a transformative and healing process for me."

The best things that ever happened to me were meeting Joan, my therapist, and having Jaime, my son. But I say Joan first because I couldn't have been the mother that I am—it's not like I'm this perfect mother, but emotionally I tend to be pretty much there for him—without her.

When I became a mother, I also became aware of the molestation. I had always recognized that something went on between my brother and me, and I always felt terrible about it, really intense, bad feelings, but when I talked to therapists, they would characterize it as sex play between siblings. Since I was sixteen, I'd gone to one therapist after another, trying to find out what's wrong with me. Why am I so miserable? Why is my life not working? I never got anywhere.

I started seeing Joan when I was thirty-five, only a few months before I became pregnant with Jaime. She said, "You were molested. This is not just play between children." It was the first time a therapist realized that I was molested. So it was the first real therapy I'd ever gotten. I started becoming aware of why I was angry, of the patterns in my family. I had blamed myself for growing myself up the way I did. I was the family scapegoat.

I felt my whole life pivot around with those words. That was the first time that I felt the possibility of healing, really healing. I knew that my life could change, so I guess, on some level, I felt a faith that I could do what I needed to do to be good mother. Even when I got pregnant, I still felt I was going to repeat the stuff that was done to me. In therapy, I started working through these issues.

One of the things that happened is I came to my therapist holding this baby. He was two weeks old, and I remember saying to her, "Now I understand that when I was a baby I was as good, as innocent, as this child is. What happened to me was done to me." I really got in a gut way that events had shaped me 'cause here was this beautiful child that was just the sweetest damn thing I'd ever seen and, oh, the love that I felt for this child . . . I thought, "I was like that once. I was like that. I didn't start off vindictive and jealous and rageful."

What do you enjoy most about being a mother?

Well, two things. One, the opportunity to watch this person develop. It's really an honor to watch his character form and to help nourish these fine qualities in him. I mean, this came out of me, this perfect, exquisite, little being. As his mind develops, I am struck again and again by the wonder of seeing this person take shape.

The second thing is to heal my own childhood. Having Jaime has been really healing for me because learning how to love him has also involved learning how to love myself. Mothering has enabled me to feel like I could heal parts of my childhood by doing for him what I wish had been done for me.

I always buy really inexpensive clothes for him 'cause I don't have money, but he's eleven and he wanted these wide, corduroy, sloppy-looking pants that all these kids are wearing now. I wanted him to have a pair of pants that he felt good about. Then he didn't wear them so I got mad and said, "All right, Jaime, what's the deal? Why aren't you wearing them?" And he said, "Because some guys made fun of me while I was wearing the pants." I said, "What did they say?" He said, "Well, they said they looked stupid." I thought about it a little bit, and I said, "You know what, Jaime? Why don't you try the pants on in a year or two when you grow and you don't have to cuff them? Maybe they'll look better. Don't worry about it now."

My mom would never have done that. She would have been all focused on the money. I really got the issue for Jaime. So, okay, I wasted my money, it's all right. When you can do for your kid what you didn't get yourself but always hungered for, that's a healing experience.

Now, Jaime and I had a really hard time. There's some bad stuff that happened that I want to recall because I don't want him to be unconscious. I want him to know what happened to him.

I took him to a therapist when he was about three because we were having a very conflict-ridden relationship, a lot of screaming on my part. Jaime's a very strong, stubborn kid, a willful kid, and has always been real intense, and I'm a real intense person, and we were constantly locking horns. We were having *big* problems.

A few years later—a couple of months after he turned five—I found a child-therapy agency. We went for four years. I was having a lot of problems. There were times when I completely lost control, I mean, I *really* crossed the line. There was one time I'll never forgive myself for, when I pushed him. I pushed him like a crazy woman. I never actually hurt him, okay? I mean, the closest I came to hurting him was one time when I was going to school. I was under tremendous pressure, and he would not go to bed. He would not stop talking, and I was trying to study, and I went into his room and took him by the arms like this, *[Gestures]* and I said, "You leave me alone!" And I actually broke a

nail on him, dug into his skin. I was horrified, and I called up my therapist, and I was sobbing on the phone, saying, "This is what I've done to
my kid! This is what I've done!"

After that, I instituted a practice with Jaime that if I ever crossed
the line again, I would owe him $10. I think I paid him twice, and I
never did it again, and that was it. I have tremendous guilt over this,
and I talk to him about it every now and then. I don't want him to my-
thologize me because then he can't heal his own childhood. When I feel
like I've hurt his feelings and screwed up, I get really guilty, afraid that
I'm ruining his life.

*Does a mother ever forget the power of young children to unleash
the furies or the terror and shame when they succeed? How does a
mother forgive herself the sins of omission and commission?*

*Maternal rage and subsequent guilt are hardly uncommon, but this
is the first time I'm hearing a mother include it as part of her recorded
story, quite apart from the cancer experience. I also notice that in spite
of the emotionally laden content and passionate delivery, Carrie hasn't
cried. I ask her how she handles her anger at Jaime now.*

Well, sometimes I lock horns with him, and all I do is piss both of
us off. I need to learn how to shut up. I think he needs me to accept him
and to hear him. I'd like to react less quickly. I tend to fly off, and a lot of
times he has to yell at me, "Just let me finish this sentence, let me finish!"
You know, he's absolutely right. I have no business interrupting him.

*This is painful material you're sharing about the dark side of moth-
ering. What about the opposite? What comes easiest to you in being a
mother?*

Gee, that's a good question. It feels like I work so hard all the time.
I love to joke around with him. I love to get silly with him. We're able
to handle things between us differently than we used to, more posi-
tively. I think I'm more consistent about validating him. I catch myself
quicker when I'm not hearing him.

I'm still learning to become an effective parent. The mother needs
someone to listen to her. If nobody's ever listened to you, it's very difficult to know how to listen to somebody else. I think my therapist
mothered me. She loved me, and by loving me, I could start loving
myself. It's just a start, but, you know, it is a good one.

Earlier you said that you didn't feel like you were getting to the whole story. Are you still feeling that way? Is it any easier to combine both the light and the dark in the story?

I guess it's hard for me to tell the story of the good things, to mix those two together.

Is that hard for you in the living, too?

Yes. One of the things that I've always struggled with is integrating the good and the bad. So, when I go back and tell my story, I still tend to tell it in this kind of split way.

It's a lifelong process for all of us to integrate the contradictions in our parents and ourselves, as well as the ones we find in other adults or our own children.

Yeah, and I've only just started learning. I'm realizing that life isn't perfect and it's never going to be. I'm much more willing to live with ambivalence, with the irreconcilable things, my own contradictory nature. I think Jaime's way ahead of me in this. He got that concept real early.

Until now, the scarf wrapped around Carrie's bald head and her pallor have been the only indications of illness. Other dramas in her life have held center stage both on and off tape. I wonder if having to face metastatic disease is once again altering her course, rolling the Sisyphean boulder back down over her.

When I was thirty-nine, Jaime was three, I decided I had to get a degree. I've always felt like I failed to do that. The place I was working at was very good to me. They were able to move me down to half-time and accommodate a very flexible schedule so I could go to school and raise Jaime, and then take me back full-time. I was getting loans and grants. I got this scholarship, which is the only thing I've ever really won, for my first semester. I was taking classes that were opening my eyes.

But I was so crazy. I didn't allow myself to breathe. I got a B+ in one course, and it killed me. I got my BA, and I pulled a 3.8, but I can't tell you the stress. . . . I felt like I had three full-time jobs. I think that that impacted both the onset of my illness and the course of it afterward.

I have mixed feelings about it now. On the one hand, I think I put myself under so much pressure, I got cancer. As soon as I graduated, four months later, I was diagnosed with breast cancer. I was so sleep-deprived and pumped up with adrenaline all the time. At the same time, I'm really proud of myself, so I don't know. It's really hard to know what the ultimate stressor is.

Carrie was first diagnosed with breast cancer after feeling something different in her "really lumpy breasts." She had a negative mammogram but continued to notice changes, was referred for a needle biopsy, and, along with the doctors, was shocked by the diagnosis. She was forty-three, Jaime was seven.

It's so ironic. I'm the kind of person who always gets anxious about everything far in advance, and this time, I wasn't. The one time I let my guard down, see what happens? I had this wonderful prognosis. It was one centimeter, considered to be very early, and I was given very good odds. But, see, I've learned a little since then, and what they call good odds is five years' survival. Who do they think they're fooling? Ultimately, you find out all this.

Carrie had a lumpectomy, radiation, and a sampling of lymph nodes, which were negative, but the mediastinal lymph nodes in the chest wall are impossible to sample. After two and one-half years in remission, she felt pain in her sternum but ignored it until a small swelling occurred. She had a suspicious bone scan but learned only later that her internist had ignored or not seen the radiologist's suggestion to follow up with a CAT scan. Telling herself it was arthritis, Carrie did not follow up until the swelling grew.

By then I knew that my symptoms couldn't mean anything else. I was getting really worried. If I hadn't gone back there, I might never have had the CAT scan. I brought a friend with me to get the interpretation because I knew that this was bad. I remember my internist, Dr. Spottswood, came in. She closed her office door and backed up against it with her hands behind her and said, "It doesn't look good." She was bracing herself to tell me what she didn't want to say. I think she was in denial herself, which is why she never scheduled the CAT scan.

It was so overwhelming. Like, I rolled up in a ball, doubled over. And I said, "Oh, my God, what am I going to do? What's going to happen to my little boy?" I thought, "Well, that's it for me. That's my life."

She said, "You have some time." I said, "Yeah, really, how much?" and she said, "Well, I have a couple of women in my practice who are still around, and they've been going for four years." I said, "Whoop-de-do, four years." I made a mistake in asking her.

What would have been a better way for her to answer your question?

I wanted her to say, "It varies so much among individuals that I can't tell you that, but I can tell you that you're not in any immediate danger, and you can make some choices." I wrote her a letter saying, "I really need to believe I'm going to live."

I had to change doctors. That's sad because I'd been with her a long time. But I can't have a doctor who has denial; I have enough for both of us.

At first, I didn't know what I wanted to do. The Tamoxifen was not working. I was in increased pain, and my chest was bigger. The swelling was pretty pronounced. It was real scary to look in the mirror and see that direct evidence. When my oncologist first told me about the stem-cell rescue, I didn't think I could survive it. I'd heard such horrible things about it.

I went to the Symington Cancer Center and worked through some really hard stuff with my counselor around fear of dying, which didn't stay worked out, but I got through a heavy dose of fear. If it had been the old days, I probably would have just gone home and said, "The hell with this, I wasted my money." But I didn't do that. I worked very hard emotionally against a lot of natural tendencies that had kept me in unproductive places in my life. I said, "I'm going to get everything I can out of this. I'm going to make it work for me." Saying that was a pivot point. This was the confirmation I needed in order to do this really frightening thing.

I decided to go ahead and follow my doctor's suggestion, the stem-cell rescue. I needed to do this because if I didn't try the most powerful thing I knew how to do and then died in a few years, while Jaime was young, I'd never forgive myself.

It wasn't as bad as I had expected. It entailed four outpatient series of CAF[1] and radiation to the area. I had a month of rest, and then I went to the hospital for the high-dose chemo. The actual hospitalization was horrible, but it wasn't as horrible as I thought it was going to be. I look back at it and say, "How did I stay there for nineteen days? How did I do it?" *[Pauses, then leans forward]*

Let me tell you something about the medical care. I was having my stem cells collected. This is after my fourth chemotherapy was over, and they were stimulating my immune system. You have to go home and self-inject the Neupogen. I could not figure out how to use these syringes, and I was giving myself massive doses of this stuff. I couldn't get the damn stuff in me, and I got hysterical because if I didn't get Neupogen every day, I couldn't have my stem-cells collected, everything would be thrown off schedule, and it would be a horror show. So I put in an emergency page to the on-call doctor and said, "I can't do this, blah, blah, blah." He said, "Well, I don't know what to tell you." I said, "Hey, you have to do better than that. You can't just say that to me. You absolutely have to help me."

I was so crazy, I was crying, and I would not let him get off the phone. He said, "Come down and meet me, and I'll inject you," and I did, and he had a hard time doing it. I said, "This I'm supposed to do myself? You're a trained man. How does anybody expect me to do this?" He said, "Come in tomorrow, and the clinic will do it, and we just won't tell the insurance company. It'll be free. Nobody's going to know about it."

When he finally saw what my plight was, he was really there. I gave him a thank-you note, but it was like, I wish I didn't have to work that hard to get this man to listen to me. Why should I have to go through this shit to begin with? I was so sick at that time. Why don't they just let me come into the damn clinic? Why? Because it's five dollars more expensive. The point is, it's not so much your doctors. It's what managed care is doing to people nowadays. It's horrific. I heard recently that Stanford is doing stem-cell rescues on an outpatient basis. Do you believe it? I thought, "The next thing you know, they're going to be doing outpatient brain surgery!"

Anyway, I've needed a lot of help, not just as a result of my physical situation but also being unable to cope because I'm overwhelmed or depressed or whatever. I would like people to be more reliable. I mean, sometimes people are key, and then, all of a sudden, they're gone. I feel abandoned. I wish I could say to people who have been inconsistent, "This is really painful when you do this. It baffles me, and it hurts me." You need people to be rock steady when you're going through something like this. You need to know who you can count on. This variable stuff is for the birds.

It feels good when people respond to my diagnosis with, "I'm praying for you" or "I'm rooting for you" or "I'm fighting with you," something like that. I felt uplifted. People at work started a fund and collected a lot of money for me. They bought me a laptop so I could stay connected by email to them. But the recurrence scared the hell out of everybody. When people responded with horror, like it was a total disaster—"Oh, my God!"—that was very difficult for me.

I went to a group last January on grief and loss. And I was the only one in there who had an illness. Everybody else had lost somebody to murder or suicide or whatever. One person said to me, "I don't know how you can do what you're doing. I can't imagine going through what you're going through." I was really upset by that. It made me feel very isolated, like I was in an especially horrible, unique position. It's a human situation! Does she think she's going to live forever? *[Laughs]* Well, yeah, she probably does. I don't want to think about this shit either, you know. But, when it does happen, you don't want to make the person feel more stigmatized.

For me, to talk to friends or cry to somebody, that makes a big difference. If I can't connect in actuality, I remember what people have said or things I've read, and if nothing works, I just hold on for dear life. Because what else can you do?

I think cancer's changed every relationship in my life because I've changed. Some people I cut out—different reasons, but I knew my energy was limited, and I decided I wasn't going to deal with them. I've been trying to be more honest when I'm hurt or angry, and that includes speaking up with the two family members I do talk to, my mother and my brother. And to be a little bit more forgiving of other people.

I confronted my brother. To this day, he denies having any memory of it [the molestation]. He did contact me after I was diagnosed. I emailed him, saying, "It would be lovely to have some connection with you, but we have to do it on an honest basis." He emailed me back, saying, "I don't know what you're talking about."

Jaime was two and a half when I wrote a letter to everybody in my family, saying, "This is what happened to me," because I wasn't getting anywhere with Ron. I said that I wanted to find a way to heal this but that I needed them to help me do it. They didn't want to. Ever since that letter, I'm not part of the family. Except for Bradley.

It's been hard for my mother to acknowledge how destructive this has been to me. Mother believes it happened without fully allowing herself to experience all the ramifications of that. She kept saying, "What would you have me do?" I said, "Have you ever said to Ron that you believe that I was molested?" And she said, "No." I said, "It seems to me that when you don't confront him in any way, it allows him to retain his pivotal position on the inside of the family and allows me to stay marginalized."

I got off the phone saying, "Boy, I really got that off my chest—where the cancer is. This pain that we're trying to diagnose right now has been much better since then. Confronting my family and letting go of a lot of the pain from my childhood has come from the irrefutable knowledge that I have no choice. It's getting it off my chest, right?

So how has having cancer and facing mortality affected you and your mothering?

When I was diagnosed again a year ago, I told Jaime right away. I was crying when I told him, and he said, "Mom, could you please stop crying?" And I said, "No, I don't think I can." So he says, "Then could you please stop making that underwater sound?" *[Laughs]* I remember even then laughing. It was very grounding.

But I can tell you cancer has not improved my mothering skills any. It's harder in some ways to cope. The hardest part is that special agony you feel when you think, "I might leave this little boy long before he stops needing me in this daily way, and what is going to happen to him?" I haven't been there for Jaime the way that I would like to be because I've been too sick. And when I'm not sick, I'm depressed, and sometimes I'm both. You're pretty much in a state of shock, and then you are under treatment.

There are times when I couldn't be a mother. When I was undergoing my chemo, I was not terribly functional. I wasn't able to monitor Jaime's schoolwork or interact with him very much. And the same thing toward the end of radiation. I was feeling lousy, and I was short-tempered 'cause I didn't have the energy reserves. Especially when I got home from the hospital, I was pretty worthless as a mother. Two neighbor families that I'm close with alternated, and then my mother took over parenting Jaime completely. I don't think I've ever been so grateful to her as I was that week. I simply couldn't function.

When I finally did start to feel better, Jaime let me know that he thought that I had been a pretty lousy mom. He made it sound like I was never there for him at all, in any way, ever. I was glad he could say it, and I said to him, "You know, you're right. I haven't been there for you as much as I'd like because I've been sick. I know it's been hard for you to realize how sick I've been, but I've been really that sick. It's important to me to be there for you, and I'm sorry that I haven't been in a lot of ways."

He can't get that. It's safer for him. So he went through a couple of outbursts, "You don't care, and you're not much of a mother, and blah, blah, blah," and that was it. I don't know whether he said everything he needed to say. I would assume there's more. He hasn't gone through any changes in his personality that are obviously correlated to what's going on with me, and I've always wondered what he's doing with it inside himself. I think we're close, but I'm aware that you don't really know what's going on. Kids are separate human beings, and they need to be separate, and there are certain ways in which I *shouldn't* know what's going on with him. I just know that it's been very difficult.

I've come to feel that Jaime has much more resiliency than I realized. He's got the ability to take a situation and become stronger for it. I think he's going to be quite a man. He runs very deep. Yeah. *[Excited]* He's very sensitive, very intense, but I think he's going to have a rich life once he learns how to master the intensity and sensitivity.

But then there's this very stubborn, rigid way about him, too. He's not the kind of person who makes friends easily, who relaxes. I want him to be a little bit less defensive, to like himself, and I worry because I don't think his self-esteem is real good, and I blame myself for that. He's a cross between his dad and me. I'm also very intense, and I can be pretty rigid. I have that same quality where you're sure that you're right about something and that everybody else is wrong. He reminds me of his dad when he does that, even though I do it in a different way.

Carrie's portrayal of Jaime sounds remarkably balanced. But she has worries related to his father. Carrie and Herman divorced soon after Jaime was born. Carrie retained custody, and Herman rarely spent time with their child. "Only a year ago did he become more involved as a parent, seeing Jaime almost every Sunday." Issues between parents are frequently exacerbated when a mother has cancer. For single mothers facing advanced disease, having to negotiate with a difficult father introduces additional anxieties.

I think seeing his father more often has been both good and bad. Good in the sense that he has to have some concept of who his father is and some kind of role model, but I think it's also been very difficult because his father will not hear who he is. I'm the one in his life who does that for him. Jaime's afraid of his father. *I'm* scared of him. He doesn't know very much about being a parent. Jaime's always feeling like he has to perform in this image of a good boy because his dad doesn't want to hear anything else. So, he swallows his anger and his personality to be with his dad.

If I should die in the next couple of years while Jaime is still young, what's going to happen to him with his father? I don't have a choice. His father's going to take him, and that's all there is to it.

Does his father support him economically at all?

Yes, he does, and of course there's all kinds of fears around that. Maybe his father will stop paying child support. Jaime's afraid his father's going to try to get custody because Herman's threatened that before. Isn't this clever? He threatens his kid that he's going to get custody because I don't know what the hell I'm doing as a mother or because Jaime's not being cooperative. Jaime said, "I'm tired of being this good little boy. I'm tired of acting the way he wants me to act. I don't care what he does." And I think, "If he can say that, I can say that, too."

I'm watching this kid in awe. I'm seeing him draw lines and say, "I don't care, this is the bottom line for me." I'm thinking to myself, "My God, this little kid, eleven years old, has got more guts than I ever had. He's going to need this if anything happens to me. He's going to need this."

I don't think he could have done that if he hadn't gone through having to cope with what I went through in the hospital. So, I think his character is being shaped by this illness in ways that are good, actually. I have more confidence that even if I'm not around, somehow he'll be okay.

I try to talk about cancer with Jaime as an ongoing process. Jaime doesn't talk about it much. He would like nothing better than to pretend that all this never happened. I want to keep it almost like a wound draining. At the same time, I don't overwhelm him with my fears. I try to incorporate it as matter-of-factly as possible into our lives. I don't think it's a good idea to impose this rigid idea of what normal has to be in order for things to be okay. Things are *not* normal, or, at least, this is what normal is now. Kids have to know that you're able to say that to yourself and to act on it in your life, even if they can't talk about it.

Carrie is starting to integrate the positive and negative, both about cancer and herself as a mother. I ask her to reflect on the overall themes and purpose of her life.

I've been an outcast in my family, and I've recreated that every-where I go. It's been tremendously painful for me, soul-wrenchingly painful. So that's been a theme for me—how to be a full member of the human race. Boy, it might be *the* theme.

The other one has to do with resentment. I tend to get into feeling victimized. So, I've been working on the way I'm harsh and judgmental toward people, toward myself. I'm trying to ease up on everybody. I'm learning the difference between feeling the feelings and having to act on those feelings. I'm softening up.

I've decided that my purpose is to develop emotionally and spiri-tually as much as possible. I've always wanted a loftier purpose, but I don't think I have a calling. Probably what I'm best at is reaching. I'm always reaching for something else and making myself better than I was the day before. I keep going. So, I think that my purpose is to develop as fully as possible and to work on letting go. Letting go of old anger and resentment and changing my patterns is a big lesson for me. There's definitely been progress since I started seeing Joan, and it's greatly accelerated in the last year with my diagnosis. I feel an understandable sense of urgency about getting rid of some of this emotional baggage I've been carrying around for so long. I have dis-covered a resiliency and a resourcefulness in myself that I didn't real-ize I had. I have more respect for myself. I guess I have more courage than I thought I had. In the spiritual, I really have a long way to go. I change so slowly.

The hardest is the fact that I might die before Jaime is old enough to take care of himself, and, even if he's old enough to take care of himself, the fact that I will die young. You know, I've always want-ed to see Jaime grow up and see what kind of man he becomes, and not just Jaime, *me*. I want the time to develop. I said to my therapist yesterday, "I really feel like I've kept myself stunted in a state of poverty, physically and developmentally." The ability is there, but I wish I had been able to emotionally take the risk to do something where I can use words in some way and also have enough spaciousness inside to help other women in their experiences with cancer.

I'll tell you something: More and more, I'm beginning to value kindness. This is probably just getting older, as well as being sick and people being kind to me and realizing how good it feels. Kindness has never been a big thing with me because I've always been so harsh and judging. But, yeah, I want to be kind.

In my group, we talk about death a lot. I've been reading about it, but, you know, it's a scary business for me. It all scares me. Being mortal would scare me, and being immortal scares me. Puts you in a bad position, doesn't it? *[Laughter]*

So, overall, how do you feel you're doing with facing your mortality?

Badly, I think. Badly. The denial is very thick, and it's hard to strip away those layers. I still have this fantasy that I'm going to be okay, that I don't have a life-threatening illness. But the chances are very, very slim that I'm not going to die young. There's a part of me that doesn't believe it in a deep way. That's what I mean by "denial." I think you lead a very different kind of life when you're on intimate terms with death than when you're putting the distance that I'm putting there.

Can you say more about that? Because you seem to be in a transformative process.

Well, sure, the story has not ended yet, so we don't know where it's going to end. *[Pauses, as if surprised]* I'll tell you what I mean. When I got diagnosed with this spread, I determined in the first few minutes that I was going to make this situation work for me. I was going to actually *use* it as a way of bounding through things that I had not been able to before because I knew deeply that it was the only thing I could do that would make my life worthwhile or bring it meaning. I'm not going to knock these walls down, I'm *jumping* over them now. I've been working at that pretty steadily. I've had so much pain in my life that to be able to let go of some of those things that have caused me pain is a great blessing. I'm much more at peace.

So, what I've realized during this past year is that there are other things that are worse than death, as scared as I am about death. There are things much worse than struggling with this kind of illness. There's living the way I used to live. Nothing could be worse than that for me.

Has there been an experience with death that has been a teacher to you?

There's a woman in my support group, she's seventy-five years old, [and] she's had this highly conflicted relationship with her husband of fifty-some years. Their whole married lives, they have this codependent, unhealthy dynamic. And her habitual stance is kind of a victim stance, very passive, like, she'll complain about something and won't do anything about it.

She reminds me a lot of me. There's a very proactive part of myself that takes control of things, but there's also a part of myself that wallows in victimhood and complains. I've always identified with her and gotten pissed off at her. She's in a terminal state of illness, and I noticed a couple of weeks ago that she was talking in a completely different way about her husband and daughters. She was in this incredibly mellow, detached place, where she was saying, "I let them do whatever they need to do, and inside myself, I do what I need to do."

I thought to myself, *My God, if this woman can get peaceful about her life and her coming death—because they're intertwined—then anything's possible.* My therapist said to me, "You should go home and write on every wall, 'Anything can happen.'" She's right. I need to do that.

That's a wonderful story.

It *is* a wonderful story. It is.

Anything can happen.

Yeah. Anything can happen.

II.

During the month following the interviews, Carrie awaits the results of some new scans. She says, "This feeling I have of detachment from whatever the results are going to be, whether I've got active cancer or not right now, is like an act of grace. You have to do what is in front of you to do, and if it's freak out, I guess you freak out. Then, the grace comes by itself."

The scans are negative. Carrie returns to work and gives me an update on mothering Jaime. "You know, you can't fix an awful life.

All you can do is deal with it." Jaime, who hasn't been doing well in school, is talking with his school counselor and going to therapy. "I'm offering him a means to get help, and he's taking it. I see that he can go to people and pour his heart out, and that's great. I'm beginning to see the positive effects of my parenting. I think I have been more successful than not. I don't think anymore that I'm passing on to Jaime that deep pain that was so much a part of my life."

I am pleased for both mother and child. But as I edit the manuscript, I am uneasy about what to include. Carrie has firsthand knowledge that "secrets make you sick" and intends to spare her child the same disease. She believes in telling the truth, first to herself, then to her family, now to her son in these tapes. I want to honor her values, but her son's needs loom larger and larger for me.

A listener in the Mothers' Living Stories Project has two goals: to provide a healing process for the mother and to guide her in preparing a product of value for her child. Usually, it is possible to achieve both without conflict. Sometimes, it is not. For the mother, the process of telling the whole story without concern for the future recipient is ideal. What the child should receive and when is another matter. Decisions can become especially hard when a mother's history includes troubling life experiences.

Carrie Arnold's childhood experience of sexual abuse is not uncommon. Other mothers bring to the recording sessions different difficult issues, past and present: family violence, mental and physical illness, fractured relationships, substance abuse, secrets large and small. For some women, healing requires throwing off the shackles of old stories and secrets—"getting it off their chest." One way to release a limiting story is by telling it repeatedly until a new perspective is achieved. This may be painful, but can also be relieving—for the mother.

But the mother's need to tell the whole story and sometimes to alter her life can conflict with the child's need for continuity, stability, and conformity. There are developmental stages during which children need to idealize their parents. To tell the children or not? When? How?

Project listeners view ourselves as advocates for the mother. We make her desires paramount, but maintain an awareness of the child who will receive the story. We try to guide the mother to tell and to time the presentation to the child in ways that will do no harm.

Ultimately, though, the listener has to let go. It's the mother's story. She will decide what to tell, when, and how to pass it on. Carrie's intentions are clear. I deliver the manuscript and suggest that she give it to her son when he is fully adult. She agrees.

Something else disturbs me: a disconnect between the highly emotional material and the absence of tears. Carrie had not wept on or off tape—she didn't even choke up when I did. Crying is not required to express emotion, but I wonder whether she ever did get to the whole story.

When I deliver the manuscript, Carrie has both negative and positive things to say and, not surprisingly, begins with the negative. "How do I explain this? I just gave up on my ability to tell a coherent story. I felt so frustrated by the limitations, that I can't really get the ultimate meaning of something. That's why I can't bear to read it. I don't want to judge it, make it into some perfect autobiography. I'm too close to it right now."

Then, after a long silence, she tells me she has not been completely honest with me. "There's an area important to my story that I did not want to talk about. It may have affected the whole thing."

I want to know more, but Carrie's tone of voice and body language do not invite further questions at this time, and I respect her need for privacy. "Any story is only a slice of life at a particular time," I say. "I don't think that there's one right life story. Look at how your own life keeps changing. Your story, like your life, is a work in progress. Perhaps you were being responsible to yourself and to Jaime by being selective in what you chose to relate and when. Trust that." Carrie nods and says no more.

The product fell short of her vision. Had the process worked for her?

"Actually, it's been more rewarding than distressing. To tell your story to somebody and have it received, really received—that in itself is intrinsically healing. Just the fact that you were sitting there listening to my story and finding it interesting is helpful because what it does is affirm the value of my story—and my value because I am my story. It means that my life has some meaning, some value, not just to me but in a human way. Also, you're telling your story to yourself, so in talking you're changing and growing.

"I'm comforted that my son has some version of my life if I won't be there myself to explain things to him. Even if it's chaotic. I'll give it to someone I trust and make sure that they give it to him. I'm not sure how old he needs to be, but I want him to know before twenty-five."

I am relieved that the process was helpful to Carrie and that she feels the manuscript will be helpful to her son one day.

A year passes before I hear from her again, this time with bad news that's delivered in a strangely excited and lighthearted voice. The cancer has spread to her ribs, and she has another bone scan scheduled soon. She had taken Jaime to his old therapist to tell him the cancer was not gone. "He won't talk about it," she says.

"The good news is that Jaime's relationship with his dad has improved tremendously. I have some relief. My mother and I have both stretched a lot. I've come to terms with her and look forward to her visits. We finally heard each other. It's been magical and inexplicable. My brother Ron, I have let go. I own the anger, but it doesn't own me."

During this and subsequent conversations, Carrie expresses interest in adding a tape because so much has changed. She has had to leave her job and is on medical disability. Then, she tells me the story she had withheld during the taping. She is becoming an artist and coming to terms with her sexual identity as a lesbian, the culmination of a secret struggle of many years. These changes she views as necessary for her psychic and physical survival, but she also realizes that they will cause havoc in her son's life. She wants to find a way to explain them to Jaime, who appears "knotted up like macramé."

Another year goes by. Carrie's cancer has gone into remission; she is ready to make a tape. Preparing for the session, I reread the original transcript and am stunned. I had held her in my memory as a woman who was depressed and anxious—the understandable outcome of recurring trauma. But unlike other mothers whose lives are in upheaval over cancer, Carrie had been mainly in upheaval over *Carrie*. Her consciousness was evolving; her transformative process was intensified, but not determined, by cancer. While recording her story it sometimes had seemed as if her entire identity was up for grabs. There were moments when I doubted her judgment—and my own.

Because of her process, perhaps because I was caught by the darkness, I had missed the larger picture of who Carrie was. Carrie said she had not been completely honest with me; I wonder if I have been honest with myself. I begin to see that her story frightened me because of some primal places where our narratives intersect. I, too, had identified with the Sisyphus myth through much of my life and had been afraid to pass on to my child the very different, but insufficient, parenting I had received. I had worked hard in therapy and, when I felt deficient as a mother, found the best help I could for my daughter to offset my inadequacies.

By the time I met Carrie, my daughter was in college and doing well, and so was I, but fears for Carrie's son easily triggered fears for my daughter, however inappropriate. Then, too, I was afraid for Carrie. I knew from experience that the idea of breaking generational patterns can backfire. A mother can change herself but still have no control over the many other forces in her child's life. Her own transformation can be hurtful to the very person who inspires her to change. If I had erred on the side of over-protection, Carrie may have erred in telling too much. But, after all she had been through, I didn't want her to be judged a bad mother. I didn't want her to feel any more shame.

I had identified too much with Carrie, so caught up with her stories of victimization that I missed the extent of her developing personal authority. The woman who several years earlier could not even choose which way to begin her story had made one life-altering choice after another. Although she claimed she had had "no choice" about confronting her family because of cancer's invasion of her chest, she did have choices and made them. Carrie's way of handling adversity demonstrates that change and healing are possible, no matter how ill a person is and even when that ill person is a mother.

Seeing Carrie more accurately, I remember an old Jewish story. Reb Zusya, a revered teacher, is on his deathbed, surrounded by weeping disciples. Zusya is trembling in fear. His students ask, "Zusya, why are you afraid? Haven't you been as righteous as Moses?" Zusya replies, "When I meet my maker, He won't ask, 'Why haven't you been like Moses?' He'll ask, 'Why haven't you been Zusya?'"

Carrie's entire life impressed me as a long journey to become authentically Carrie—open, unashamed, free. Having cancer reinforced her determination to get there before she died. She was going to free herself. But, with her new confidence and new consciousness, the forward thrust now snagged on the rock on which her son stood. She felt her needs pitted squarely against those of her child. She was intent on transforming her own life, but she was unsure how to do it. And, how could she tell her fourteen-year-old son, who had already had his share of suffering, who—like all children—wanted only to have a healthy, "normal" mother?

Carrie's new dilemma heightened the questions that had been a subtext throughout her story. What price must a mother pay to become a full human being while her child is young? What price must her child pay? How does the merciless split between the selfless-mother ideal and the selfish-mother judgment change when a mother is seriously ill? What are the limits of maternal protection?

Carrie would probably agree with Deena Metzger that "the best protection is truth."[2] But, this mother had already experienced that telling the truth can wreak havoc, sometimes tearing apart a web of relationships that, however frayed, might otherwise support both parent and child, especially during illness.

Many child-oriented advisors would say to Carrie, "Wait until the child is grown. You don't have to shake up things now when your son is so young. Or, if you do, at least don't let him know about it." But what if waiting is not possible because there may be no future? What if the mother believes that she must change her life in order to stay alive?

But Carrie was unstoppable. And her choices at each point along the way were consistent. For her, healing her life involved nothing less than confronting the past and the people who had caused her to suffer and continuing to make dramatic changes in herself and the way she lived. As I prepare to meet her, I finally feel that I have a grasp on the issues, for both of us.

Carrie arrives on a warm August afternoon. Her brown hair has grown back in salt-and-pepper curls, softening her perpetually worried look. Her eyes hold less fear than I remember. However, her intensity is unchanged. It's been almost three years since we recorded the last chapter of her story, but she moves quickly to the purpose for our meeting, acknowledging some anxiety about the taping.

I begin the tape by saying, "This is an update for Jaime about some important things that have happened so that he has a better understanding of what's going on for her right now."

CARRIE

Okay. I'm sort of in the midst of a revolution inside myself. I've been wrestling with my sexuality ever since I've been a teenager and really haven't wanted to deal with it. The shame that I had ever since my brother molested me has made it harder for me to deal with the fact that I find myself attracted to women. Okay, I always have, but what's happened is it's become imperative that I deal with this in a forthright manner and *say* it. I don't know how to start living it. So, I'm poised on the brink of—yeah, I guess I *am*—declaring this to be the case for me. . . I'm just going to pause this for a moment.

This is the first of many times Carrie will use the pause button while she gathers her thoughts, deals with her anxiety, and asks for my advice.

So, this is a fraught moment because I'm really aware that Jaime has very negative feelings about anything homosexual at all. His father has so many. *I* have so many. I've internalized so much of that stuff myself. So, that's where I'm at.

It sounds like you're going through the hard process of coming to terms with a part of who you are.

Yeah, I am, and I don't know how to be in the world in the truthful way that I feel like I now need to do and what impact this is going to have on my relationship with Jaime and with his dad. When we were together, I told Herman that I was attracted to women, and he could not *ever* put that to rest. I've felt so much pressure over the years from him not to say anything. My fears are that he's going to . . . get *nuts*! And start yelling and saying all kinds of horrible things to Jaime about what I am and how I don't care about anybody but myself because if I did I'd keep it to myself.

What do you want Jaime to know about why this is so important for you and why it's not a selfish or careless thing?

Because I don't feel like I have an emotionally viable choice. I feel that if I want to live, I have to *really* live. I can't push it down because it's like my life force. I'm not ready to die, I guess, is what it is. It's very connected to the art.

In the last couple of years, there's been a tremendous upwelling of stuff related to art. I used to do stuff when I was younger, and then it got put away for twenty-something years, and I felt a great loss. I pushed it down the same way I pushed the sexuality down. And I *know* they're linked. I think art's a part of my life force, part of my creativity. I think sex is, too. I can't have one without the other, and I can't change the way I'm made. "Don't ask, don't tell" doesn't work.

It seems as if you've already paid a very high price in suppressing so much of yourself.

I *have*. The art has a frantic feeling to it. *[Gesticulates rapidly]* It's been pushed down for so long that it's . . . it's overwhelming. I've never been a fast worker, but it's coming out of me like there's a need. . . . I've done two pictures since Sunday. I want to be at ease. And I don't know how all this is affecting Jaime. He knows that I'm drawing. He knows I'm very absorbed with it. . . .

What do you love about drawing? What is it like for you?

It's a great joy to see something take shape. It's making the inchoate tangible—like, I'll see something, and I'll have a feeling about what I am seeing. And what comes out on the drawing is all mixed up with love because I love what I'm seeing. Or I'll start to love it as I'm drawing. It's joyful to take a blank piece of paper and make it beautiful.

It's wonderful to hear you talking about joy. When we first met, you were suffering so much. It's beautiful to see how you've changed inside to be able to experience that kind of freedom. On some level, I would think that Jaime is also feeling it.

I don't know.

No, you don't, and I don't either. Kids want all the attention, and they want their parents to conform in certain ways, but they may also come to recognize what a good thing it is for them when a parent has gone through as much as you have in your life and come through it to have joy.

The suffering has opened the doors, I think, to joy. I mean, you can do two things with suffering. You can wither, or you can expand. I know that suffering is a honing thing for me. Yeah. Suffering has been a way to grow. It seems like I've had to do an awful lot of it just to grow a little bit, so sometimes, I wonder about the proportion of suffering to insight.

Is there something that you would like to say to Jaime about what you've learned about living through this that might be helpful for him in his own life?

Yeah. What I am learning is that the only good thing about suffering is if you can become a better human being from it; otherwise, it's no good at all. Since I've been dealing with the metastatic cancer, I've been making conscious decisions to walk the edge where growth takes place. I'll pull back, but I always find myself on my own personal edge, which is the only one that counts.

Actually, going after joy is a courageous act when you've had so little self-esteem. I'm becoming aware of how little joy I've allowed myself to have—partly to punish my mom or my brother, to say, "See what you've done to me, you've ruined my life." There's still a thrill in that, but more and more, I'm beginning to feel that it's better to go ahead and have happiness and stop trying to punish them. I'm recognizing that I have a choice; I can let myself be happy. I'll get into a bad place, and sometimes I can say, "You know, I don't feel like doing this. I think I'll go and take a walk." I'll start drawing something, or I'll do *something*. I can switch the tenor of what's going on a little bit. But the main thing, I think, is to keep going, *just keep going*. Keep putting yourself back on your feet.

You've certainly been an example of that.

Yeah, I guess so. I used to feel that I was pushing the stone up the mountain, and it kept rolling down. I have to keep going, and it's hard, but I don't feel the Sisyphus myth is really what I resonate with any more, and it's a major change.

Do you have a sense of what story or myth you're living now?

Well, what's my myth? My myth . . . *[Thoughtful, then brightens]* Today I did a drawing. You know the chalk cliffs in England? Well, I saw a picture in *National Geographic*, and I *loved* it, and I whipped it out in one morning! It's a flat piece of land that drops off in a sheer cliff, then there's the ocean underneath it. It's a moonlight scene . . . and I had an image when you asked what's my myth of walking the edge of the cliff. I guess that's the way I see myself—walking the edge—because that's where all the growth takes place. Right now, I'm doing that. I'm pushing the limits of how I define myself with the art and with my sexuality.

It's not surprising that there is a connection between the two, both of which involve your senses and life force. Maybe part of the lesson in that—for Jaime, too—is the importance of internal freedom, of not cutting off parts of yourself.

Yeah. Oh, man, I've been so tied up in knots. I see Jaime tied up in knots. He's got a lot of struggle. I think it's hard for Jaime to break free and be buoyant. I see him as heavy a lot of the time, very serious. He does get silly sometimes; I'm maybe one of the few people who sees that part of him. I guess I want Jaime to have more joy. I think that's where his growing edge could be.

So, do you want to say something to Jaime about your desire not to hurt him as you're struggling with your own identity issues?

Yeah, I don't want to hurt Jaime, and I think this will hurt him a lot. He makes all kinds of negative remarks about gay people. I think he really doesn't *like* that. For him to think that his *mother* is that abhorrent thing . . . So what happens if I actually do have a relationship with a woman? Can I take that step? And what effect will that have on Jaime and his dad? How will they see this? It's really hard to think that what you are in essence is something that's hurtful to your kid.

Is there something from this situation, if you do move forward, that you think Jaime can grow from in positive ways, even though it will be confusing?

I always feel that we grow by encountering the truth. I can't help but think that what's basic and necessary to me is going to help him also because they work together, and that he's paying some kind of a price right now, just like I've been paying a price. But it's what he has to go through to get there that I worry about. How can he know that what I'm saying is true, even though I feel that deeply in my life? All he would know is: "My mom is fucking my life up, you know, she's really fucking my life up." I want him to have some support. I don't think his father can support him in this because his father has so many feelings of his own.

I stop the recorder, thinking it might be helpful for Carrie to reflect on what she wants to say about Jaime's dad. She tells me, "I don't want to undermine his relationship with his dad, but I don't want to undermine something in Jaime that needs expression. I want him to know that I really struggled with this, and I'm hoping I did the right thing." I sense at this point she might be ready to speak directly to her son.

Okay. So, Jaime, I'm going to talk directly to you even though it feels weird.

The subject of your dad is very much in this conversation, and you and I have had some talks about how your dad finds it hard to deal with certain aspects of you that are important to your sense of yourself. And I *really* would like for you to be able to be who you are in the most full and glorious sense and not have to pretend to be a certain way with your dad or to tiptoe around his anger.

I also hope for you to free yourself from the conflicts that you have towards *me*. I think it's been real hard with us at times, especially when you were younger, before we got therapy. But, even now, I don't think I'm an easy person to live with, and I think that you've got your share of stuff to work out with me. My wish is not only that you free yourself from your father's clutches but from my clutches, too—that you separate from me in a way that's healthy so that are your own person.

Another thing that I wanted to talk to you about was how sad I am that you and I have been so isolated from my family because of my brother molesting me and my needing to stay away from them because I felt so unprotected in their presence. Unfortunately, I've carried you along with me in that because there really wasn't any other way.

I've told you that when you get older, you might want to get to know individuals on my side of the family on your own. I want to say again that I'm split on this. There's a part of me—which is not the higher part, it's this human part—that wants you to be loyal to me and to not want to get to know people who have hurt me so deeply. Another part of me, my higher self, wants you to do what you need to do to become a full human being. I want you to feel free to find out who these people are, and to have relationships with them if you want to, and to not feel tied by guilt.

Here's a big issue in my life: forgiveness. I have to tell you that I don't know a whole lot about it. I've struggled with a lot of resentment, and forgiveness is the other side of resentment. My natural tendency is to hold onto grudges and to anger.

So, who do I have to forgive? Well, I have to forgive my family. This is *really* a struggle for me. I think I've paid a very high price for wanting to punish my family. It's trite but true. My resentment eats me up. So, I'm actively struggling to not feel resentment for *my* sake because it makes *me* so much less. I'll be happy just to stop resenting people. If I could make it to forgiveness, that would be gravy. And I want you to know that to whatever extent this is impeding your life, I'm sorry for it.

Is there anything that you need to ask forgiveness for from Jaime?

Asking for forgiveness. *[Big sigh]* It's hard. *[Begins to weep]* Okay. You know, when you were little, I was so overwhelmed. I just couldn't cope, and I hadn't had enough therapy, and I didn't do a very good job. I used to get in these rages with you, and I don't know if you remember, but I know that it affected you. It's really important that you remember it, I think, so that you can dig it out of yourself. And I want you to know how sorry I am for the anger, and, I don't know, I just feel really bad. *[Crying]* I feel bad about it because you were always such a very sweet little boy, and I wasn't very loving to you sometimes. But I do love you. I do love you very much, and I want you to know that. That's all.

Carrie cried for a long time, and I was choked with sadness—for her suffering, for her son, for all parents who struggle to forgive themselves. When she had collected herself, I asked whether she had any closing messages for her son.

I know what I want to tell Jaime. For a long, long time, my life didn't feel like it was worth living, and it was filled with pain—enormous, gut-wrenching pain—and it doesn't feel that way any more. It's hard, and I struggle, and I get depressed sometimes, and sometimes I wish I could end it because I'm tired of feeling all these feelings. But life is a rich thing for me, and especially if I cannot be there to pass this on myself, what I want Jaime to know is, you don't give up. Keep struggling. Keep finding a way to make it start feeling good. It means you're going to have to give up certain things in yourself that you're real attached to. I've been very attached to my righteousness and victimization, and I've had to start giving those things up in order to feel the richness and beauty of life. So, I guess my message is, "Don't give up, and don't calcify. Don't harden. Keep yourself open, and get the help you need to become a happy person or a person who at least values life."

I want Jaime to see the positive things he gets from horrible situations, not just the pain. Even my early death, I now realize, could give him strength and resourcefulness. It might cause him to do something with his life that he might not otherwise do. Like, a nurse I talked to became a nurse because her father died when she was so young. She really gets connected to people. She honed that gift because she was so distraught by what happened to her when she was a kid. Out of that loneliness and pain came a great nurse.

So, Jaime, know that you may not always be able to see right now, as a child, how this seed is going to grow, but have some faith that something wonderful will happen from it. I have more faith in myself and in something beyond myself than I used to. I often feel like I'm getting just enough of what I need to keep going. There are definite times in my life when I feel guided or supported by something that I can't grasp but feel. You have to have that faith.

As Carrie ended this chapter of her story, I had an image of her standing at the edge of a cliff after a long, arduous journey, looking down on the huge boulder she has finally dropped. She is buoyant, ready to make another leap. I wondered if Jaime would ever understand what his mother had borne, how she had moved from fighting for her own life to teaching him to fight for his to letting him have his own life, separate from hers. Then, I remembered: He will have the tapes.

part THREE
Living Legacies: Being with Dying

THIRTEEN: WHEN THE TIME COMES

I HAVE COME to the country to write about death. With me always are the voices of mothers I've come to know: "Just let me get them through high school. Just give me another three, seven, ten years." Swept along by advancing illness, these women cling to markers of survival like trees that will save them from drowning.

What does it mean for a mother to let go before her work is done? If very sick mothers, like Tina, should have the right to stay alive even when they experience themselves as a burden to their families, what about the other side? Do mothers ever have permission to stop treatment? How do doctors, family, and friends respond when they do? Navigating my personal river of loss helps me bridge what is impossible to know firsthand.

In 1989, my eighty-one-year-old father wanted to die. The bone metastases from prostate cancer had reached the point of intolerable pain. He was no longer able to tend to himself. Broken bones from a fall provoked the final medical crisis. He lay in the hospital bed, unable to move without excruciating pain, and refused surgery. With my sister and me standing by, he told the oncologist that he wanted to die. "I need something more for the pain," he said. We had coached him to say the words that would give his doctors legal permission to increase the morphine until a coma was induced. Fortunately for my father, the oncologist agreed to support his decision.

But what about mothers still raising children? I am not talking about assisted suicide or euthanasia but rather refusing aggressive treatment, demanding nothing but palliative care to relieve pain and grant some quality of life. How do we feel, say, about a twenty-nine-year-old mother whose story has barely begun?

It is three years earlier, I am on my way to pick up Gloria Moore, a young African American woman who wants to be a nurse, who likes cooking, singing, and playing with her four children, nine months to nine years old. It's been less than a year since she was diagnosed with inflammatory breast cancer, a rare but aggressive, advanced form of the disease.[1] Gloria has already completed recording her life story with one of our listeners [2] but still wants to be interviewed about mothering through illness.

When I arrive, her cousin, who has come over to baby-sit, lets me into a tiny two-room apartment filled with the sounds of children's activity. Gloria is at the stove, preparing a bottle for the baby, who is propped on the sofa between two large pillows. She turns to greet me, but the baby begins to cry, and for a minute, all three of us just stand there. Gloria starts to move before lines of pain crease her face. She stops herself and says, "I can't pick him up, my side hurts too much." She nods to her cousin, who reaches for the baby. The morphine is clearly inadequate.

Gloria slumps into the passenger seat as we drive to a nearby office. Her eyes momentarily close beneath a baseball cap, visor cocked to the side over her bald head. She hugs an oversized, iridescent-green sports jacket to her chest. When we arrive and settle into the armchairs to begin the interview, she continues to shiver.

"My body is cold, and I stay cold a lot," she explains. "I can have two pairs of socks on, sweatpants, a T-shirt, a sweatshirt, and I'm still cold." Although it's seventy degrees outside, I turn on the heater.

Gloria recently had a mastectomy, believing it might relieve the pain in her breast. There is not much hope of arresting the advance of the disease, which has already spread to her chest wall. Chemotherapy is not working. The doctors are considering a bone marrow transplant, a second mastectomy, and removing her ovaries to reduce estrogen production in a last attempt to suppress tumor growth. They have drawn up the battle plan, but I see a gravely wounded soldier longing for sleep.

She was misdiagnosed two years earlier, when she first sought medical attention. "I wasn't listened to by the doctors when I told them something was wrong," she tells me. "I had a lump, and I was hurting. My great-grandmother and aunt had breast cancer in their thirties. I knew my body, and I kept telling them there was something wrong. They wouldn't give me a mammogram, said I was too young. I got pregnant 'cause no one told me not to. My breast turned hot and swelling. Red, burning. I couldn't stand the pain. There was something under my arm, too. Finally, I found a doctor who did a biopsy and told me I had cancer. I trust her. She gives me a fifty-fifty chance of making it."

I ask Gloria why she thinks she was misdiagnosed. "It's mainly because of Medi-Cal. When you're poor, it's hard—no matter what color you are. You could be white, Chinese, black, green, blue—if you don't have any money, you don't have any money, and you can't get services. Like now, my doctor was telling me that Medi-Cal wouldn't pay for a bone marrow transplant." She thinks for a minute and adds, "We're not rich, but we're rich with love and trying to understand things."

Gloria tells me about her mother's death of a brain aneurysm at the age of twenty-two, when she was six. "I know one day I'll have to die, but I always thought it would be when I was old. I didn't want my kids to go through the things that I went through, as far as loneliness and depression, wishing that I could have died with my mother. I was just heartbroken when she died. For a long time, I felt I didn't have anything to live for. I was always sad. You know, I could be playing, and I would start crying and say, 'I miss my mother, I want my mother.' She had no choice but to leave me, but that changed my life. I got into trouble a lot because I didn't want anyone telling me what to do.

"As I got to be a teenager, I grew out of it. I had wished that I had more sisters and brothers so that I wouldn't be alone, so I always said to myself that I would never have just one child. Then, when I started having my own kids, I was like, 'I have a lot to live for now.' I know my mother loved me, but I made a promise to myself that I would never leave my kids, no matter what, like my mother left me."

Gloria fulfilled her wish to have a large family, but she is reluctantly transforming her hope of raising her children to another one: that they will be raised together. "It's hard for anyone to take four kids.

My grandmother and great-grandmother are still living, but they are ill," she explains. She voices her desire for the children's father and his mother to take them. "I want to use the tapes to make a will and decide what to do."

Speaking to the children, Gloria affirms her desire to live, but her growing acceptance of death is also evident. "I'm twenty-nine years old, and this is not my choice to leave you guys behind. Remember I tried to beat this cancer. Remember I loved being your mother. I tried hard to live. It was just that I got this disease, and I couldn't beat it. But I'm going to try to stay here as long as I can."

Gloria talks about battling the disease—"If I die, I'm going to go down fighting. That's all I can say"—but I see little fight in her. I say, "It's obviously so hard for you now," and she agrees and takes it further: "Having kids makes me fight harder, but it doesn't help me cope any better. You have some mothers with cancer that can still move and take their kids places and do a lot of things. But I wasn't that lucky. I can hardly care for them. Cancer is a lot of pain. I'm trying to deal with it, but I'm tired.

"Sometimes I don't feel like I'm going to make it at all. It hurts. My stomach cramps a lot from the chemo. I don't eat. My body's worn out from chemo. I was already anemic. Sometimes I have to have the heater at ninety degrees in the house just to get warm." She shivers and hugs the jacket closer. "You know, you have to worry about everything. I could have peace now if I knew for sure my kids would be well taken care of, if I knew exactly how they'd be raised, who would love them. If I wasn't a mom, I wouldn't try to fight as hard as I am now."

Gloria reaches for a tissue as tears roll down her face. "I wouldn't go through the bone marrow transplant. I wouldn't worry because I have nothing else to leave behind in this world. Everybody gives me support to keep fighting. When I first found out I had cancer, my cousins would tell me, 'Stop crying because there's people worse off than you.' Yes, people are worse off than me, but I did not expect to get sick. So, yes, I'm going to cry about it."

She puts her head in her hands and sobs. I hit the pause button and wait.

"Then, sometimes, I catch myself telling my aunt and family, 'I don't know if I'm going to be here too much longer,' because that's how I feel. I said the other night that the Lord gave me a boy because I guess He knew I wasn't going to be here much longer. I had three girls. My family tells me, 'Oh, be quiet, you're not going anyplace.' But they don't know how I feel. They're trying to make me have a positive attitude." Gloria moves slightly and winces, points to her side. "This is where it hurts me."

On the return trip, she speaks about the people in her church, how no one lets her talk about dying or gives her permission to stop treatment. I want to say, "Gloria, it's okay to surrender," but I stop myself. I'm peripheral to her life and aware of how easy it is to undermine a person's will to live. Instead, I nod sympathetically, and after a few minutes, her head drops for a nap.

Thinking about Gloria's situation hurts. It makes me angry at the injustices of poverty that delayed her diagnosis and treatment, angry at the doctors who may be trying to make up for negligent medical care by overtreating her with surgeries and protocols that will most likely do little to prolong her life. I'm angry at the people who deny her reality in order to protect themselves. And I'm frightened—for Gloria, for her children, for all young women, including my daughter.

Memories of my father's dying weave in and out, too. I realize that I held my tongue with Gloria partly because of my own bias toward release, a result of the anguish, impatience, and guilt I felt when the death he desired—rapid, painless—didn't happen. My sister and I stood on either side of the bed while the doctor increased the morphine drip and then departed. My father smiled, closed his eyes, and waited. And waited. And after a number of hours, he awoke with a start to gasp in pain and outrage, "Why am I still here?" The oncologist had left for the weekend; the on-call physicians would not increase the drip. We had lost control.

My father's death, the first I had attended, taught me that death holds the same mystery, drama, risk, and discovery as birth. And dying can be a long, hard labor. Stopping treatment and ramping up the meds do not always insure a speedy delivery. I also saw how far I was from knowing how to support a dying person and decided it was time to face my fears and learn about one of life's greatest experiences.

I began attending workshops on critical illness, death and dying, and healing, and I participated in hospice trainings from various traditions. The more I learned, the more I understood that no one can predict the power of the survival instinct; no one can know in advance one's response to the ethical, psychological, and spiritual knots that can appear during the dying process. Study, training, and practice are valuable, but being with dying is an altogether humbling apprenticeship in which there are no experts. Still, we can think about death, speak about it, and try to be aware of our emotions and judgments so as not to impose them on others.

When Gloria wakes, I carefully try to hold both sides of her conflict: her stated desire to fight and her equally strong impulse to quit. I tell her I believe that either is a valid choice and her choice alone. But I'd like her to realize that she has the right to let go if she wishes, even at twenty-nine, even with four kids.

Gloria had not yet entered her dying time, but death was there, the silent witness goading me to explore my reactions. I was glad that I had learned enough to contain my own biases, but I could not counter those of her family, which were causing her to suffer more. Almost everyone seems to feel that if the ill person refuses more treatments, however questionable the effectiveness or high the risk, she can be blamed for her own decline. For a mother, the added implication is that she is failing her children.

Family members, friends, and other cancer patients understandably want to avoid talking about death. Most of us worry that doing so will undermine the will to live, will be a burden to the sick person, or will unleash more grief than is bearable for everyone involved. We don't want to be reminded of the unthinkable, which ill mothers represent. That mothers can die before children are grown is dangerously close to what is generally considered the worst death, when children die before their parents. In all cultures, people reel at a reversal in the expected order of things.

What is unthinkable is unspeakable, as Gloria found and as the many mothers in our project have repeatedly stated. But silence magnifies fear, increases isolation, and drains energy. Ill parents who can't talk about their feelings or who find their tentative forays at honest communication rejected are not well equipped to help children talk about their own. Parents who are isolated during crises are less able to mobilize resources for themselves and their families.

I have spoken with many people whose mothers died during their childhoods and whose families responded with a conspiracy of silence. Silence kept their mothers from acknowledging encroaching death and rendered them unable to express to their children the words of love, concern, and advice that could have brought some consolation. Silence kept the children in the dark about what was happening and unable to talk to others about what they were experiencing. Both the children and their mothers suffered unnecessarily because everyone avoided the subject.

Connie, whose mother died thirty-two years earlier, when she was five, says: "I would have killed to receive a manuscript or set of tapes or even a letter, a note, *anything* from my mother. It would have changed my life to have known something about her, to have read or heard her words of love for me. I knew nothing. No one talked. No one talked about it when she was sick. No one talked about it when she was dying. Or after she died.

"I have a few random memories. I remember her making me hot chocolate in the kitchen once. I remember her putting me to bed once. I remember that she had sweater-and-skirt outfits and pearls that they wore in the sixties, but that's it. The day after she died, the Goodwill truck came, and everything went. We weren't allowed to talk about her. Everyone would start and then stop. You know, they would sort of say, 'Oh, she was such a great woman,' and then sigh and trail off.

When someone dies and people *do* talk about them, it's always in the most glowing terms. Years later, someone who had known my mother told me, 'Well, you look like your mom, but you have nicer skin. Your mother had big pores.' I was so excited about that detail because it was the first honest, unfiltered statement someone had ever made about her. It wasn't candy-coated: 'Oh, she died, we can't say she had big pores.' I ran to tell my sisters."

Robin was eleven when her mother died of breast cancer. She wrote to me: "Who a parent is is a core part of who their children will become. Without the personal knowledge, memories, and guidance of a parent lost to illness, there is a gap left that will never be filled. Years later, relatives told me that the thing that hurt her most was that there was so much more to teach me that I could not understand at the age of eleven. At least some of my mother's pain could have been alleviated if she had been given a way to leave her legacy for us to receive when we were ready."

Children need to know what is happening around them in terms that are appropriate to their age. Most parents need to unburden their hearts and tell. Unfortunately, what a culture deems unspeakable seems shameful, setting up the ill for self-reproach. Our belief in medical science and in technology's unlimited ability to control nature makes humiliation the lot of those whose diseases cannot be cured. And there are some new twists.

Growing scientific evidence of the body-mind connection and of lifestyle factors affecting health have spawned alternative philosophies and healing practices, some of which may influence the prevention and treatment of illness. However, there is a downside to the belief that we can make ourselves sick and, with the right attitude, make ourselves well.[3] Emotions and thoughts are but one part of the cause of or recovery from disease. Still, it's hard to stop believing in the god of control. The sicker people become, the more desperate the need to believe. Those who can't control the disease often suffer feelings of failure and guilt that are passed on as a dark legacy to children, who, in turn, assume responsibility.

Many mothers newly diagnosed with cancer believe, and are told by others in both overt and subtle ways, that they must have done something wrong. They waited too long to have children, they neglected to breastfeed, they were too angry, depressed, or stressed. They weren't emotional enough, or they were too emotional. Women whose cancer recurs after some years in remission feel that they let everyone down by failing to defeat the disease. Perhaps they didn't meditate enough. Ate the wrong diet. Had too much treatment, or too little. And dying mothers—often after suffering years of arduous treatments, living in pain, and with no realistic hope of recovery—desperately try one aggressive protocol after another, even when they clearly want to stop. They are afraid that they might be accused of not trying hard enough to stay alive for their children, that dying makes them selfish.

Who is giving these messages? Many of us. Well-meaning family members and friends become cheerleaders to the dying of any age: "Don't stop fighting, never give up, don't let go." Oncologists are sometimes the ones to push the hardest, not always because they believe that the extreme treatments will help but because they cannot accept defeat.[4] For mothers with dependent children, the pressures are intensified, internally and externally.

One mother told me that her doctor was "miffed with her" because she had refused a stem-cell rescue. "They all believe, 'Keep trying, keep trying,' but I don't believe in it. The oncologists have an agenda to give out chemicals no matter what. The chances of a bone marrow transplant working for me are slim to none. A doctor I saw at Stanford admitted that was true. It makes your last time worse and may drive you to the grave sooner. It would be more damaging for my kids to see me as a vegetable. I'd rather live three months less and have good, quality time."

In another twist, advances in early detection and the proliferation of services like support groups, however welcome, can be spun to the detriment of the patient, pushing both facts and feelings underground. Overly upbeat and hopeful messages from cancer organizations tend to obscure a number of unpalatable facts. Jude exulted that cancer is now a chronic disease and that women are *living* with cancer. That is true. But Jude added the words "not dying with cancer." Unfortunately, that is false. Women are still dying of cancer and in large numbers; an estimated 275,000 will die of the disease in 2005.[5] Breast cancer is the leading cause of cancer death for American women between the ages of fifteen and fifty-four, prime childbearing and childrearing years.[6] And there are nearly 250,000 women under forty living with breast cancer; close to fourteen hundred die each year.[7]

Advances in medicine have led to overly optimistic messages, whether motivated by politics, economics, or psychology. To cite one example, the omnipresent public-service message that early detection of breast cancer saves lives is, as Musa Mayer points out, not false but simplistic. The message helps many women overcome their fear and get screened but lulls them into false security.[8] Some cancer activists remind us that all the upbeat hype deflects attention from seeking the causes of cancer or a cure.[9]

Many parents of young children continue to die from many cancers and other diseases. All want to be treated as alive until they die. They don't want their hope or will to live undermined, but they also want their darker feelings acknowledged. And sometimes, when treatments are no longer effective, when the disease has spread beyond control, they might want permission to let nature take its course.

Is there ever an acceptable time for a mother to die? What does it mean for her to let go before her children are grown? How can she find some peace?

Dr. Ira Byock, hospice physician and author of *Dying Well* and *The Four Things That Matter Most,* has worked out a schema describing the developmental tasks of dying.[10] Among them are tasks that the MLS project has facilitated from the beginning through our living stories. These include a life review, the telling of one's stories, the transmission of knowledge and wisdom, and expressions of gratitude, love, and forgiveness. Mothers in the project typically touch the five messages Dr. Byock and many hospice workers believe help the dying separate from their loved ones: "Forgive me. I forgive you. Thank you. I love you. Goodbye."[11]

Negotiating the final separation from those we love and from life is daunting under the most favorable circumstances—having lived to old age, having sufficient resources, having good medical care and pain control, and being at home, surrounded by loved ones. *Dying Well* is filled with moving stories in which men and women of various ages and life situations have found, with the help of hospice, a way to enjoy quality of life and dignity in their final months. With one exception.

During a telephone conversation with Dr. Byock, I remarked that the only person in the book who didn't seem to die "well" was a young mother. She fought to the last inch of her life and suffered immensely because she could not bear to leave her children. If death requires the dissolution of our roles and release of relationships, those defined by mothering may be the hardest to relinquish.

A compassionate man, Byock spoke carefully. "I know what you mean," he said. "I've had to rethink what it means to die well so that we don't set up some new ideal of a good death. I've come to think that dying well is dying in your own way, whatever that is."[12]

I appreciated his words, having already seen so much needless damage done to women by standards of perfection in childbearing and childrearing. And now we have "the good death," although most physicians will acknowledge that a good death is not always possible. Just as not all lives are well lived, not all deaths will be positive experiences. I was thinking of Gloria and mothers whose suffering can become unbearable. I was also thinking of myself and other caregivers who want to do the right thing for a dying person.

What helps any of us do the work of letting go? An eighty-four-year-old listener, Virginia Jouris, said, "It's not just about the dying, it's about the living. Are you even present for life? Some of the young moms are so busy trying to do anything to stay alive that there is no life left. A desperate approach to the situation is not necessarily a positive approach. But who can judge? You do the best that you can. You do what you do. Nobody knows the right way. You don't kill hope, but beyond a certain point, hope for a miracle or cure becomes grotesque. The mother needs permission to let go so that she doesn't have to fight to the very last breath."

And yet. Some mothers will fight to the last, and there may be dignity and meaning in that, too. In the Old Testament, Rachel refuses to be comforted as she dies in childbirth. Scholar Aviva Zornberg writes that Rachel's refusal, her insistence on remaining conscious of her children's suffering, constitutes the work of faith in this world, a "painful radiance," "a tragic optimism."[13] I wondered whether I would meet a mother who personified such faith.

The central task of dying is letting go, which is also a core task of parenthood. In some ways, parenthood is a bulwark against loss and death. Children tie us to the past, ground us in the present, continue us into the future. While raising dependent children, parents, too, depend on their youngsters: to confer purpose, value, and identity, and to connect them to life through bonds of responsibility and love. But parenthood is also a constant lesson in letting go, in loss. Our extended dependency insures that we form intense attachments. The process of living insures that there will be significant leavings. Parents raise children to release them to their separate lives.

Children look to parents to show them how to live, how to love, and how to go on after loss. The culture offers parents little guidance. Storyteller and psychotherapist Clarissa Pinkola Estes says: "Yet love in its fullest form is a series of deaths and rebirths. . . . To love means to embrace and at the same time to withstand many many endings, and many many beginnings—all in the same relationship. Our culture courts death but doesn't dance with it with grace or wit—as do other species."[14]

Deena Metzger explains that our cultural response to death is polarized. There is utter denial at one end, and at the other, an extreme, sometimes perverse fascination with the images of violent death that assault us every day: Columbine High, earthquakes, kidnapping, war. But there is no real meeting with ordinary death—the one that will most likely happen to you, me, and the people we know.[15] In America, death always seems to happen to someone else somewhere else, anywhere but in our own homes.

We may never be comfortable with the idea of mortality or be able to comprehend the end of physical life. But ignoring death makes it more dreadful. We need to invite death into the room because it's usually better to court the part of us that is terrified than to be throttled by it. We need to become acquainted with the dying process because parents and children alike will eventually face it. We need to accept what we can't control and control what we can, which is to insure that those left behind are not overburdened and utterly unprepared financially and emotionally. We need to invite death in to ameliorate the suffering that *not* facing it causes the ill and dying, who may be the people we love the most. By acknowledging death, talking about it, and planning for it, we can soften the hard facts of life for our children and enlarge our sense of life's value and preciousness.

Still, there is never a good time to lose a mother. My own mother died at the age of eighty-four, having lived in a nursing home for years with senile dementia. I had released her long before, but my grief when she died was no less acute, and I was close to fifty. "Come back!" I wanted to say. "Just let me ask you all the questions I never bothered to ask. Let me tell you how much you meant to me."

Every once in a while, my twenty-five-year-old daughter, who is living on her own, reminds me of her need for me. A few months after the 9/11 attacks, I suggested that I fly to Chicago, where she was living. I hardly got the word "fly" out of my mouth before she said, only half joking: "No mothers in the air now! No mothers in the air!"

If not at fifty and not at twenty-five, how can a mother's death be acceptable when the children are fifteen or three? And what does that mean for mothers who have reached the point where they must let go? These women have grappled with the tasks of dying, as we all must. But they have had the additional challenge of separating from young children, recognizing the magnitude of the loss to themselves and to the offspring they expected to raise to adulthood. The horror and the gift of cancer for them is that they are confronted with teaching their children about a life that is large enough to include mortality. What can we learn from them?

We begin with Leona Reardon, whose ability to choose to stop treatment, to release her child, and to be conscious and whole in her dying stunned me. Before meeting Leona, I had not realized that dying people could be active participants until the very end. I had not known that even when a person has decided to stop all treatment or has received a terminal prognosis, and even when immersion in symptoms progresses and the body fails, the person can continue to contribute to family and community, sometimes for many months. I had not understood that a home in which death is a presence can be filled with living or that the acceptance of imminent death can make one's time richer. Leona was the first in a series of women to show me my uninformed assumptions.

Fourteen: "A Soul on Vacation"
Leona Reardon

LEONA REARDON TELLS me she has just tried and rejected an extreme alternative treatment even though she understands the consequences of that decision: There will be no other treatment options. "I've decided to stop taking everything that's going to make me sick. I'm not going to do anything that is going to be arduous or painful. I've concluded that this is a lost battle. I've watched people use up life chasing after things that don't help them. The strain of trying to survive has become harder than letting go. You'd better come soon."

In starting the project, I had known that confronting mortality could help us live more fully in the present. But I needed a teacher, and I found her in the project's first Mothering Through Cancer support group. Leona had been a regular participant until she became too ill to leave home. At one of the last meetings she attended, she said that she had created a book to help her three-year-old son, Gabriel, talk about her illness, as well as videotapes and other documents as a legacy for him. She and her partner, Claire, had also put together an extensive support network. Leona told me she'd be happy to share what she had done and even offered to help the project by doing some fundraising. Her overture was a surprise, the first of many. I knew she had a fast-moving colon cancer.

The night before our interview, I awake at 2 AM from a dream that some horror is going on in the next room. I don't know what it is, only that it is dangerous and dreadful. My fear of death has entered the house.

I ring Leona's doorbell the next morning with both anticipation and dread. Claire greets me and leads me into a modest bungalow filled with the smell of simmering soup and the sounds of women working. We enter a bedroom at the end of the hall, where Leona is lying propped up on a stack of rose-colored pillows, facing a bureau covered with an array of family photos. Her face is pinker and her body smaller than I remembered. The only signs of illness are the medications on her nightstand and her slight grimace when she moves.

We have two hours before Gabriel returns from preschool, and so we begin.

When the tape recorder is set up, I ask her why at this point in her life she would be willing to grant an interview. Her answer is simple: "I've had a good life." Eyes shining, voice clear and composed, in spite of childhood polio leaving a serious limp; a home far removed from her South African family of origin; being socially marginalized due to her identity as a lesbian and convert to Judaism; and now, at forty-four, dying of cancer.

LEONA

I feel that I have had a fabulous life. The only thing I haven't done is as much community service as I would have liked. This interview is a way for me to address that. It's been pretty clear to me in talking to people that I have experience that other people find useful. The women in the group didn't have as extensive a support system, some didn't have *anything*. Not only didn't they have it, but they didn't think they *could* have it, and they didn't know how to do it. They think that they don't know anybody, but it's almost never true. And they don't know how to ask.

Having the support that I had has enabled me to prepare my family. I wish the project's help with recording my story had been available to me when I first got sick. It's fundamental for mothers to be supported.

Leona adjusts her position, sips some water, and begins her cancer story.

It first presented as an ovarian cyst. When they found that the cyst was cancerous, they looked around and found a tumor in my colon. Who knows how long it had been there? Colon cancer doesn't present symptoms, or people don't catch the symptoms, and by the time I started chemotherapy last year, I already had secondaries in the liver. It was a very quick progression from "This is not a big deal" to "Oh, geez, this is a very big deal." I thought at that time that I would die within five years, and I tried really hard not to. My family wanted to believe that I could overcome it, but the survival rate of colon cancer with secondaries is, like, one percent.

One of the major issues for me when I was first diagnosed was that Gabriel was so young. He was actually a little shy of two and three-quarters, a baby, really. He didn't have a lot of mechanisms for coping with this. I had talked to him when I was first diagnosed. He knew that we were upset, so it was important for him to participate in the process. He had been very, very upset about me being hospitalized, so I said to him, "You know, it seems like you have a lot of worries. Why don't we make a book about this?" And he was thrilled. He said, "Yes, let's do that, but the first page has to be a picture of you throwing up."*[Laughs]*

I had started him in September in a preschool, and the teacher had sent him home at one point with a storybook called *When Mommy is Sick* that she had been reading to him and that he wanted to read over and over again. Books were a way to make his worries concrete so he could get a handle on them.

We went together to the store, and he picked out a notebook, and then we bought stickers and some cards. I said to him, "Do you think these are good worry pictures?" Mostly we bought pictures that he picked out. Then I got out magazines and family photographs, and we spread them all over the table, and we got scissors and glue. He wanted a picture of me throwing up, so I cut out a picture of me, and we made a little drawing, and it was very graphic. *[Laughs]*

I said to him, "Okay, so here's the picture of me throwing up. What would you like to put on the next page?" He wanted to put his worries on the next page. He picked out pictures of frogs and bats and scary animals, and I made a drawing of a scary worry for him, and he gave me the noises, "This one says 'agggrrrrr,' and that one . . . " Then I said, "What do you think we should do about these worries? This is a lot of worries." He said, "Well, we should make you better." And I said, "Well, how do you think we could do that?" He said, "With glue." So we did a little picture of that with flower stickers.

I wanted it to be *his* book about when I'm sick. It's not slick and understandable. It's a two-year-old's attempt to cope with this. He still drags it out and shows it to people: "This is my book. I made this book, and this will help you understand Mommy's illness." He said to me recently that we need to do some more work on it, so it's been a great tool for him. It's something he has added to in ways that make no sense to me but obviously have some meaning to him.

When I went for surgery, I explained to him that I would be going to the hospital but that he could come see me. Then, I had taken him with me to register where they do the pre-op stuff because I wanted him to know where I was. Claire brought him to visit two or three days later. He was totally freaked out until he realized that he could make the bed go up and down, and then he was fine. It was a rocket ship, and it was cool. I was so seasick when he left, but, you know, he loved it. So I cut out a picture of him and put it on the bed, and he said, "Gabriel came to visit Mommy in the hospital, but he didn't bring his worries because they didn't deserve to come." So we didn't put any worries on that page.

I brought him with me to the oncologist, not for the first visit but after so he knew who she was, and I also brought him with me to chemo. He was really worried about chemo—he thought they were going to hurt me. So I took him with me, and then he caught on that chemo was really a place where you go and you sit in these big recliners and watch *Snow White* and, hey, you know, this is very cool. . . .

By making the book, Leona was helping Gabriel create a story to hold him through the illness. I was curious about what had impelled her to begin preparing other stories to hold him after her death.

It started because as a parent, the only thing you can do is prepare your child for life, and if they screw it up, they screw it up, and it's not your fault. But you have to do your best to prepare them for the real world, however you interpret that. And so, when I realized that it was likely that I was going to die soon, I started working hard on ways to prepare Gabriel for life without me. I felt that was my obligation as a parent to make death normal, to have the kinds of conversations that one doesn't normally have with a three- or four-year-old because, you know, it's sad, but it really is part of his life. I feel a responsibility to make the transition as comfortable for him as possible. I don't think it will be easy, but I think that there are a lot of things I could do to make it less traumatic for him.

I have always written Gabriel letters because I was forty when he was born, and I thought the chances are pretty high that I could die before he was forty or before he thinks to ask questions that I now ask my parents. When I was diagnosed, I realized that writing letters wasn't enough and that I needed to start thinking about conversations that I wasn't going to be able to have with him. Also, I realized when I was on chemo that I had no brain, and whereas I could lie on the couch and talk into the camera, I really couldn't write, and I didn't want to. I was tired.

One of the things I thought right away was, "Geez, he's so young, he's not going to remember me." I borrowed a camera and made videotapes because I wanted him to know what I looked like and what I sounded like. I didn't have a plan, but I had things I wanted to talk about. One of the things I really want him to know is that he didn't make me ill, that he can't do anything about it, that it isn't his fault, that however often and passionately he has wished that I would die in the last year, I know that he loves me.

There were things that I know about his father I wanted him to have access to. He'll know Claire, and Claire has certainly been a parent to him. But he doesn't know his father, and if I die, he won't have that biological connection.

Kent Nerburn wrote a book called *Letters to My Son*, which I had bought a while back before I was ill because I figured there would be things that men wanted to talk to their sons about that I hadn't a clue. And indeed there are. I wanted to talk to him about what it means to be a Jew. I also wanted to talk to him about the fact that he's a Jew, and the rest of my family is not Jewish, and why we made that decision for him. It comes from Claire's Jewish background. When we were deciding to have children, we agreed that we would raise our children as Jews because that's how we lived but also because we figured Claire would have the kids. And then, when *I* was pregnant, I started thinking, "Oy, we really have to think about this in a different light."

War was something I wanted to talk to him about. When you have a son, you think about that. I do, anyway. I wanted to give him a history of my life because I've had a fabulous and interesting life. I was born in Africa, grew up at the end of the British Empire, and saw the British Empire disintegrate. It was real to me; it wasn't a piece of history. These are things that I think he probably won't be interested in until he's in his thirties or forties. I figure Claire will know when he should get them.

I realized that I was making tapes about issues that were important to *me*. I had made tapes about a lot of adult subject matter, but I wasn't going to be around when he was a teenager, and that's a really difficult time, and I wanted to acknowledge and talk to him about that. And I hadn't done anything for him *now*. So I started making audiotapes of stories.

I started with stories that he likes now as a three-year-old, and they've been sort of getting older. We're reading nursery stories now and just starting to read chapter books. I'm going to read him *The Flame Trees of Thika*. It's something that reflects my life and that Claire wouldn't think to read to him because it's about a child growing up in the part of Africa that I grew up in. I probably will do *Treasure Island*, I'll do Sholom Aleichem . . .

I started reading stories on tape to him so that he can have my voice. I have given him some of the tapes already so that this isn't something that happens and he thinks, "Oh, Mommy now lives in my 'radidio,'" *[Laughs]*, that he understands that this is a tape. We've done some videotaping together. He's seen those, and he'll have those. I left the other videos with Claire. I put them in the safety deposit box, and I have told Claire to get them copied so if we lose one set, we keep another set somewhere else.

I have written him letters for life-cycle events because I think that children are really resilient, but they get to their bar mitzvah or wedding or graduation, and the grief recurs. "Oh, God, I wish Mom could have seen the baby or met my wife." So, I bought him a present for his bar mitzvah. I bought him a *tallis*[1] because I couldn't think of anything else that wouldn't be totally out of date by the time, that wouldn't embarrass him half to death. It was very difficult to figure out, you know, do you go with the magenta, or do you go with the traditional blue-and-white and hope that . . . Oy, who knows?

And I wrote him a story. There's a *midrash*[2] that when God spoke at Sinai, each of the people heard the voice of God as the voice of that person's mother—God spoke in each person's mother's voice so that the people wouldn't be afraid. I've always really loved that. So I wrote that I had bought him this *tallis*, and when he wraps himself in it, he should know that I am there and that I want to participate in that event.

Leona momentarily whispers and becomes teary, the only time during our meeting. She pauses briefly, then smiles.

I said to him, "You know, I hope that you will hear my voice as part of the service." And who knows? He'll be thirteen, he'll be thinking . . . Oy, who knows what he'll be thinking? He may be thinking, "Oh, my God, you bought the blue one. Do I have to wear this?" And Claire will say, "Absolutely," because that's what she's like.

Have you written any other letters?

I did one for his bar mitzvah, one for his graduation from high school, one for his marriage if he chooses to get married, one for the birth of his first child if he chooses to have one, and I think that may be all. I wrote to him about events I thought would be times when he would miss me. I know that when I was pregnant, the first person I wanted to tell was my mother, before anybody, even though I knew my mother would be appalled—and she was *[Laughs]*—but, you know, it was this totally irrational thing.

I wanted to write to him about who I think he is and what I think is important. He's incredibly bright, but college is not important to me about who he is. I care whether he's kind and compassionate and self-supporting. Recently, I told a woman that I used to work with that I had done these things, and she said, "What an interesting *process* to write to him at these ages when you have no idea who he will be." And I said, "Yeah, I know, I really won't." "But how wonderful because in those letters, you are revealing yourself to him in different ways." I hadn't thought about it like that. It was a nice way to put it.

You've put together things that most people don't think about. Did you come up with these ideas on your own?

When I was pregnant, I was conscious of the fact that one's children are unique and separate people. They don't belong to us. I was aware that it was a privilege to raise a child and an incredible responsibility. When we chose to have a child, we made a commitment that we were going to put this child's needs first. And it seemed apparent to me when I became ill that he needed this kind of preparation. He needed somebody to make his life bearable in the absence of both his biological parents. I realized at a certain point, he's no worse off than a lot of kids who were adopted. In some ways, he's better off because he's actually known me. *[Laughs]* I don't know if that's better or worse, who knows. . . .

About six weeks ago, I started having Gabriel see a child psychologist, not because he seems disturbed but because I felt that he needed a safe place to act out whatever traumas he was experiencing. And one of the moms from Gabriel's playgroup put together a meeting with the psychologist, Carl, so that he could talk to them about how they and their children could support Gabriel, which I felt was an incredible gift. He was going to be a pain in the ass sometimes; I didn't want him excluded.

Hordes of people went to it. I did not go, but apparently it was very informative for a lot of people. I remember having this discussion before I was ill—one of the moms said to me that when they watch the video of *The Lion King*, they always fast-forward where the dad dies. I thought, "Why?" What a bizarre thing to do. But I know that some people can't cope with death, and they don't want their young children to deal with it. God knows, it wouldn't have been my choice, but I have made a point of making use of things like that with Gabriel. "What did you think when Simba's daddy died? Simba wondered, 'Where did Dad go?' What do *you* think happened to him?"

I've met many mothers, family members, and health professionals who become anxious about preparing a will or legacy, thinking it will hasten death. It sounds as if you haven't engaged in that kind of magical thinking.

Well, Gabriel does that for us, he's very good at that. *[Laughs]* I guess I think about that. "If I do this, I'll die. . . ." Right. I understand that feeling 'cause when I was diagnosed, I really did think, "I am going to die." And I kept thinking, "Oh, boy, you mustn't think that way because if you think that way, you *will*." Eventually, I gave up on that. I finally came to, "Okay, if I don't die and I do an ethical will or whatever, what's the worst that can happen? I'll have an ethical will—terrific. If I do die, I'll be prepared, and I won't have this anxiety to cope with on top of everything else."

I started making the tapes with the idea that Gabriel and I would sit around at sixteen or seventeen, and he'd say how completely off the wall I was to raise these issues, and we would laugh about it. That thought helped me when I made them. Maybe it will help others, too.

Most people can't do this alone, but they can do it. I say to people, "Okay, so if you don't do this and you don't die, no big deal. But if you don't do this and you die . . . whew." Everyone who can gets health insurance. They don't *not* get health insurance because they might get sick. It seems like the same thing. I mean, all this hysteria about Princess Diana, but the thing that I kept thinking was, *Here's a woman who has two small children and didn't get to say goodbye.*[3] And I did. I can say with all honesty I am not worried about my child. What an incredible gift, you know.

Leona is clearly unusual in her ability to face death and to leave behind a child without excessive worry—and to prepare without help. I ask her what she thinks that ability is due to.

I think two things. When I die, my child will still have a mother that he's had since birth, so that's a big part of it right there. I would be much more beside myself if I did not have a partner who was a woman because wonderful as dads are, I think young children need a mother.

And the other part of it is: I have done as much as I can do to make this an okay experience for my child. I have prepared him as well as I possibly can. I have prepared my family because I realize that it's not just about preparing him. It's about preparing other people.

I wrote a letter to my family recently, talking to them about funeral arrangements. I have arranged to die at home. I want Gabriel to have access to my body for as long as he wants because if he chooses to go to the cemetery, I want him to be clear that when they bury me, I'm not there, I don't live in my body anymore. If you spend any time around someone who has died, you really get it that the person is gone, and I want him to know that. But if I didn't prepare my family for that, they would be shocked.

I also realized that Claire and I have talked to Gabriel a lot about what is happening, about what happens after you die, but I hadn't said to my family, "What we've told him basically is when you die, you don't come back." He's very magical about that: "I'm going to make you come alive again. When I grow up, I'm going to be magic." I have been very clear with him all the way down the line that you couldn't make me sick, and you can't make me well. When people die, they do not come back.

The other thing that I wanted my family to know is that I have said to him, "When people die, we don't really know what happens. Some people think you have another life, some people think you go to heaven, some people think whatever." I said to my family, "He may talk to you about these things, and if you want to tell him what you think, feel free, but make sure that he knows that this is what *you* think. This is not the definitive answer. I want him to know that we don't know."

Somebody offered a while back to give us an aquarium for Gabriel, and Claire said, "Just what we need, something else to take care of," and I said, "No. We should do this because the fish will die, and Gabriel gets to practice being sad. Indeed, the fish died, and he wanted to see the body, he wanted to touch the body, he wanted to have a funeral, he wanted to sing *Happy Birthday*, he wanted to say, "Fluffy, you were a wonderful fish. I love you," whatever. And the first funeral he goes to isn't mine, and that, I think, will be very good for him. Maybe he'll decide not to go to the funeral. One of the things that his psychologist said is that we should follow his lead—with all of the children. I've known the kids in his playgroup since they were born. It was a baby group originally, one of those only in the Bay Area, where all the moms are Jewish lesbians. *[Laughs]*

You talked briefly with me on the phone about losing the battle with cancer. What does Gabriel know about that now?

I feel really good about where Gabriel is right now. I'm *sure* he knows that I will die because he came to the door yesterday morning and said, "Oh, Mommy's dead," and I said, "No, I'm not, we told you we would tell you," and he said, "Oh, thank God, because you are very important to me."

So, he knows. I have always answered his questions, and I have never gone beyond what he has asked. A couple of nights ago, he said, "Mommy, how come we eat in your bedroom now and you never go to the table anymore?" I said, "Well, it's hard for me to get up and sit at the table for a long time." And he said, "How come?" "Because it makes me very tired, and I don't feel very well." I don't tell him that it hurts because I know he worries. So I said to him, "I want to eat with everybody, and it's easier for me if we eat in the bedroom." I stayed with why we don't eat in the dining room. He was quiet for a while, and I said, "Is there anything else you want to ask me about that?" And he said, "No." So, fine.

He has said off and on over this year, "Are you going to die?" Initially, I said to him, "People do die of cancer, but I am trying really hard not to, and some people don't, so we don't know." I've always said to him, "If it changes, I will tell you." More recently, he started saying, "Are you going to die *soon*?" And I have said to him, "No, I'm not going to die soon," because if I die in two weeks, it's a long time for him and I don't want him sitting around being anxious. I have said to him, "If Mama and I think that I'm going to die soon, one of us will tell you so you won't be surprised." I'm Mommy, and Claire's Mama, and we get confused, and he never does. His psychologist said, "There may come a point where you can't tell him. You need to not make that promise." So I've switched to, "*One of us* will tell you."

You've made a decision to die at home. Many mothers feel that they want to protect their children from seeing so much suffering. How have you reconciled that for yourself?

First of all, you can't protect your child from life. Dying is part of living, and that's a risk every child takes when they're born. My decision to die at home was based on the fact that it would be logistically very difficult for Claire if I were in a hospital. She would either have to shlep him back and forth or find childcare, and I thought that was an added stress that she didn't need.

Another big part of it was that I feel that if you prepare children, they can cope with death. What is really traumatic, I think, is "Mommy goes away and doesn't come back, we don't see her for days, we don't know what happened, we don't know where she went." I have said to Claire, "When I die, you will be very busy. If you have someone come and take Gabriel out to play or whatever—because he's going to be a drag and also because he's going to need to go out—you need to prepare him so that he doesn't come home and find that I'm not here anymore. You need to say to him, 'So-and-so's going to take you to the park. When you come home, Mommy may be gone.' Then, give him the option: 'Do you want to stay until Mommy's gone, or do you want to go now and take your chances?' Because he can say that."

I'm really fortunate that my child is very good at articulating what he wants. Children don't lie at this age. And about this kind of stuff, I don't think they ever lie if you give them the opportunity and they feel like they won't be censured.

Is there more you still feel you need to prepare for Gabriel?

There is always more. I have a tremendous sense of peace because I realized somewhere along the line that there would never be a good time. I went about thinking, "God, this is so terrible, my child is so young, this is such an awful time to die," and then I thought, "Yeah, but if he were older, he would be entering puberty, he would be getting bar mitzvahed, he would be getting married, having babies, getting divorced. . . . So, at a certain point, I realized that there is never going to be a good time, there would always be things undone because there just *are*.

What I have done—and I think this *is* important—I have been able to prioritize what I wanted to do. I made Gabriel the priority, which I think was hard on Claire, but I know it was the right thing to do because Claire and I have had fifteen years together. She knows a lot about what I think, and he doesn't. So, I did everything I wanted to do for him first, and then I did what I wanted to do for Claire. I'm still in that process.

This is something that parents may want to do. I have talked with Claire extensively about the fact that we parent in very different ways. They're complementary, but I do different things than she does, and I have different strengths. I have written down for her a lot of the conversations that we have had about parenting because I know that she will forget.

I watch them bicker. When I was first ill, they were just bickering up and down, and I thought, "I'm never going to be able to die because these two will kill each other." *[Laughs]* And then I realized they had to learn to work this out, and they have. That's just part of their *meshugas*[4].

One of the most important things that I have said to Claire about parenting is, "Make him a partner in how you parent him. It's inevitable at some point, he is going to turn around and say to you, 'You're not my real mom.' Whether I died or I lived, he was going to say that." And I have said on tape to him, "Don't think that for a moment. Mama is your mother, and you have to live with that." But I have also said to

Claire, "The more you make him a partner, the less difficulty you will have with him as a teenager. He's going to withdraw because teenagers do, and he's going to hate you and think you're an idiot because that's their job. But if you give him a sense of responsibility for the family that you build with him, he's less likely to withdraw completely, and he's more likely to come back." What do I know? I've never had a teenager. *[Laughs]*

You've told me that doing all this preparation for Gabriel has had a ripple effect in your family.

I started because of Gabriel, but it has expanded in ways that I couldn't have imagined. I realized I needed to talk to my family about things for Gabriel, and then I realized that I just needed to talk to my family, especially because my family doesn't want to talk about it. Claire has gotten to do a lot of grieving with me, which is, in some ways, very wonderful. It has opened up an incredible dialogue with my family and also with people I worked with and people at the synagogue.

I wrote and sent the same letter to my family. Then, I wrote a letter to each of them individually about what they've meant to me. I was going to leave those letters with Claire to give to them, and I realized as I was writing that one of the things that happens when people can't talk about this stuff is they don't get to finish their process. So, I have sent the letters to my family and said, "If you have things you want to talk to me about, now's the time." Especially my mother because I know my mother has issues that she will never talk to me about if I don't open them up. I was able to write a letter and say, "I think this is an issue. If it is, I'd like to hear about it."

One of the things that Claire and I have gone back and forth about a lot is how much my family should come visit. I have been very adamant with Claire. I am not going to tell anybody, "No, you can't come and do what you need to do," even if they've been here a zillion times, because I know you can't finish things with people after they die. Except my mother because my mother would be here every other day. *[Laughs]* I have come to the conclusion that my family of origin has as much claim on me as my family of choice. I've told them, "My priority is Gabriel and Claire, but if you want to come . . . "

Aside from the benefits to others, what has it been like for you to do all this preparation for Gabriel and your family?

It was very exhausting, and I had to force myself to do it some-times, but it's also incredibly rewarding. I feel like I have had a much more conscious process than I would have had otherwise. I feel like I really will be a part of Gabriel's bar mitzvah. I will be present in other significant events in his life, whether he wants me there or not. The other wonderful thing is that I have gotten to say to my teenager all of the things I wanted to say without being interrupted and without having to listen to the back-chat. However erroneous what I have said might be, I've gotten to do it.

I've also been a lot more conscious of the changes in Gabriel. When I was first diagnosed, I was beside myself. I remember saying to Claire, "How will I ever leave that baby?" and "My God, what will I do?" And now I look at him, and I can see the baby that he was, and I can see the man that he will be, and I can also see the child that he is now, and I don't think I would have been able to do that if I hadn't gone through this preparation.

I would add that it's been very healing to do it all, it's given me a greater sense of control. It's a way of coping and of integrating the concept of death into life. Everyone's going to die, we may as well be prepared. It makes death less frightening.

What would your advice be to other parents who might be consid-ering recording their stories and legacies?

I think it's incredibly important to do. I would say to people that you need to say the thing that is the most important about your child in a way that your child can go back to.

Although it's really about me because I don't know who Gabriel will be, I have done it with him in mind always. One of the things I wanted to say to him that he can't understand now is, "Whatever pres-sures come to bear upon you, there's an integrity to who you are that will give you the answer. You are responsible, ultimately, for what hap-pens in your life."

Somebody said to me, "He will go back to these at different times and will hear them differently when he's a teenager than when he's in his twenties." That's true. I have always been aware that my child lives in a world that I will never enter. He lives in the future, and I live in the past.

How do you know something like that, Leona? Is it from your religion? From meditation?

No, I've always been this way. I just know it. When I was a child, I figured that I was a soul on vacation, and really, from very early on, I thought, "Oooh, God, you had better make use of this lifetime because you are on vacation here, and if you don't pay attention, next time around, you're going to get creamed 'cause this is such a good life." When I was first diagnosed, I thought, "Oy, I really didn't pay enough attention, and now it's too late."

I think that cancer is another aspect of life, and I feel very fortunate. Lots of people don't get to say goodbye, and I have, and I feel incredibly blessed that that has happened to me. I think that a lot of people feel incredibly resentful, and they should. I happen to have done that in my twenties around having been disabled, so I didn't need to do it around cancer. I would encourage people to make peace in whatever ways they can with whoever they need to make peace.

Leona keeps coming back to the importance of having a support network and even a medical advocate—someone to help negotiate the healthcare system.

I think the most important thing is for the person who's ill to have an advocate, preferably not a family member so they don't have that investment, and that the physicians honor that relationship. I have people set up hospice care and stuff for me and call Betsy's office [Leona's oncologist] and say, "Leona wants this or that or the other thing, and you need to make the call." And Betsy's office has been very good about saying, "So-and-so called. Is this really what you want?" and then going ahead and doing it.

I had polio when I was about Gabriel's age, so I didn't need a lot of help dealing with doctors. I'm not frightened of hospitals. I know how to cope with medical people. My father is a surgeon. My brother's a cardiologist. My other brother's a GP. I'm not intimidated. I know they're people. Like, I know what they look like in their underpants. That's made it much easier for me to talk to them.

I think physicians need to be much more respectful. Although all of my medical practitioners—except this one gynecologist, who I got rid of right away—have been incredibly respectful. I have been able to say to them, "This is what I want. What do you think we can do given that this is what I want?" And when I want changes, I have been able to say, "Well, you know, I changed my mind, and if I want something else, what do you think we should do?"

I have had Gabriel participate in a lot of my medical care, and Betsy has been very good about allowing that. I would explain to him what she was doing, and she would engage with him. I think that's the most important thing—some sort of sensitivity.

Especially with kids, I think it's vital to set up a support community so it doesn't all fall on your partner and your partner is then isolated. I said to Claire very early on, "I do not have cancer. We as a family have cancer, and we need to present it to people this way, and we need to cope with it as a family," and we've done that.

Initially, I didn't know what to ask. I needed help getting rides, and that's how we came to have a meeting. This woman who I knew through the synagogue for years but who wasn't a close friend said to me, "I will schedule rides for you. I will make all the telephone calls. We need to have a meeting. There are a lot of people who want to help you." Zillions of people came to the house—I was astonished—and Claire and I sat down and said, "Gee, what are we going to tell these people?" And we made up a list of things, like getting Gabriel's baby furniture out of the basement.

The group has taken on a life of its own. They have come up with phone trees and email lists. Some are members of my family, but there are people I used to work with, members of my synagogue, people I didn't know very well. There's a woman I used to work with who came the last three weekends and grouted my shower and brings me lunch. I never thought of Leslie as a very close friend. She called me and said, "I understand that you have a team. I want to be on that team." I said, "You have two small children." She said, "I have help. I want to be on that team." She's been over here in her underpants cleaning the shower. Go figure.

The hardest thing for people to do is to ask for help, and I think the crucial thing is to ask somebody to be the asker for you. Find somebody in your church or your child's preschool or your whatever and say to them, "I need somebody who will schedule what I need and who will ask people to do it." If you can bring yourself, or even your spouse, to ask that one question, then everything else snowballs from there. When people say, "Well, let me know what I can do," they mean it, but they don't know what to do. Who would have thought this woman would come and grout my shower? It's very hard for me to set up hospice care. It was not hard for me to say to one of the people in my group, "I need someone to call hospice. Here's my health card, take care of it." And it's not hard for her to do it.

Most ill parents don't recognize what a gift that is to other people, and they don't understand how rich their experience can be once the network is in place. My support network has come up with things that I would never have thought of in a million years to do for us. They thought to meet with Gabriel's psychologist, and it will serve him.

The other thing is that this group of people who didn't know each other will continue as an entity after I die because Claire and Gabriel will need them. They have become involved with him in ways they never would have. It's a real gift to your children and to your family to provide them with that kind of support. People will look at Gabriel years later and know that they had a part in making this easier for him. It's a continuity. The people that are here are remarkable, but I think it's not as remarkable as it seems. Most people want to do something. They hear you have a situation which they are very glad they don't have. You give people an opportunity to participate in ways that are very rich for them.

So what for you has been the hardest part of being a parent with cancer?

Claire and I have not had nearly the kind of time alone that we would have liked to cope with our relationship and our sense of loss in terms of each other because Gabriel is there. Claire wakes up in the night and cries, partly because it's the only time she has when she's not busy.

I have felt guilty about the amount of time he's had to spend away from home last year because we wanted time alone or because I couldn't cope with him and Claire wasn't available to be here all the time. I haven't been well enough to be with him. I've been impatient with him. Part of the reason I started the morphine patches is because I was in so much pain that I was not a good mommy. I was ready to give him to the gypsies at any moment because he's loud, he's a three-year-old, he needs attention, he wants to talk, and I just wanted to kill him. That's another way in which people need their support system. People will come and sit in the garden with your kids. People who don't even know you will do that.

I think that each person's journey is unique. The hardest period of time for me was a month of absolute terror, and it had nothing to do with Gabriel. I would wake up with this adrenaline, and it would go on all day. I would hyperventilate, I was in a constant state of terror, of physical flight. The mothers' support group was incredibly important to me because, when I started your group, I was in the middle of that month. Talking to other parents brought that [terror] down to a manageable level. It went away. It was about a lot of things that I think I have made sense of, and one of them is I was afraid that death is not the end. I have come to some kind of peace about that.

But the hardest things for me, I think, I learned from having polio, not from having cancer. What's made cancer easier for me is that I was disabled so I wasn't shocked by my own vulnerability. I understood the frustrations that ill people have. I am not afraid of this situation because it is not unfamiliar. I have always known that I would die.

Cancer has not been nearly as difficult for me as being a disabled teenager was. God, that was miserable. Especially at the time that I was growing up—nobody talked to me about the fact that I had polio. We never mentioned the word. I would see myself walking down the street, and in the reflection of the window, I would recognize myself by the clothes I was wearing because I didn't know that I walked like that. I was just walking.

There was a certain point in San Francisco at which it was fashionable, politically correct, to be disabled, and it drove me nuts. When I was a teenager, I had two things that I had to deal with that have gotten easier as I've gotten older. One was that I was classically beautiful, and people project all kinds of personality traits onto people who are beautiful. I also had polio, and people project all kinds of other things onto disabled people and on people who are ill. Those have been the most difficult things for me to learn to deal with graciously.

One of the things I learned early on with cancer was I had to learn to be gracious. It was important to me when I knew I was ill to not be a pain in the ass because, as a hospice volunteer, I had seen people do AIDS lots of different ways. It was important to me to do this well 'cause there's lots of bennies you get out of doing it well, and I wanted those.

But I learned that you have to learn to be gracious with people who don't get it, in whatever way they don't get it. The lesson for me has been to not just shrug those people off and say, "You know, those people are a pain in the ass, and I don't care about them." I have been very fortunate in that the person who does the coordinating for me has dealt with a lot of those people so I haven't had to.

Has being a parent influenced your treatment decisions in other ways—for example, by having more treatment than you would otherwise have had?

No, I don't think so. I wasn't sure that I was going to do chemo when I first was diagnosed. Here's the reason I never went back to see the gynecological guy: My first question to him was, "What if I decide not to do chemo?" And his response was, "You have to do chemo!" and I thought, "Okay, I don't have time to educate you in how to listen, and we don't need to have any more discussions." I decided that I would always regret it if I didn't do chemo and I became sicker. My benchmark for deciding about treatments has been, "If I die and I don't do this or that treatment, will I feel that I should have?" You can second-guess it, I suppose, but why bother? I'm really not into torturing myself. At a certain point, you have to say, "You know, this is not worth it any longer."

I was told five months ago that the chemotherapy had not been successful, and I said to the oncologist, "Okay, where do we go from here?" She said, "It's up to you," which, thank God, she's willing to do. She said, "I wouldn't recommend more chemotherapy because it's not working and also because you have a terrible reaction to it. There's surgery that people are doing that's experimental. There's something else that's experimental that I don't know much about, but I will find out for you. There's a second string of chemotherapy that you could do, but it probably won't be very effective."

I had all this information, and I went to Mexico, and I thought a lot about surgery. I thought, "If I could live a little bit longer [to] where Gabriel would be that much older . . ." I decided that my measure was: Will this be a quality of life for my entire family? Will I and my child and my partner benefit from this, or will this be a burden to them or to me? And that's how I've made the decisions. I might have made different decisions if I hadn't had another mom to take over. I don't think it would have made any difference to the outcome.

I have rarely met a mother free of guilt, especially when it comes to caring for herself. Mothers with cancer have an additional burden. How have you handled it?

I have been fortunate, partly because I have a partner who's a woman. The expectation isn't there that I will take care of the family. I've taken care of Claire, and she's taken care of me. That's made it easier. I think it's much harder if you're a parent because there's that insatiable need that children have, and then there's all that guilt that parents have, even if they're doing a terrific job. I feel terrible that I won't be there for him, that I had a child so late in life. You name it, I've got it. But I don't think you can sustain that. I am grateful for having Gabriel even though I haven't been with him very long. I know that being a parent completes one's life in a way that nothing else does. When Gabriel was born, I remember thinking that I had fulfilled my purpose.

Has anything good come out of the experience for Gabriel?

Oh, yeah, I'm sure it has. Cancer is one of those experiences we call a golden fucking opportunity. *[Laughs]* First of all, he gets to live without my negative aspects, it's quite wonderful. I won't be there to nag at him and bitch at him and complain about him. I think that it will make him a more compassionate person. When I was pregnant, I said to Claire, "You know, if this child grows up to be kind and self-supporting, I will feel that we have done a terrific job." There's not much more you can expect. I care that he's happy, but you can't do anything about that. People make their own lives. But I do care that he's kind, and I think you can teach people to be kind.

Have you come to any understanding of suffering through your experience of illness?

In forty words or less, "Oh, God, I don't know." I mean, yes, of course, in some ways. I have thought about that a lot because of having polio.

Gabriel asked, about six months ago, "What does God actually *do*?" I loved the question.

First of all, I don't think that God takes away the pain. I think it's God's job to provide the wherewithal to cope with the pain. The issue to me is not, "Where was God in the Holocaust?" but "Where were the German people? Where were the people of Europe?" I feel the same way about cancer. The sense that I make of the suffering is suffering is part of life. Life is hard, and then you die. *[Laughs]* You make it what it is.

I hope that we will figure out cancer. But there's an epidemic in every generation. It used to be consumption, then it was whatever it was. And every mother lost a child. I know that I would go mad if I had lost a child. I can relate to my own mother in that. If this were Gabriel, I would be a basket case. But people die, and we forget that. Biologically, once you have reproduced, life doesn't care about you much more. Like when you're pregnant, everything is going to the baby because that's what life is about—continuity.

At this point, what do you hope for yourself?

I have said that as long as I can communicate and I'm not in pain, I am willing to linger about and be a perfect nuisance and burden to everybody. But the moment I'm not able to communicate or that I'm in significant pain that we can't control, I do not want heroic measures to be taken.

I hope that I get to know the answers to all the things I've always wondered about. When I was a child, I used to think, "When I die, I will know what happened to the princes in the tower."[5] I really want to know who shot John F. Kennedy. And I have always thought that when you die, the mysteries of the universe become clear so I hope this is true. I've been watching Stephen Hawking and all his black holes on TV, and I have been thinking lately, "Gosh, I wonder if this stuff will become clear to me soon?"

When I was a child in Kenya sitting in the ocean, I had a glass in my hand, and I was picking up water out of the ocean and pouring it back in. I remember thinking, "When I hold the water in the glass, it's a particular entity, and when I put it back in the ocean, that entity is still there in its entirety, but I will never be able to reconstitute it." That's what life is. When I die, I think that I will go back into the ocean because the laws of physics are that energy is conserved. I can't think of any reason why it would be different for people than it is for anything else. I will become part of the available energy, still there, but I won't be reconstituted in this form.

So, Leona, it's time to ask you "the Barbara Walters question." How do you want to be remembered?

Oh, God! *[Peals of raucous laughter]* I hope that people remember me the way I am, and I don't know what that is really. But I hope that however they remember me, it's the way I *really am.*

When I had done all these tapes, I realized that there were people who still live in San Francisco who knew me in that time between leaving home and getting together with Claire, and that I was a different person in a lot of ways. I contacted some of them and said, "If Gabriel's interested, would you be willing to talk to him about what you remember of who I am?" and they said, "Yes." Recently, I said to one of them, Edie, that somebody told me not long ago, "You've been such a role model for me about disability." And I said to Edie, "I thought, 'Oy, you should have known me in my twenties.'" She knew what I meant and laughed because I was so *not* a role model for people with disabilities in my twenties. I was furious and rude and ornery, and I'm glad that there's somebody around who remembers that, who can say to my son, "God, what a pain in the ass she was."

Two hours have passed. Leona seems energized, and I feel more alive than I have in weeks. I thank her for the gifts of time and wisdom. She thanks me for the opportunity to do her "community service." As we talk about the project's future, Leona remembers that she has not helped with fundraising. She invites me to look at an altar by the bedroom window, on which she keeps a set of muslin bags.

"Make a wish," she says with a half-smile. "Write it down—something that you want to happen, like money to come to the project—and put it in one of the bags. Then say, 'It's in the bag,' and let go of it."

No one knows why bad things happen to people, especially to children. Nor do we understand the long-term effects on children who suffer great loss and hardship at an early age. Crippled in childhood and resentful and bitter as a teenager and young woman, somewhere along the way, Leona transformed her wound into an offering that would help not only her own child and family but also the larger community.

Leona was at peace with dying in a way I had not imagined possible. In understanding how to include death as a part of life even with young children, she taught everyone around her a lot about living. She seemed to know a great secret of life: None of us is replaceable, none of us is replaced. Those who suffer great losses early in life can heal, as she had after polio. As Gabriel would after losing one of his beloved parents. She knew that her death would not be the end of the story—and that her son would have his own separate journey and his own narrative.

Just as there is no one formula for living well, there is no one right way to die. But Leona showed a way for all of us—especially for parents of young children—to face death with wit and wisdom by preparing for it and by giving what may be the greatest gift of all: one's complete presence.

After this interview, the project began to serve other women in their dying time. They have lived with dying, as they have with illness, in different ways. Some used denial to protect themselves and their children until it was too late to do anything but the most minimal preparation, but what they did do brought healing. One was so distraught by what her children would face in the future that she could not protect them from her own emotional chaos. Others were so frantically trying to stay alive that they sacrificed their quality of life and had little time left over to spend with their children. The majority succeeded in finding a middle ground. They accepted the inevitable, relayed the truth, and released their children to the care of others, yet held onto hope—hope for time to heal relationships, for a pain-free death, for their children's well-being. They were able to continue their parenting by recording messages of love and creating memories for their children. In so doing, they found a measure of personal peace.

FIFTEEN: "IN YOUR BEST INTEREST IS PEACE" ANNETTE NISEWANER

"THERE'S A MOTHER WHO might be ready to record her story. She doesn't have much time and is only now beginning to acknowledge it. It might be a matter of days. She was just hospitalized again, and I don't think she'll be going home."

"What about the children? What's the family situation?"

"Horrendous," continues Marion, an oncology social worker at a local hospital. "There are two girls, both teenagers, and they're at each other's throats. One is almost eighteen and wants to live on her own. The younger one threatened suicide last year when it seemed she might have to live with her father, from whom she's been estranged. I don't know the details."

"Are there other family members or friends?"

"A few, but they're at a distance and not too involved. There's a neighbor the girls are attached to, a Mrs. Herman. They like to hang out at her place. But she has no rights in the situation. It would be great if you could help Annette to do this, just great."

I am not sure how great it would be. It would be great *if*. If the mother wants to make a brief tape since it's already clear that she will probably not be able to record a life story. *If* there is time to help her think through her words to children who are unprepared for losing her, who don't know where they will live after she dies or with whom, who are already in turmoil. And *if* I can find a listener who is both available and up to dealing with the challenge of recording among the interruptions and noise of hospital life.

I swear—and then try to analyze my disturbance. The later a

woman comes to us in the course of her illness, the higher the stakes for everyone involved in making the tapes. Ever since we began serving more women with end-stage disease, I have become acutely aware of the special challenges. The mother will know that her words might be the last ones she will speak to her children, and she is aware of the way in which they might remember her. What she says and how she says it might have an extraordinary impact, especially if communication has been limited or troubled. The fact that there might be no time to pre-pare Annette or help her think through her message puts increasing pressure on the listener.

But there is something else, something more personal. I had al-ways connected directly to the mother, and through her stories and love imagined the children. In Annette's case, I don't have a photo, and I've never heard her voice. My allegiance has turned toward the two young girls. I am uncomfortable with this unusual shift. I'm swearing because I am angry with Annette. *What was she thinking?* I wonder. *Why hadn't she prepared them or arranged for guardianship if the fa-ther was unsuitable?* I realize that I am projecting onto Annette my own wounds—as a child and as a mother. I still sometimes hurt from having had a mother who failed me in many ways. I still get angry with myself for ways in which I failed my own child. As I calm down, I turn my attention to what the project can do for this family. If it seems right for Annette to make a tape, if she can open her heart to her children, perhaps there can be some healing for all of them.

I call Michael Ann Leaver, who agrees to work with Annette. There have been many blessings in doing this work, and one is the listeners themselves. Whatever the situation, however messy, scary, or sudden, I have always found one of them—always, it seems, the right one—who says "Yes." Michael, a nurse familiar with hospital routines, calls An-nette and sets up a visit for the following day.

Annette is tired when Michael arrives, explaining that she hasn't slept well because her roommate wants the television on all night. Mi-chael explains the taping process, but Annette remains cautious, unsure about making the recording. Every minute seems to sap her strength. After some consideration, she decides to do it and begins by explaining why she is making the tape.

"It was suggested as a gift to give to my children, Heather and

Beth, for them to have and remember me by." She then directly addresses her daughters. "The other reason is that I love you both dearly, and I know that when I'm gone, when you're gone from each other, even if it's temporary, it would be nice to listen to something and have each other's voice and remember the fun times and the special moments we shared together. Okay?"

"*When* I'm gone," not "if." Annette is beginning to accept her death even while intimating that there might be time to make other tapes, even time for the girls to make some recordings of each others' voice to ease the impending separation.

There isn't time. Annette dies several days later. After conveying the news, Marion tells me that, in spite of Annette's terminal prognosis, "everyone was surprised because she wanted so much to stay alive for her daughters and looked so strong and beautiful." Most surprised and distraught are Heather and Beth.

During the following weeks, Michael prepares the gift box for Annette's daughters. The box contains the tape, instructions for preserving it, and a booklet explaining the project and the context in which the recording was made. On Christmas Eve, she delivers the box to the neighbor, Mrs. Herman, who in turn is to give it to the girls. In a follow-up phone call, Mrs. Herman tells me that they have already separated. She hasn't seen Beth, who is living with her father, and eighteen-year-old Heather, who is now living on her own, has angrily refused the box: "My mother didn't want to do this." But Annette *did* do it. She did choose to speak from her heart to her children. She spoke with great intensity and care, looking inward, often with a smile. In the beginning of the tape, she answers some of the questions that had plagued me about her.

Annette

My overwhelming sense in the last three years has been to protect my children, to protect you, Heather and Beth, from having to cope with more trauma than necessary. When your father left, that was a trauma, and then that I was ill and in the hospital was also a trauma. So, I didn't go into a lot of detail about the illness with you guys—or even with my doctor for my own sake. My focus was to get well, and

I wanted you girls to know that. And, although I was ill, critically ill, I was strong and able to carry on pretty well, and I didn't have a lot of side effects, so I was really lucky. And then I was lucky to have you guys because it was a lot.

You know, we always would cuddle at night—okay, we slammed some doors and that sort of thing, but we got away from the illness as much as we could. Then I got well, so there were a lot of good moments during that stage of illness. And then, when I had the recurrence, I was angry and I was upset, and it was a lot harder for me to protect you from my sense of hopelessness about cancer and illness in general. It's been . . . a challenge. And it's been a challenge for you guys, too, at school, at home, with your friends, with other adults—your dad.

Of course I remember you, Heather and Beth, at different stages in your lives as very different people, and it's been fascinating to see how you've developed and changed and how I've developed and changed with you. I think a lot of it has been really positive, and I think a lot of that is because you're both very talented, strong-willed, intelligent, curious kids that are willing to stick your necks out for what you believe in and find out why some things work and some things don't, even if it's at your own expense. And this is very courageous, and it's helped our family to pull together.

So I'm glad that you guys cause a little trouble now and then, *[Laughs]* raise a little rabble now and then, have your little conflicts. It's a way of learning. I wish it was easier on the furniture and the doorjambs, *[Laughs]* but maybe you'll learn carpentry, too! And meanwhile, there have been so many beautiful things that have come out of it—I'm sure every one of them is remembered by you. And your cousins and niece and now your *great*-niece, all of these people will be important in your life, just as I have been important in your life, and I won't stop being important. I'll always be there for you to turn to as a memory. You can create out of that memory whatever you want, and I hope that you will remember that I always loved you, respected you, honored you, even when you spit in my face or when you slapped me and pushed me, and I think that's part of growing up. I think it would be nice if *your* kids didn't have to get that. . . .

But there are other parts of growing up, too, like museums and concerts and trips across country and friendships. These are all aspects that make you who you are, and I'm proud of you to explore these different areas, and I hope that you will keep enlarging them to include new areas, new friends, new people, new substitute mothers.

I've done mothering for some of your friends, and I'm sure there are plenty of friends of yours whose mothers will put an arm around you when you need it. Don't hesitate to ask, they're there for you, just as anyone else is. Including your father and all the people who you might have some animosity toward, some difficulty relating to. But all of this is in your best interest. It teaches you, and then you can teach others, and it helps you to be a giving, loving person to join with other people. And that's what healing is all about.

The more we can join together and take care of each other, the more healing we'll have in this world. The more we pull apart and we're angry and resentful, the less peace we'll have and the more conflict and turmoil, whether it's on a personal level or a national level. So, keep that in mind. Keep in mind that in your best interest is peace. And, in my memory, please try to share that peace with each other and with the people around you and in your world and make it manifest.

I love you both. Bye-bye.

The first time I listened to the tape, I heard how anger was part of this family. The mother's anger when cancer reappeared, which reflected her hopelessness and despair. The girls' anger at their father's leaving and at behavior we can only guess at. Their anger at their mother even before cancer, again for reasons known only to them. Additional anger at their mother for getting so sick and now for dying, which they expressed through aggressive acts toward her, each other, and themselves. Anger may have felt safer than terror at the impending abandonment, especially in the absence of open discussion. No wonder Heather rejected the tape, which had become symbolic of her mother's final departure.

All I could do was light a candle in Annette's memory and pray for Beth and Heather: May the fierce and willful natures their mother celebrates become their strength rather than their undoing. May they one day, and soon, listen to their mother, who had finally acknowledged the limits of anger and silence and turned instead toward the possibility of peace.

Annette's story was the shortest recorded by the project, but in some ways, it was also the hardest. I listened to the tape many times before I heard her message. She was releasing her daughters, giving them a way to carry their actions and feelings without self-recrimination. I also felt her struggle to forgive herself as she explained how she had dealt with her illness and acknowledged that her protective efforts were partly for her own sake.

As Annette became more real to me, I understood how my initial judgments had served to protect me. They defended me against reopening my own wound of maternal failure. My daughter was becoming a strong, young woman who trusted in me. But there had been much harm from which I had not been able to shield her—my bouts of anxiety, the pre-divorce war zone, the post-divorce minefields, and my difficult adjustment to the economic stresses and loneliness of single parenting.

One morning, I awoke weeping with the wish to do it all over again and realized that Annette had not had what I have had—the luxury of years in which to step out of single-parent madness, the time to consider whether protective acts were helping or hurtful, and to whom. She would not be able to reconstruct a relationship with a young adult, to begin the long process of reviewing the mistakes and losses of the past, and to revise them, one hopes, together. When I grasped what this mother had accomplished in twelve minutes and twenty-seven seconds without preparation, I was humbled. I grieved for her. And I forgave myself.

Sixteen: "I'm Just a Ball of Fire"
Reiko Garcia

PROFOUND SHIFTS IN CONSCIOUSNESS and character can take place even moments before death, bestowing blessings on the dying person and her family. Sometimes changes at the end are not salutary. There are devoted mothers who turn their faces to the wall, refusing to leave a message for their children, refusing even to see their children.

In some instances, a mother's responses to illness and dying exacerbate her worst qualities. Undone by the inability to protect her children from loss, she may leave them unprotected from her own emotional maelstroms. Reiko Garcia is one of those mothers. She voices what many people feel while immersed in illness but don't say for fear of pushing others away.

Reiko had felt like a changeling in her traditional Japanese family, which thwarted her desire to talk openly and express intense feelings. She fell in love with Flamenco music, moved far from home, and married a Spaniard against her parent's wishes. Passion was the hallmark of their marriage. They loved hard, worked hard, played hard, and fought hard. Their son, Yuri, was born, and for a time, life was good. Then, when she was thirty-six and Yuri five, Reiko was diagnosed with breast cancer.

"They found a spot on a routine mammogram, so they did a biopsy, and it was cancer. The next day, my primary care doctor told me I was pregnant and asked if it was good news, and I think I was hysterical. But the initial prognosis was not so bad. It was a small tumor in the breast, and it didn't appear it had spread. The lymph nodes were clear. I got opinions from different doctors. Some felt I should abort.

I was just a few weeks pregnant. One group felt I could continue with the pregnancy. I really wanted this second child. I had suffered a miscarriage, so when I found out I was pregnant again, it meant so much. My instinct told me that I could have this baby, and I did. I have absolutely no regrets.

"Once the baby was born, I said to my doctor, 'I want to nurse him for three months before I start chemo. I remember feeding him for the last time, and that was very hard. I cried. Then I started the chemo, and during that time, everything was okay."

Three years after baby Ken was born, cancer returned. Shortly thereafter, Reiko heard about the project and joined one of our focus groups. She enveloped me in a hug that almost knocked me over and did the same with the other women. Her affection was so genuine and magnanimous that we responded in kind. When Reiko introduced herself and said the cancer had metastasized to the brain and eye and that there were new spots on the liver, everyone in the group wept with her.

Almost two years later, she tells me her life is still under siege. Nevertheless, she wants to be interviewed about her experience of mothering during illness. We decide to meet in her home, a small, stucco bungalow in a blue-collar neighborhood.

When I arrive, Reiko embraces me warmly and then looks stricken, waves her arms at the disarray of papers, toys, newspapers, and laundry in the living room, and blurts out, "I'm just a ball of fire!"

She is. Her emotions smolder, flame, subside, and rekindle, sometimes within minutes. Nevertheless, it is not hard for me to listen to the hot words. There is nothing hostile in Reiko, no cruelty or malice. Her anger is an outlet for her pain, aimed more toward herself and life than anyone else.

This is just who Reiko is, but the way she is is very difficult for her. She knows she doesn't have the tools to control her emotions, especially anger, or to help her children manage theirs. "I'm not very good at dealing with my anger because I just . . . I scream. If I can find somebody to listen to me, it really helps."

For the next two hours, Reiko talks practically nonstop; it seems to do her some good. She releases frustration and fear, desperation and wrath, beginning with her family's reactions to her illness.

REIKO

I never felt I was loved growing up. The reason I felt I was never loved is my parents never said they loved me. Of course, they expressed their anger. I was not abused, but I think I grew up feeling very angry. I'm a very emotional person. I have to talk to somebody when I'm upset about things. I think talking really helps. I am the black sheep of the family. I don't know if it's my culture, my family, both . . .

When I was first diagnosed, my mother's sisters were in town, and they were getting ready to go on a cruise. [My mother] would come to me and say, "Don't tell your aunts about your cancer because they would be upset, and they wouldn't want to go on the cruise." I haven't been able to let go of that. I'm forty years old. I have a lot of ongoing issues with my mother. It has not been resolved.

All the grandchildren gravitate toward their grandfather, but my father doesn't speak English. There's a lot of things that he doesn't do. My father lost his father when he was nine, but he never talked about it. He never talked about any emotional pain.

My brother never talked to me about my illness, never showed any compassion. I remember, he gave me a ride to the hospital one day. I sat there, he never talked to me. I hate the silent treatment. He's always been like that. I had a difficult time with him growing up. I guess a person never changes. A lot of times, I thought maybe illness brings the family together, but it didn't.

I don't know how anyone can be at peace. I don't ever question why this happened to me. I'm just angry that it *has* happened to me. I have to search very, very deep to find some positive. I'm so angry at this illness, about the whole situation. A lot has to do with the stupid insurance. I wanted to see a specialist who was willing to biopsy my eye, but my doctors and friends wouldn't support it. They said the procedure was too controversial with unproved benefits. I fought the insurance companies and lost. I had to deal with it alone. I think a few things could have been done that could have prevented this illness from worsening. If everybody was doing their thing, if my own oncologist was to back me up to seek treatment with this specialist, my illness would have been contained in some way.

I'm angry about my whole life being disrupted. You know, I look at other women, at anybody walking on the street, I envy them because they don't have to go through the things that I have to go through. Half of my hair is out, half of my hair is not out. I hate the way I look. I look at my body. . . . My body is filled with scars, and there's hardly a day that has gone by that I don't feel the effects from chemotherapy. There's always pain. My fingers are getting numb. I would do anything to have a day that I could feel good and forget about my cancer. Everything I read has to do with cancer. It's with me all the time. It's a twenty-four-hour deal.

Oh, I have a lot of things to be angry about. I'm angry because I can't enjoy a Christmas without worrying, *Is this going to be the last one? The Nutcracker* was so beautiful and so moving, and I couldn't even enjoy that. There's always something behind me that says, "Gee, if I was dead, I would not be able to enjoy it."

I hate to say it, but "shitty" is a perfect word for it. I feel so shitty all the time. I'm not comfortable driving any more. I don't *want* to drive. I feel I don't want to go through any obstacles to achieve something that gives me pleasure, to see a movie. If someone wants to take me, I jump at the opportunity. I hate trying to find a parking space. I don't want to drive at night. When do I have time to go during the day? Ken is in school three hours in the morning, and a lot of time I'm going to the doctor. I mean, I'm disabled.

I want to get some therapy, even a massage. I don't have the resources. Other than having to deal with the illness is the financial situation. I feel bad because I don't have a life-insurance policy that I would leave for the boys. Social Security took a lot of stress off me because we didn't have enough money to buy food. Now at least I know I can pay for my food. If Yuri wants to take a swimming lesson or drawing class, we can send him.

A family has good times and bad times together, but I feel a lot of our times have been bad. We're really restricted because of my disability. When we go to the aquarium, I get very tired. I really need to go home or sit down. I want to go to the soccer games. I'd love to volunteer in the kids' classrooms, but I can't. Any type of outing depends on when I'm going to have chemo. I feel the family is not whole. And to have the children see me going through what I have to go through, it's terribly painful.

I get angry with my husband because I pretty much deal with this whole thing alone. He feels he supports me. He feels the pain that I'm going through, but I feel a lot of anger toward him. If we could afford it, we could go to some counseling and really get the issue out. I feel he's never done enough. I feel he's never supportive enough. In spite of my illness, I get no help from anybody. I do my own laundry. Somebody has given us some housecleaning services, or else I would still be cleaning the house. I feel he's very lazy. My doctor said, "I've seen people as sick as you are live a long time with good quality of life," and I said, "Well, don't tell my husband because then he's going to think I'm going to live a long time." *[Laughs, then sobers]*

I don't know. He is not a bad person. He doesn't go out and drink, he doesn't have buddies. He pretty much cooks dinner every night and cleans up, but then the children also need to be cared for, the clothes need to be washed. I don't know who can do it. He takes them for bike rides, playing hockey, he's been telling Yuri stories at night. But I feel so much anger toward him, I don't know why. . . . Well, don't send a copy of this tape to him. I have a hard time telling my husband that I love him. You know, we talked about how much we loved each other in those romantic days, but now . . . now I'm beginning to be like my mother. I don't know if that has to do with my mood changes.

I'm thinking that Reiko's mood changes might be caused by the tray full of medications standing on the sideboard or the tumor that is invading her brain.

The things I want to do, I'm going to do. I want to go to Japan. I want to go to the opera. I want to dance. I'm not going to wait around for it. Because of the disability money, I have said to my husband, "I want to have some fun with it." He said, "Oh, no, we've got to pay bills." I said, "What if I had paid my bills and then the doctor said to me, "Hey, Reiko, you have a few months to live?"

I think that's one of the things my husband doesn't understand. I don't know if he realizes the seriousness of my illness. I feel there are times when he is not with me emotionally. Every woman I talk to almost feels that their husband is the same way. I guess I want him to listen to whatever I say and do whatever I say. But that's impossible. I've said to him, "I get much more support from my women friends," and he said, "Well, they don't live with you." *[Laughs]* Which is true, which is true. He has to live with me, and I do complain a lot. I'm not able to let go of a lot of things. I expect a certain way for things to be done, and I don't like compromise.

A part of it is I'm not at peace myself because I'm not able to let go. I get upset over a lot of little things. I think I would be happier if I could let go of some of the not important things. I don't meditate. I don't know how. I don't ask for help. It is very hard for me to ask. I'm irreplaceable. This is why it's so hard. I see losing a mother as a very devastating, tragic experience. Because of this trauma, how are they going to deal with it? Their father is going to be really stressed because he's going to have to raise these children alone. My husband would probably remarry, which doesn't bother me; I'm just hoping it will be someone that will love my children.

That's why I hate this thing. It really would help me if I could just find peace. I don't know if it's possible to let go of the feeling that my children will not be cared for. It's just too hard for me.

I hope they would be happy and feel loved, be emotionally well-adjusted. I'm hoping they would grow up to be normal kids, normal adults. My hope for the children is that someone will help them if something was to happen to me. I mean, not just the daily care but emotionally. Someone who would understand them and help them through. I think my husband's family would be able to do that. His family is a really wonderful, loving family, and I know Yuri will be in good hands, but . . .

If something was to happen to me, I worry about Yuri. I know he would be cared for, but it won't be by me. My husband's family would move back to Chicago so they would have to deal with losing their mother, and they'd have to deal with a new environment, friends, school. I don't know how I could be at peace and feel Yuri would be okay. Yuri would *not* be okay. I couldn't let go of that fear of Yuri not being able to deal with things. I feel he would be traumatized by it.

So I don't even know if I can help them because I feel that I'm such a mess. I'm not organized. I just feel I'm like a ranting, raving maniac.

Reiko is not the only mother I've met whose concerns center on a child she sees as particularly vulnerable. She seems willing to speak about what many parents are reluctant to acknowledge—that feelings toward their different children vary.

Ken is three and a half. He's very happy. He is not aware of my illness. I don't know what to do with Ken yet. I don't know if it's too early for me to talk about my illness. I don't think he's ready for it. We had a dog that died a few years ago, and he has no concept of what dying means. He would say, "Mommy, is Clover still dead?" So now I'm trying to tell him dying means that somebody has gone away and they don't come back. I think he would have an easier time dealing with it than Yuri. The little ones are more adaptable. But Ken just seems to be a very happy child. He likes to take care of himself.

Yuri is the complete opposite. Yuri is eight and a half. He is a very quiet child. He's like my husband, shy. Yuri will talk about other things, but when it comes to emotions, he will not talk. He internalizes things. He seems to be a very private person. He never, ever asked me any questions. He loves to draw, and in school they said, "Draw something about your mother." He was drawing a few figures and then wrote: "Illness. Tired. Cancer." [Sighs] It's extremely difficult for me. He is my great concern if something was to happen to me.

I feel a very strong bond toward him because he and I used to hang out together for five years before the other guy came along, and we would have such a nice time. After nursery school, we would go do things, just me and him. I really miss those moments. As quiet as he is, I feel very close to him. If I could ever feel that Yuri will be okay if something happened to me, I think I could deal with my illness easier. It's not that I don't love the second one—I never regret having Ken—but it's a different relationship. Because every time something happens, my initial reaction is about Yuri.

My way of dealing with it is to let everybody know so they can be aware of the situation, but then their life is like a fishbowl. So if there's anything Yuri does at school, they're going to look at him and say, "Gee, it's because his mother is sick, that's why he's acting out." I don't think the poor kid can have a normal childhood because of my illness.

For a while, we thought he was dealing with it okay because he never expressed it. Through denial, I thought, "Gee, maybe this kid is really coping quite well." Then he started acting out, and you have to wonder, "Does it really have anything to do with the illness?" But then, around the time I was going into the hospital, we got phone calls from teachers that he's been really, really angry in school. Now, when he's frustrated and angry at something, his nose starts to bleed. I said, "Yuri, what do you do when you are angry?" He throws things; if it's a pencil, he'll break it. You know, that's how he deals with anger. I try to encourage him not to do that, maybe try to talk about it instead.

I gave him a journal. I said to him, "Yuri, if you don't want to talk to me about it, write down your emotions. Write down your feelings," and he got really upset. He snatched the book from me. He went into his room and said, "I do not want to talk about my feelings," and he cried. *[Sighing]* I wish there is a way to get across to Yuri that we can have a chat because I find talking really helps relieve my frustration, my depression. Maybe not for him. That's why it's so hard for me to understand or help Yuri. Because he's completely the opposite.

A friend from his class, Gene, his mother died from breast cancer. Yuri never talked about it. I heard about it from the teacher. Then, recently, maybe with all the group therapy he's been going to, he has opened up to me a little bit. I had to go into the hospital for the procedure, and we were talking about it in the car, and I said, "How do you feel about me going to the hospital?" and he said, "Not very well . . ." and then he started to cry, which is very, very unlike him. So he said, "Mommy, what if you don't come back, like Gene's mother?" And with tears in my eyes, I said to him, "Yuri, I'm very happy you're talking to Mommy about it. There is reason to be concerned." And then, in the past three to four months, he said, "Mommy, it doesn't make me feel very good when you're lying down. I feel much better when you're up and about doing things."

I feel relieved when he opens up. There was a little book I found for kids who have a sick parent, and I thought he would be really resistant. But then he sat next to me, and he was interested, and we went through the whole thing, and so I'm seeing that maybe there are ways to handle it, but not directly asking him. But I don't know the technique. I was being forceful. I insisted. Painful, very painful. *[Grows agitated]* When you're feeling so yucky, what do you do? I don't know how to do it. It's very confusing, very scary.

Having children and cancer and worrying about not being able to see them grow . . . it's a pain. I can't even describe it. I don't think anybody can imagine how hard it is. I can't imagine the pain of what a child has to go through. It's more than anyone could bear, losing their parents when they are so young. What I think would help me is to try to find an adult who grew up without one of their parents. Maybe someone could share with me their experience growing up, what they have to go through. Maybe it's not that bad after all.

During a break, Reiko tells me that she doesn't want her sons to hear what she has taped so far, but she does want to write or audiotape her story for them. I let her know that I'll help her whenever she's ready. I ask if she has talked with Salazar about the possibility of her dying and perhaps preparing together.

No. No. We have not talked about it. It's too painful to talk about it. I think if I had the courage, I would better prepare myself. I have not prepared at all. I have not labeled any of my things. I don't have my will drawn up. I started writing a journal—I have two entries in it. It was very hard for me to do because I knew when the children started reading it, I would be gone. I didn't have the courage to go through with it. I remember trying to call the Neptune Society when I found out that it had spread to the liver. I just couldn't bring myself to do it. . . .[1]

At least my mind is sane, and I'm still able to make plans for myself, but on the other hand, there's the denial. I thought, as sick as I am, maybe I don't really have to worry about it. I think once I'm given the death sentence, then I'll want to be prepared, but my instincts tell me I should start doing some of these things now, like you said. But I've been dealing with this whole process for such a long time that it's hard.

I feel like I'm just wired. I'm not focused. I just feel like I'm a ball of fire. I'm not as crazy as I was. I don't get emotional every . . . but my life is just . . . I am not at peace with myself. I am petrified.

Reiko wants to help her children but doesn't know how. She knows she should prepare for dying but can't. It's as if she realizes that both the cancer and her emotions are spreading like wildfire and will not be contained, that her insight about her brother—"I guess a person never ever changes"—applies equally to herself. As our time together draws to a close, I try to help her focus on the few things that have eased her pain and panic, even momentarily. She mentions her son's nursery school, which "really, really pulled together" for her, a healing circle of women "who cared for me," and a breast cancer support group, which "helped me to talk about things."

Whenever I'm upset, if the support group is not available, I have to talk to somebody. Writing a journal. Listening to a tape at night. Sometimes, I take a pill to calm me down. When they found the lesion in the brain and then in the liver, those two pieces of news were more than I could handle. I think the antidepressant helped through that time because I was beginning to have hope again. But then part of the side effects from the antidepressant, I think, was yelling or getting very anxious, so I weaned myself from it.

Now death comes through my mind all the time in a different way. I know eventually I'll die, probably from cancer. Now I don't know if it's healthy for me to be hopeful or not to be hopeful. There's reason to be hopeful, and then there's also reality. I mean, statistically, I should be dead. But, of course, you're not a statistic. I think I've learned to cope with my illness a little bit better than before. Maybe emotionally, I feel a bit stronger. It doesn't make it any easier.

Because of cancer, I felt an outpouring of love from people, not very much from my folks and brother. But that's the only positive thing. I mean, I have said to myself, "God, now I can go to my grave saying that at least I felt loved." But I don't need to get cancer to feel loved, you know.

I return to my office feeling heartsick. I hope that Reiko will be able to leave something for her sons but know she can't do it now. I decide to help her apply for a scholarship that might pay for massages and other healing treatments. I encourage her to use her journal and our telephone conversations as emotional outlets. Reiko and I continue to exchange calls, holiday cards, and affection. The conversations are lengthy and often end in tears, with Reiko telling me how important the contact is.

About a year after the interview, I receive an elated message from her. She seems to be rallying with "the first sign of positive news in nine months." Although the disease is still active, the liver tumor has shrunk a bit. "I'm doing chemo and Japanese mushrooms. I'm volunteering every other week at Ken's school. I'm praying, I'm just praying. I love you, and God bless."

Five months later, I call Reiko, who immediately tells me that she is upset, suicidal. *"I started writing a little, it seemed to help. Another time, I wrote a letter; it helped me calm down. The tumor in my brain is growing. I screamed at the kids. . . . "*

Another treatment regime, another rally. I speak to Reiko following her long-awaited trip to Japan, which has lifted her mood immensely. *"It was fun! I haven't had any fun in a long time."* The doctors say there isn't much more treatment to try, but Reiko remains in relatively good spirits. *"I'm eating seaweed,"* she laughs. *"I'm going to try to make a video and audio for the kids. A friend is going to help me."* She tells me about one of Yuri's homework assignments: *"What makes you cry?" "If my mom dies." "What does your mom do?" "She rests."* Reiko laughs again. She reads me the latest Mother's Day card from the child *"who never talks." "Dear Mom, I wish you didn't have cancer."* This, Reiko says, is a lot from Yuri.

After a lapse of a few months, I learn that she has deteriorated, both physically and emotionally. A member of Reiko's support group calls and asks me to help Reiko make a tape or letter. She is dying. I call several times and leave messages with machines and family members. It is too late.

Reiko died at home just after Christmas, two and a half years after we met. An oncology social worker who attended the death told me that things had disintegrated completely. *"Reiko screamed and screamed, not so much in physical pain but in desperation and rage. She was cantankerous and difficult. She threw things around, she threw herself out of bed, she tore at the sheets—much of it in front of the children. It was awful for Salazar and the boys. This family will need a lot of healing."* My colleague paused. *"What irony. Before Reiko died, she shared one wish: that her kids would have good memories of her."*

Reiko went out, as she had lived, with great passion. The form of her defeat may have been as much due to brain metastases, hormonal fluctuations, and medications as to her temperament. It was not a passing that anyone, including Reiko, would consider desirable. Still, it was her death, the only one she could have.

After Reiko's funeral, I sat for a long time with the irony and with a Dylan Thomas quotation: *"Do not go gentle into that good night. Rage, rage against the dying of the light."* Such a grand sentiment. How differently the call to battle reverberates in the sickroom of a mother *who wants to create good memories for her children, the witnesses to and prisoners of her war.*

I continued to puzzle over Reiko's preoccupation with Yuri. Temperamental differences aside, I would have expected baby Ken, who had arrived with cancer, to have been the object of equally grave maternal concern. Perhaps Yuri was the child of Reiko's heart because he was also the child of her health. As Reiko acknowledged, she had been more attached to Yuri because of their intimate years together. But part of the attachment, I believed, was also to the happy, hopeful story that had been theirs before cancer invaded their garden. Maybe Reiko felt Yuri's pain more and feared more for him because she knew what both of them had lost.

The desperate concerns Reiko felt for Yuri and for herself seemed fused. She couldn't imagine her son's ability to recover from losing her any more than she could imagine herself recovering from the cancer that had shattered their lives. Reiko knew she was not going to be cured. That knowledge and that panic stymied her ability to create a story for herself that could hold the end of her own life alongside the continuation of her child's, separate on his own path. Reiko had been caught in what Arthur Frank calls a "chaos narrative," "whose plot imagines life never getting better," where "the suffering is too great for the story to be told."[2] The only outcome she could imagine for her beloved son was similarly disastrous.

However, when I listened to the original tapes, I heard humor and laughter, which I had forgotten. I also heard a request that I had neglected to fulfill: "What I think would help me is to try to find an adult who grew up without one of their parents. . . . Maybe it's not that bad after all." Reiko was trying to create a narrative that would not include her but would project a hopeful future for her motherless sons.

Although we can prepare for our eventual death while we still have our faculties and health, ultimately, we have no sovereignty over our children's minds, dreams, or recall, just as our own parents could not control our memories of them. The news, however, is not all bad. That a parent will be remembered is rarely in question. Even when a mother dies early in a child's life, the child will gather dream and memory fragments, photographs, and tales of the parent to create an enduring portrait. The conversation with a parent, no matter the conditions or timing of loss, continues throughout a child's lifetime. In psychologist Louise Kaplan's words: "No voice is ever wholly lost."³

Still, in a situation like Reiko's, how a parent is remembered is of concern. Last acts, last words, and traumatic events are powerful in a child's life and can have long-lasting effects. There are no guarantees, but memory can be kind. While the movie of childhood wounding replays through the years, so does the reel of other, happier associations. As one mother said after reviewing her life: "It was healing . . . to realize it's not the big things that leave the big impressions. It was very insignificant small things. . . . The little pleasures. The small blessings." Defense mechanisms, too, help children cope and manage loss. A certain amount of forgetting is necessary to get through life.

Reiko knew it would have been best for her sons had she been able to record her story. I wish I could have told her that one way or another, they will probably tell themselves stories of her made up not only of the worst nightmares but also of their best memories. My hope for Yuri and Ken is that over the years, they will forget both the screams and the terrible silence that followed. I hope they will cleave to other memories of their mother's passionate nature: the generous hugs, the openhearted declarations of love, the joy she found in music, and the courage that took her to Japan and the strength to volunteer in the classroom though profoundly ill. Eventually, they may learn to hold all of who she was with kindness.

SEVENTEEN: "MAKE EVERY DAY COUNT"
DOROTHY GREENWALD

BY THE TIME I have my first telephone conversation with Dorothy Greenwald, her ovarian cancer is advanced. She received the diagnosis two months earlier, along with her physician's prediction that she had only three weeks to live. Dorothy immediately changed to a doctor who is "much more open" and willing to enroll her in a clinical trial. She says that her main tasks now are to heal herself and her relationships. "I want to give as much as possible to others."

Dorothy maintains hope for "licking the illness" but says she is moving toward peace with the fact that she might not make it. A single parent, she has already become far too ill to care for her twelve-year-old daughter, Nicole. Having lived almost full-time with her mother since her parent's divorce years earlier, Nicole now stays with her father and stepmother. "She visits me once or twice a week. It's been hard," Dorothy says.

The separation is a painful necessity, which this mother bears by focusing as much as possible on the positive. She says it is a miracle that she is still alive and that a miracle has happened between her ex-husband and herself. The divorce and aftermath had been acrimonious, but that changed when Dorothy was diagnosed. Cooperation has supplanted hostility, for Nicole's sake. Dorothy says there has been true healing in her relationship with her ex-husband and his wife. "We've become loving friends."

Despite extreme weakness and the presence of a nurse's aide, Dorothy is ready to greet guests. She opens the front door and wraps her thin arms around me. I am taken aback by her appearance because her voice on the telephone had sounded so strong and hopeful. Her body, wrapped in a chenille bathrobe, is emaciated, with the exception of a round belly distended with fluid, making her look five months pregnant. She is no longer able to eat solid foods. "But I'm still here, fighting," she says, smiling. Her skin stretches tight across delicate facial bones.

I assume that Dorothy will want to return to bed, but she invites me to sit at a dining room table laden with the supplies she continues to use for drawing and painting when strength allows. Her hands are exquisite, with long-tapered fingers. Clear, glowing eyes never break contact.

Dorothy, too weak to write, dictates answers to our pre-interview questions: What are the reasons you have chosen to participate in the Mothers' Living Stories Project? What benefits do you hope to receive?

"I would like to make this as a gift for my daughter and also for my own healing. I want to reflect and look back and make sense of my life, to look at my strengths and weaknesses, to see how strong I was. I want my daughter to know me as a woman. This is something I can do for myself and for someone else—to make every day count. I would also like to help other women."

After I leave, I drive down the street, park again, and weep. I think about the cruelty of life that separates mothers from their children. But I move rapidly from my identification with Dorothy as a mother to myself as a child—the child who had longed for a mother who, however physically present in the same house, was never emotionally available.

Since the deaths of Leona, Reiko, and other women I knew, I had begun to think of my mother. The hardest part of my grief when she died was that I never really knew her story and now never would. By the time I was ready to listen, she had sunk into senile dementia. Eight years into doing this work, I see that by helping ill mothers tell about their lives, I have been doing a lot more than healing my wounds as a mother. I have been giving myself the stories of love and wisdom that I wanted to receive from my own mother. Each of these women is giving me a gift, a piece of a narrative to help me rebuild my own.

Most mothers record their life stories with the intention that their children will receive the tapes when they are adults. Many make an additional tape in which they speak directly to the children with content and tone more appropriate to the children's current ages—"just in case." The mothers we served made their decisions about what to record and when to give the tapes without consulting their children.

Dorothy has her own ideas. By the time volunteer listener Betty Stone meets her, Dorothy has told her daughter about the recording, and Nicole has told her mother exactly what she wants. She wants to know about her mother as a child and what it had been like for her at Nicole's current age, twelve. She wants her mother to speak about the illness that has already forced their premature separation. And she wants the tapes *now*.

Involving her daughter in this joint project seems to be a brilliant stroke for both of them, bridging the distance and allowing more control. Making the tapes gives Dorothy a way to be known as a woman by her daughter, to share her essential self. Through the recording, Dorothy is able to remain an involved parent, capable of meeting some of her daughter's needs.

Dorothy and Betty have two brief sessions together, three days apart. After each meeting, the tapes are delivered immediately to Nicole.

DOROTHY

One of my earliest memories is that when I was lying on a blue chenille bedspread as a little baby, and the sun was coming in, and I was feeling such bliss, I knew that my purpose was to come here to bless. I perceived my purpose.

When I was a little girl, Nicole, I had a rabbit. And I loved that rabbit. You know that I love rabbits still, and I like to draw them. The rabbit is a deep symbol of many things. You think of the rabbit of Easter time, the time of renewal. The Easter bunny brings the eggs. But the rabbit is also a certain kind of knowingness and intuitiveness—it celebrates the intuition. Other animals eat the rabbit, but everything gets eaten eventually, you know.

My mother had seven children, and I got kind of lost in the shuffle. I was next to the youngest. It was tough because my mom didn't have the energy or the strength to give each of us the individual attention that we needed. But I loved my mother very much, and I know that she loved me.

We would go to the farm we had, Nicole, when I was a little older, every summer and on the weekends. I loved those summers because Mom would read fairy tales to me. We would go down to the stream, and there was a little lean-to. It was called the "*Hansel and Gretel* hut," and she would tell me stories there by the stream.

That's where I got my love for fairy tales. *Beauty and the Beast,* that's one of my favorites. Because we all have a little bit of Beauty and a little bit of the Beast in us, and we have to come to love and accept both. You can't transform anything without loving it. That became part of my graduate thesis, Nicole, the stepmother in myth and fairy tale, and why we're so negative toward the feminine in this culture.

As an older child, I'd go down by myself and play in the water. And that's where I would build houses for the fairies out of stones with leaves in them. The next day, I'd come back, and I knew that they'd been there.

So I never want you to give up your belief in the fairies because there are many, many things that exist that we know nothing about. Unfortunately, intuition is one of the senses in our culture that is very much put down. We believe that we have to look out all the time rather than looking in. We see each other that way, too. We have so much conditioning to get over. But that's part of our journey, to find that everything is already within.

I had friends and school and so forth. But cliques hit in sixth grade, and I was bewildered. And it got worse in seventh grade. Sometimes, all of a sudden, you'd be excluded from friends that you'd had before. Now I understand it as part of an age where kids are trying to understand who they are. Nicole, they're moving a little bit away from their families and forming new friendships with their friends. I think that some kids didn't know how to be part of a group and also have another friend.

I was much younger than everybody else, so that interest for me in boys came a little later. It changed probably in ninth grade. I got awkward. They'd have these parties, just like you do, and dancing. You'd wait for a boy to ask you to dance, and it was pretty awful.

One time I went to this party, and I had a pink silk dress that Grandma had bought for me that was really beautiful. It wasn't a boy-and-girl party. It was an adult party. Some man came up and said, "Oh, yes, and you are nine." And I was thirteen. I dissolved in tears. After that, my mother, your grandmother, took me to a seamstress and had a beautiful dress sewn for me. Blue, royal blue wool that fitted my figure exactly and was like a princess style so it was flowing, and I loved it. Then I went to a party with that dress on. And, you know, those guys didn't pay much attention to me. Thirteen-year-old boys aren't that interested in girls, either. Or they *weren't*. But it was okay because I knew that I looked good. I thought it was beautiful, and I felt so happy in it. And I was confident. So I learned something from that. I learned about your own knowings inside. Nicole, remember that the things that help you connect to your knowings will make you stronger.

Someone once said, "You can't control your reputation." If you give a talk, Nicole, or you do a piece of work, there's going to be a hundred people that will see it, and some people will love it, and some people will hate it. You're not responsible in that way for your reputation because that's made by other people's judgments, and you cannot change those opinions. But you *are* responsible for how you behave and what you do. And what's inside of you. I've been through many difficult things, and at least I can look at myself in the mirror because I never lied or tried to hurt someone, and I tried to always understand. Even with that divorce, I don't have anything that I'm ashamed of.

In the past, I've let other people determine my worth, and that's been a mistake. I felt if my art was no good, I wouldn't do it. And I realized that you have to keep doing it. Some things you're going to love, and some things you're not going to love, but you have to keep showing up for it even if it isn't perfect. And the things that I've really put that effort into, and gotten rid of those no-good voices, have worked, especially carving. So, like Leonardo or Michelangelo, you have to carve out from a stone what's real and what's vital, and you let go of the other stuff.

When I was your age, I wish that I had heard, "Dorothy, what's wrong? Talk to me." Someone to have comforted me, to have praised my art. Each of us is special, and yet none of us is special. I want you to know that whatever I didn't get as nurturing, I vowed that I'd try to give to you. I wanted you to know that you could grow and flower and be who you are. Of course, I've not done that perfectly, but I've really tried, and I keep trying and will keep trying all my life to listen to you and to accept you, to accept who you are at this moment. I accept you, I love you deeply.

It was one of the best things that ever happened to me—to become a mother. I think it was the biggest gift I ever had. It added a richness and depth to my life. Nicole, you're a great blessing to me. I hope that I can be a blessing to you. And I hope that this tape will be a blessing to you.

You were a wonderful baby, just wonderful. Your dad would carry you around and sing to you. I had made you a light box that threw beautiful shadows on the ceiling of color and patterns as it revolved. You started talking fairly soon, and your first words were "Dada" and "Mama" and "light." You loved light, and I hope you always keep that word. Always turn toward the light when things get tough. Because you are very much loved.

Nicole, you have a very artistic and deep nature. When I would look into your eyes, I would see the universe almost. I think that you have a spiritual quality to you. When you were little, you would tell me, "I've been here before, Mom," and I believed you.

Are there things, Dorothy, that you've learned through your experience about how to cope when things are tough that you'd like Nicole to know about, too?

One of the things that has taken me a long time to learn when things are tough is to talk about it and not keep it stored up inside. Because it helps to put it out in front of you and see. I've been too private in some ways. And it's really helped me to talk about what's going on. Not with everybody. You have to choose the right people for that. I hope that you, Nicole, can learn this, too, not to keep stuff stuck inside you. I hope that I can help you to do this as we go through my illness. And find a good friend or your dad or your stepmother or the people around you that love you who will listen to you and honor you and not tell you: "Don't feel what you're feeling."

Prayer helps a lot. I think that we're loved much more than we ever know we are. I think that we've already come here with love, and I think that when we were born, we were surrounded with love. Connect to that, connect that to God. God is within you, Nicole. You've already been blessed by being here, just by showing up. And if things don't work out quite right, you've got to keep trying. And, if you do that, generally, you'll get stronger. Our challenges make us stronger. I have faith, and I hope that, Nicole, you can find that, too, whether you decide to be Jewish or Christian or whatever. I'm sort of eclectic, I'm kind of everything because I think that there are many ways to truth.

I have, over the years, been quite healthy, actually, and so this illness came as a big shock. Nicole, as you remember, in November, I was not feeling well. And then I landed in the hospital in December for two weeks, and they thought I was going to die and gave me three weeks to live.

But I'm still here, and I'm still alive! I've started the chemotherapy, I have put myself in the hands of the people at Columbia Hospital because I feel that they're supportive now. One thing that I've learned from this—that I'm *learning*—is to trust myself more, trust my body, believe in the healing powers of my own body.

It's hard. Because I don't get to live with you. I don't get to take care of you. I don't get to come to your things. It's very hard for me sometimes. But I work to accept it. I work to keep a positive attitude. I'm on the [clinical] trial, I think that there's great hope for this, I have great hope, and when I get down—which I do, Nicole—then I look at that, and I bring those fears up to the light, I put them out in front, as I've said before. I've talked to people, and I have wonderful support, I have wonderful friends that love me and care about me and will listen and are praying for me. And I believe in the power of prayer, and that helps me a great deal.

I want you to talk, too, because I know this is very difficult for you. It's difficult for both of us. And the thing that *hurts* me is that I feel that I'm causing you suffering. But I'm doing the best that I can, Nicole. I want you to know that. I'm doing the very best—to kind of bring up the fears and look at them and bring them to the light when they come and not get stuck in them and to keep going forward. And that's my challenge. So the most important thing is that whatever happens, I want you to know that I love you deeply. *Whatever* happens. And, if I don't make it, I want you to know that my prayer is that my life has been a gift to you because you have been such a gift to me.

But I *am* going to make it, and that's all that I'm thinking about now. I'm putting everything I have into it. I get weak, and I get very tired, and that's part of the chemo now. And I get tired of being tired, but again, I have to just accept it and go with it, and then my strength comes back. And when I look at it that way, I'm so grateful for the strength that I have to get dressed in the morning, to take care of things that I need to take care of. I'm grateful for Bernice, the lady who comes. I'm grateful for everything. This has actually filled me with more gratitude for my life than I've ever felt before.

There's a little part of a song that seems to be coming up into my mind. It may sound silly, Nicole, but it's from *Oklahoma*,[1] which I think you and I saw together.

When you walk through a storm
Hold your head up high
And don't be afraid of the dark
At the end of the storm is a golden sky
And the sweet silver song of the lark.

Walk on, walk on
With hope in your heart
And you'll never walk alone
You'll never walk alone.

Dorothy died one week after these words were recorded. Her voice, her arms around me, the sunlight in the dining room, and her sorrowful luminous face stayed with me. In her, I had seen a maternal vision of "tragic optimism" that reached all the way back to the biblical mother Rachel.

In the few months she had between diagnosis and death, Dorothy was able to heal embittered relationships, care for herself and her daughter, speak truth to a child without overwhelming her, and maintain hope for living while preparing to die. Knowing what she could and could not do for her daughter, Dorothy gave herself permission to put her focus on her healing at the same time that she ensured her child a loving and stable home. And she made every day count.

EIGHTEEN: NEW STORIES OF MOTHERHOOD

SOMETIMES, WHEN GRIEF becomes too much, I walk toward the Berkeley hills and keep going until my view expands and I am surrounded by silence. Ten years have passed since I began listening to the stories of mothers with cancer. Many of the women have died. Others struggle on with illness and children. I have carried each voice, each story, with me. Now, I listen to the entire chorus. What has been learned from so much suffering and loss?

I return to the questions that have guided the work: How do mothers diagnosed with life-altering illnesses reconstruct their lives and raise their children in a culture that denies sickness, death, and the underside of motherhood? What helps them live with a shattered narrative? What will it take for mothers to be seen as complex human beings? And, I add: What has changed for mothers with cancer since I first asked those questions?

Sick parents are more visible today, and some of their needs are being met some of the time. Some parents can find support groups or resources for themselves and their children.[1] A few books and national organizations address the special situation of younger women with breast cancer, some of whom are mothers.[2] Other books, videos, and online resources exist for ill or disabled parents wanting to help their children.[3] Several even speak to issues from the ill mother's perspective.[4] Studies and articles about the impact of cancer on families are more plentiful. Mothers occasionally appear in movies and on television, spurred in part by pharmaceutical ads using mothers and by media stories about high-profile individuals, like Elizabeth Edwards, Stephanie Spielman, and Melissa Etheridge, sharing their experiences with breast cancer.

Changes may be due to increasing recognition that breast cancer is not only an older women's disease and that people are living longer with many cancers because of earlier detection and more effective treatments.[5] Awareness has also grown due to the proliferation of illness narratives and more public discourse about illness, healing, end-of-life issues, and preparing wills, advanced directives, and legacies long before old age or illness.

There is still a long way to go. It remains difficult to know the number of parents of dependent children living with cancer. Neither the American Cancer Society, the National Cancer Institute, nor any other national cancer organization is able to provide an estimate, which means that services and resources are sketchy and uncoordinated.

Although cancer is seen more as a chronic disease rather than "a death sentence," both image and reality are slow to change. We're a long way from knowing how to prevent or cure most kinds of cancer or from offering less debilitating and mutilating treatments. Meanwhile, the safety net has been largely dismantled, and the numbers of medically uninsured and underinsured keep climbing,[6] with devastating repercussions for families when illness strikes. Dialogues about illness and death at the community level are still limited, and most of us do not prepare for the inevitable.

Though mothers with cancer may be slightly more visible in the media, portrayals of them are limited—stereotyping them as noble mothers, dying heroically. Even in the resource-rich San Francisco Bay Area, many mothers I speak with still feel unrepresented in the larger culture and under-supported in their own communities.

Some things have changed for the better, some not. But behind the statistics and images are human beings who have to get up each morning and face another day. The mothers I worked with were living their stories when cancer came and interrupted the narrative line, throwing them into varying degrees of crisis and chaos. As Sara said in the focus group, "Be sensitive. These women are on edge." She implied more than frustration or anxiety. The disease forced the mothers to a precipice of uncertainty, threatening their lives, their ways of living, and their relationships with their children. Their experiences were usually uncharted, messy, moment-to-moment. In Jude's words: "It's all happening at the same time!" And mothers had to cope on all fronts simultaneously. They responded, each in her own way. Tina would have said, "They just did what they did."

The mothers needed what their children needed:

- protection from overwhelming stress,
- a secure and predictable environment,
- permission to talk truthfully about the things that matter and the things they fear,
- channeling feelings into constructive activities,
- practical and emotional support,
- a way to make sense of the situation and find meaning and hope, and
- the certainty that somehow they would be cared for and valued as full human beings in spite of changes brought by illness.

Mothers especially needed to find safe places to express their thoughts and feelings about cancer and to explore the long-term consequences on their lives. Some women needed a different kind of discourse than talking about illness or emotions. When asked if she had a message for the community, one mother said: "Don't be afraid of us. When we go out into the real world, we don't want to talk about cancer. We can still talk about normal things."

But the cry for compassionate listening reverberates through the stories. The mothers wanted people in their lives who were not afraid of their situation, who could hold whatever it was they had to say without fixing, advising, arguing, or fleeing. When they felt heard, they could often move from a sense of chaos and loneliness to coherence and connection.

For many mothers, illness was an initiation, a profound turning point. They temporarily lost the sense of their own voices and the thread of their stories. "You reclaim your story by finding your voice, and you find your voice by telling your story," writes author and philosopher Rabbi Marc Gafni. "A single thread can lead us back."[7] Over the ten years of the Mothers' Living Stories Project, only a few women turned down the opportunity to tell their stories, including their cancer narratives, with the help of a trained listener.

For those who chose to participate, recording their stories served multiple purposes. Taking time each week to focus on their lives before and after cancer was a way to reflect on what had happened, to integrate the experience, and to reconstruct a narrative in light of it. Talking to a compassionate listener was an antidote to isolation and anxiety. Doing something for their children strengthened the bonds with them and offered a way to carry on parenting through illness and after death. Knowing that they were doing it, in part, for their children, also diminished concerns about selfishness or guilt. Caring for self and caring for others were inextricably tied together.

One way to go on after loss or trauma is to make sense of the experience, to reassign value and meaning to one's life. Telling their stories helped mothers make sense of the cards they had been dealt. The process was not always conscious, transformative, or, as in Reiko's case, successful, but each mother made the attempt. Even mothers like Lorraine, Julie, and Leona, who did not feel the need to reconstruct their conceptual frameworks after illness, found that reviewing their lives and preparing a legacy spurred them to grow and deepen.

Engaging in the storytelling process helped to return identity, stability, and hope. It also encouraged mothers to expand their vision. One mother said, "You go through all this stuff, [and] you're just another person with cancer. You turn into cancer, you lose your identity, but, goddamn it, you have a whole story. [Reviewing my life] put it into perspective in a really good way. It gave me a chance to feel cancer has been a hard part of my life—but only a part. I'm not just cancer. I'm this person."

Everyone's view becomes constricted during a crisis. At times, mothers became temporarily caught up in the struggle to cling to life and to protect their children. Who wouldn't? Yet, every mother needed a sense that her own story was larger than her illness, than others' projections onto her, than current conceptions of motherhood or mortality. Some mothers began to see not only their individual lives but also life itself differently.

Diana: "The kind of suffering I've been through pales in comparison to living in Sarajevo, or during the Holocaust years in Eastern Europe, or Cambodia."

Diana: "There are tragic deaths, there are tragic lives, but death itself is not tragic."

Julie: "I have this deep sense of life, death, life, death, and the cycle and the process and the naturalness of both."

Dorothy: "Each of us is special, and yet none of us is special. . . . Everything gets eaten eventually."

Janet: "You think when things happen to you, you're the only one they're happening to. I took it all so personal. . . . When I think about other people going through worse, that sets me back on an even keel. I just have to put things in perspective again."

Leona: "There's an epidemic in every generation. It used to be consumption, and then it was whatever it was. And every mother lost a child. People die, and we forget that."

Seeing the bigger picture did not take away the pain. But, when mothers were able to perceive a larger scheme of things and humans' minuscule place in it, something eased for them. They could glimpse the preciousness of their lives and of their stories. They could better accept what had happened to them and use it to good ends.

However, almost every mother would happily return the "gifts" of cancer, agreeing with Julie, who said to her child: "I would have preferred ignorant bliss to a deepened soul from cancer. And I would have wished the same for you. But those are wishes, and the reality is that you get what you get . . . and that's what we got."

What we do with what we get seems to be what counts. Deena Metzger first introduced me to a term that speaks to the mothers' challenge: *amor fati*—the love of your fate. "Every one of us must go through the process of soul-making to become who we are," explains Metzger. "You need to love and accept your fate because your suffering shapes your soul and makes you aware of what truly matters. How we meet our fate is ultimately the only thing that matters because we can't change it."[8]

"Accepting your fate" is not synonymous with fatalism, with romanticized suffering, or with passivity. In its simplest terms, *amor fati* means surrendering to the story you are already living. And then choosing how to meet it.

Tina expressed this: "About the only part we can change or influence is how we feel about it." Sara said, "I can only control what I can." Lorraine and Janet used religious language, "handing it over to God." Religious or secular, mothers at times met cancer by acknowledging their limits, loosening the grip on control, forgiving themselves for being ill and for what they couldn't do, doing what they could, and appreciating what remained.

Having an enlarged sense of life and of their own stories also informed the way some mothers thought about parenting. They realized the importance of talking to children honestly about cancer and preparing them for real life and for death, whenever it might happen. Seeing her own journey sometimes allowed a mother to perceive her children's separate journey as well, not just as a forced rupture caused by cancer:

Carrie: "Kids are separate human beings, and they need to separate. There are certain ways in which I shouldn't know what's going on with him."

Julie: "She is her own person. No one person can hold up another."

Leona: "Our children are unique and separate people. They don't belong to us. My child lives in a world that I will never enter. He lives in the future, and I live in the past."

A mother's life is intertwined with her children's lives, but she can't direct their fates any more than her parents could control hers. Children are not just characters in parental plots but authors of their own narratives. The mothers sometimes came to realize they couldn't protect children from their own suffering. Children, too, will "get what they get."

That insight initially was a cold shock. But seeing their children as individuals on their own paths helped some mothers relinquish guilt about children's pain and have more faith in their developing strengths, in the loving capacity of other caregivers, in a world where renewal can follow death. These mothers could give a message to their children that I believe is a great gift: "You are your own person, you are on your own path, and you will be all right."

And some found peace in the process of dying. Leona: "I can say with all honesty I am not worried about my child." The presence of another mother helped. But the work Leona did to prepare herself to surrender, not only to her own fate but also to her son's, was critical in helping and then releasing him.

Falling down and getting up are intrinsic to living and to raising children. Some mothers recognized the limits of fear-driven mothering.

Diana: "I wanted to cushion their young lives. . . . My thinking has changed. To probably take a hundred-and-eighty-degree turn. . . . They are learning about having to push themselves through something that's hard."

Janet: "You want to protect your kids from everything, but you can't protect them. Sometimes we feel that kids can't take things, but I think we have to give them a little more credit."

Carrie: "I don't want him to be unconscious. I want him to know what happened to him."

Leona: "You can't protect your children from life."

Cancer pressed the mothers to an edge, where they had to reconsider their lives and their mothering. The stories they told themselves about cancer differed—it's a gift, a curse, a wake-up call, a teacher, an incentive, a tragedy. There is no one-size-fits-all story to guide us through life or to help us face death. Yet, no matter the story told, almost every mother grew in consciousness and wisdom through her cancer experience—sometimes because of it, sometimes in spite of it, but always without acknowledgement and support from the larger culture.

Mothers do not raise children, become ill, or revise life stories in a vacuum. Every culture organizes the experiences of death and dying, childbearing and childrearing. It defines the "good death," the "good life," and the "good mother" and presses those aspirations upon women while simultaneously creating the less-than-ideal conditions in which they rear children.

Mothers living with cancer are simply mothers who have become sick. Like all mothers, they internalize the dominant culture's ideals, with subcultures having a tempering effect. They then experience the disconnect between the romanticized expectations and the truth of their experience. Bumping up against the discrepancy without understanding the cultural context can lead to anything from vague discomfort to serious confusion, self-blame, and guilt.

Earlier, I made the point that sick mothers are caught between the prevailing motherhood myth and the taboos surrounding illness and death, having to carry our fearful projections about the dark side of life. Not only could the mothers not see their experiences mirrored in the culture, they also had to reshape their stories against a motherhood myth that recognizes neither women's life-giving strengths nor their vulnerability and mortality.

When I became a mother in 1977 and shortly after entered the field of maternal and child health, feminist scholars and mothers were beginning to deconstruct the prevailing myth of motherhood. Exposing the underside of the mothering ideal, they revealed images of mothers to be stereotyped and sentimentalized. Mothers were assigned responsibility and blame but lacked moral authority. Anything other than a complete focus on the child was considered selfish. Mothers' personhoods were neglected, the work of mothering was devalued.[9] The outcome for many women was overwhelming confusion, guilt, and defensiveness.

Over a quarter of a century later, there are shelves of books and websites addressing these issues.[10] Some women openly acknowledge ambivalent and angry feelings about their children and the conditions of motherhood, and find support in mothers' groups and parent education classes. But these women's ideas and feelings about the subject have not penetrated the larger culture. Shockingly little seems to have changed in the ways mothering is culturally valued or supported or mothers are perceived. "Mommy Lit," a dismissive term encompassing the recent books about and by mothers, points out the ways mothers are not yet taken seriously.

Mothers with cancer represent every condition in which women are raising children, with illness making everything harder. Raising children during extreme situations exacerbates, and therefore illuminates, much of what is wrong with contemporary conditions of motherhood.

While more fathers are involved with childrearing, most mothers still bear—or feel they bear—the primary responsibility. They feel blamed when things go wrong and under-appreciated when things go right. Maternal guilt, ambivalence, and frustration are still popular topics in magazine articles and on TV talk shows. More women are gainfully employed, and some are earning more equitable pay in better positions. But whether wearing white, blue, or pink collars, many mothers, juggling multiple roles, are unable to reconcile the conflicts among their own needs, the demands of children, and the burden of too many demands at home and on the job.

And that's for the lucky women. For many families with children, socio-economic conditions have worsened. In a country that equates personal worth with wages, the work of children's caregivers is still devalued, including, of course, the unpaid work of mothering.[11] Worst of all is the situation for the truly powerless unemployed, underemployed, and homeless mothers, including those raising the 12.9 million American children living in poverty.[12]

In the stories of mothers with cancer, alongside the passion and commitment most mothers feel for their children, intensified by the threat of separation, I witnessed many of the same difficult issues made worse: Struggles with taking care of themselves and asking for help; single-parenting stresses; isolation and loneliness; anger at partners for not doing enough; the paucity of resources, including money; concerns about being selfish or neglecting children; conflicts about how much to work outside the home; guilt for anger at children; exhaustion; confusion in talking with children about difficult issues or understanding their teenagers; frustration at never having enough time.

I heard the dark side of the mothering myth revealed in the impossible expectations many mothers have for themselves, followed by a double dose of guilt and feelings of failure—first for being ill and then for being ill mothers. Some mothers, like Irene, wanted to be "this more perfect mom" because they didn't want to be remembered in a negative light. Illness exposed other conditions that made their lives as mothers even harder and more frightening: lack of access to medical care or social services, problems with health or disability insurance, concerns about toxins in breast milk, the food and water supply, the air.

So internalized is the cultural devaluation of mothering that, in a cruel twist, some women only came to understand their importance as mothers when their lives were threatened. Tina: "I used to think that my importance as a mother was what I did, and I've come to realize that my value as a mother is just being me, just being here. That's a hard thing to learn." Essential questions are raised: What is the value of a mother? What is the essence of parenting? If a mother doesn't fit into the cultural story of what a mother is, what is her worth, her story? How is it that some women avoid the emotional pitfalls of the myth? What will it take for us to see and treat mothers as complex human beings?

These women's individual stories highlight what has become increasingly obvious in recent years—the lack of a sustaining story of motherhood. Women need stories that reflect the truth of their experiences and desires, that nourish them, and that initiate them into the complexity of the entire mothering adventure, including illness and death.

The prevailing myth of motherhood, reflecting both the suppression of feminine powers present in the ancient motherhood myths and the denial of death, is a story lacking imagination, soul, and passion, which are the heart of and most needed in the mothering enterprise. Fortunately, what has been pushed down in a culture often rises up. The mothers' stories are an important contribution to an enlarged story of motherhood because they explode the current myth and even much of the literature on mothering.

On one hand, these stories highlight the themes—including the multiple complaints—of modern motherhood. Who better to lament the conditions of mothering than women trying to raise children without cultural support while living with serious illness and the possibility of death? On the other hand, their stories are much larger than any conditions or complaints. While revealing holes in the institution and the myth, they are also filling in the suppressed parts of the motherhood story. They break silence and then restore pages that have been torn out.

Each of the individual stories reveals an aspect of a mother's struggle to live a whole life. Taken together, they portray a motherhood in which women are simply human, and it's good enough. In all these ways, the narratives of ill mothers, however extreme and marginalized, are revising the larger motherhood story, perhaps paving the way for a new one. The humanity and power of mothers and the nurturing capacity in both men and women has yet to be valued. When it is, who knows what new stories we will be able to live by?

Epilogue: Walking On

ONE OF THE REASONS I came to this work was to understand how to face my own mortality and be with seriously ill and dying people. I feel grateful that I am no longer afraid to enter a sick room or hold the hand of someone who is dying.

I have yet to completely integrate illness and death into my own story or make meaning from the suffering I have witnessed. But I know my work with these women has been worth the trip. Over the years, some mothers have said to me, almost apologetically, "This work must be so hard for you to do." I want them to know that being with them has been a blessing and a great gift. Those of us called to serve the critically ill for whatever period of time are neither angels nor saints, as we are sometimes referred to. While assisting others, we are also serving our own needs: for learning, meaning, healing, redemption, connection, and all manner of ego and soul gratification. I have received far more than I have given.

There are unresolved complications and loose ends in the story of any human being's living and dying. Most of us can only understand the decisions, mistakes, and accomplishments of our lives in hindsight. In parenting, too, there are no guarantees; we err and learn as we go. Another reason I came to this work was to heal the parts of my life concerning the two most important women in it.

At the beginning of the project, my daughter was seventeen, almost on her way to college. My mother was in a nursing home, just months away from her death. Although physical separation from both was inevitable, emotional separation would take much longer. I still carried a heavy burden of pain and guilt over past failures as both a daughter and a mother and didn't know how to put it down. I had not been raised with a healthy model for recovering from trauma. The one I had absorbed from infancy was this: Living stops after illness or loss. In spite of years fighting this example, a part of me was still in hiding, clinging to pain and the past.

The mothers showed me another way by allowing me to observe how they were coming to terms with what life had dealt them and their children. My healing process entailed accepting that what happened happened; it was part of my life. It also meant discovering gifts in the events that had been wounding. The story that injured me the most—my feelings of failure and impotence as a mother after my divorce—gave birth to empathy and wisdom that I could then pass on to other mothers, made concrete in the project. The irony is that my finest gifts were born in the event that had hurt my daughter, the person I love most. Accepting my fate has necessitated accepting my daughter's pain, for which I bear some responsibility. It has also meant forgiving myself, recognizing that I did as well as I could at the time.

Through directing the project, reviewing my own life, and telling my story, the wounds began to heal. I can finally hold my own suffering differently—because I have told my own story enough times, and it's been held by loving hearts. Contact with the mothers, prayer, meditation, hard work, and time all helped me to finish grieving and let go of the past. Perspective on my story and the events that shaped it and hope for a different way of being slowly overcame self-blame and regret. I have reclaimed my voice and my passion for life.

Laying the burden down or finishing a story inside of us does not mean we're done with the past forever. Some psychotherapists say that past traumas remain with us but we learn to carry them differently. I prefer the metaphor of a garden: I have taken the boulder that was weighing me down and placed it among the other stones in my garden. I move the stones around to rearrange the design, to make art of what is there. The boulder has found its proper place in the overall pattern of my life.

To acknowledge my own fate brings with it the startling recognition that my child's fate is her own. I did not have this awareness of our separate journeys at the project's inception; it is far more a product of my experience with the mothers than of the passage of time. Accepting that my daughter has her own story quite apart from mine means I can finally let her have her own suffering without trying to fix it, talk her out of it, or agonize over it. It is a hard-won position of maternal respect rather than control or enmeshment. It is also a position of faith—in myself, in her, in life.

Facing my mortality, my demons, and the fact of my daughter's separate journey has made me a better mother. Doing my best is finally good enough, which offers my daughter a way to see herself as good enough, simply by being. I have shed the delusion that I can protect my child from life or propel her in a direction of my choosing. I now gauge my mothering against Leona's more attainable yardstick: I would like my daughter to be kind and self-supporting. She is. Therefore, I'm a successful enough parent.

Being with the mothers has changed my perspective in ways that feel life-altering and irrevocable. I have come to renounce idealized notions, and that includes "healing" and "wholeness." Anything—birthing, mothering, dying—can be spit out by the culture as some new, impossible standard. As a recovering perfectionist, I have decided to settle happily for a wholeness that includes brokenness rather than striving to become "perfectly whole."[1] I'm becoming content to live in the pieces rather than seek a perfect peace.[2] The mothers have been exemplars.

Psalm 90 has both guided my work and become a touchstone for savoring the moment: "Teach us to number our days that we may attain a heart of wisdom." Initially, I believed that the heart of wisdom was knowing that our days on this earth are numbered. Now I realize that facing death is not an end in itself. The knowledge of death must serve life by helping us taste the sweetness of each day and make it count. However, the heart of wisdom must always include the willingness to see all of life and still bless it.

I know that I am ready to start a new chapter in my life, and that to do so, I must once again let go. The mothers helped me release my daughter, my mother, my guilt, and my tendency to live in the past. Now, after almost a decade, it is time for me to let go of them.

I have cared deeply, though differently, for every mother I've known through the project. Even those I met for only a few hours left an imprint. The mothers remain with me as internalized voices that communicate at unexpected times. I often hold imagined conversations in which I ask them for help—sometimes with the writing, sometimes with living my own challenged narrative. Mainly, I turn to the women who have died but continue to stay within me as powerful guides. Sometimes it has felt as if I'm living with ghosts, ghosts I love.

All of the mothers are a part of my interior landscape, but Tina Salomon came to hold a prominent place. Perhaps it's because she was the first woman with metastatic disease whose life story I recorded in its entirety. My relationship with Tina and her family extended over five years. Perhaps it's because, in spite of great differences between us, Tina and I shared self-defeating tendencies toward overwork, perfectionism, and control. We took too much responsibility for everything and everyone and then resented it or felt guilty. Perhaps my deep connection to Tina was rooted in our need to learn the same tough lessons.

After Tina signed off on the story, it became our habit to speak by phone every few months and sometimes meet for lunch. Tina would fill me in on her life and ask about mine. We grew closer.

Throughout the next years, Tina endured a barrage of drug protocols and a number of hospitalizations for pneumonia and congestive heart failure. No matter how sick, she resolutely timed her release from the hospital to coincide with the first day of school, usually against doctor's orders. "If I'm in the hospital, the kids will start off the year on the wrong foot. I'd like to see people and be part of the living, breathing world." During every brief reprieve, Tina would help out at Nathan's school, prepare some piece of Mark's forthcoming bar mitzvah, or take trips with Jack and the boys.

Meanwhile, I found myself praying for her every morning, dreaming of her more often, and identifying more with her even as our contact diminished due to her advancing disease and my expanding project responsibilities. During our telephone conversations, Tina would update me on the status of her children and her marriage and describe her increasingly frequent medical "episodes" and the insults of aggressive experimental treatments. Then she would break down: "This always happens when I talk to you. . . ." Her voice would trail off.

I began to wonder if I had come to represent leave-taking and loss.

Perhaps it was time for me to back off so that Tina could focus exclusively on living as fully as possible as her time became more and more precious. I wondered if I needed to do the same for myself.

My work life, and with it my relationships to mothers who were seriously ill and dying, had continued to intensify. Accumulated exhaustion, commonly known as "compassion fatigue," was taking its toll. I recalled that Tina and I had both suffered serious back injuries caused in part by our refusal to acknowledge physical limitations or extricate ourselves from traps of our own making. It was that very obsessive drive that, rightly or not, Tina blamed for her cancer. Here I was once again, sick with overwork and ignoring the danger signs, just as she had done. Had I learned nothing about valuing my health from these years of being with the mothers? Tina, close to death, was more a part of the living, breathing world than I was. I knew all this but was having a very hard time letting go.

As if in answer, I had the following dream:

I am an overnight guest in the Salomon home, where I have been helping out. The children are sleeping peacefully somewhere upstairs. I enter my room, which is narrow and dark, and as my eyes adjust to the shadows, I notice that a window has been cut into one of the walls and left open. The light is on in the other room, which I recognize as Tina and Jack's bedroom, and I can see that they are there. I think I should close the window but remember that Tina always attended to every detail. She must want me to look. I turn on the light in my room so they will know I'm there and then stand as still as I can and watch.

Tina's gorgeous red hair has been shaved, and her scalp is exposed. She is wearing only a white, silk slip that barely covers her flat chest and scarred stomach. She and Jack face each other, whispering and laughing. I cannot hear what they say. Jack kisses Tina's lips sweetly, tenderly. He lifts his hands to caress her bare shoulders, playfully fingers the delicate straps, and begins to slowly lower the top of her slip. I tiptoe into the shadows, turn off the light, and walk toward the door, closing it as quietly as possible behind me.

Just before waking, I think: I have finished my work here. I have learned what I came to learn. Life goes on. Life and laughter continue through the unspeakable pain of life-threatening illness and dying. Life goes on after trauma, tragedy, and loss. So does love.

ACKNOWLEDGMENTS

I needed the help of a veritable village to write this book and was blessed to have one. I am deeply grateful to individuals too numerous to mention who have made the Mothers' Living Stories Project and this book possible.

Any thanks must start with the many mothers I have met through the Project. You have each honored me by inviting me into your lives and by trusting me to carry your stories into the community. Whether or not your own story made it onto these pages, your spirit and love did, inspiring and holding me through a seven-year labor. I am especially grateful to the mothers and their family members and friends who gave moral and financial support along the way. Out of respect for your privacy, I will not name names; you know who you are. I hold you in my prayers.

I owe a debt of gratitude to the volunteer listeners, who are the heart of the project, my sisters in recording mothers' stories. The original group includes: Marianna Cacciatore, Carol Charlton, Eleanor Coffman, Maurine Gordon, Virginia Jouris, Michael Ann Leaver, Leah Maria Lewis, Betty Stone, Karen Zeldin. Carol, Eleanor, Maurine, Virginia, Michael, and Betty have been listeners for seven years, Karen for four. You have become teachers in the work and my dear friends.

The MLS Steering Committee encouraged me to write this book, sustained me with wise counsel through times when I faltered, and gave generously of themselves over many years. I am indebted to Edd Conboy, Hillery Jaffe-Urell, Maurine Gordon, Dale Ogar, Susan Sands, and Gale Uchiyama.

I greatly appreciate the support of our national advisors over the last decade. I thank you for your contributions to the project and your service to the community: Shelley Adler, Deborrah Bremond, Ira Byock, Carolyn Pape Cowan, Philip Cowan, Rabbi Amy Eilberg, Rabbi Nancy Flam, Sadja Greenwood, Marsha Guggenheim, Annette Hess, Lynn Humphreys, Nancy Iverson, Jill Lacefield, Rohana McLaughlin, Leslie Medine, Deena Metzger, Eliska Meyers, Cynthia Perlis, Natalie Compagni Portis, Maureen Redl, David Spiegel, Debu Tripathy, and Cherry Wise.

Projects don't exist without money. Kristina Flanagan, Eva Chernov Lokey, John Kerner, Jill Lacefield, Carole and Dale Landon, and the Bay Area Affiliate of the Susan B. Komen Breast Cancer Foundation are angels. Period. The biggest angel of all is my dear friend, Kit Neustadter, who, while coping with cancer, gave me a room of my own in the redwoods, meals, and financial and emotional support through the last two years of writing.

My attachment to the mothers and my desire to honor their lives created special challenges in revising and cutting. In an act of supreme generosity, Laura McAmis, a member of my writers' group, read this book in its many drafts repeatedly and cheerfully, making insightful suggestions with each reading. The other group members, Mary Ganz, Michael Ann Leaver, and Carolyn Shaffer, were dedicated and tremendously helpful editors at various stages of rewriting.

Susan Rawlins was a superb editor for the final manuscript. She was brilliant, incisive, and exacting, delivering feedback with both honesty and sensitivity. Susan's open heart to the mothers and to me made her red pencil less painful.

Other readers and friends who offered valuable suggestions and support include Marjorie Bair, Libby Colman, Daidie Donnelley, Mary Felstiner, Cindy Hyden, Hillery Jaffe-Urell, Paul Kaufman, Annette Lareau, Wendy Lichtman, Jean McMann, Rochelle Nameroff, and Judith Schmidt.

Along the way, a number of remarkable individuals gave spiritual guidance that influenced my writing process and my willingness to persevere in the face of so much suffering. I thank Deena Metzger, Pilar Montaine, and rabbis Amy Eilberg, Nancy Flam, and Stuart Kelman. Sue Austin, Lenore Goldman, Alexandria Hill, and Andrea Jepson were generous and steadfast volunteers, consultants, and coaches.

I could not have written this book without the gifts of space and time provided by writers' residencies and informal retreats. I offer my gratitude to the Anderson Center, Hedgebrook, the Mesa Refuge, and especially the Ragdale Foundation, which gave me exactly what I needed to write for four summers in a row. Thanks to the Friends of the Lake Forest Library in Illinois for a fellowship supporting a Ragdale residency. Karen Gray's retreat allowed me to begin the book and find solace from grief in beautiful West Marin. The Squaw Valley Community of Writers sharpened my editing skills and encouraged my work.

Dorothy Wall was an instrumental guide in preparing the book proposal. Felicia Eth is a terrific literary agent—savvy, persistent, tough, and kind, with just the right balance of truth and hope. Thanks to the good people at Seal Press for taking a chance on an unknown author and a difficult subject and for their passionate commitment to this book: Jill Rothenberg, senior editor; Krista Lyons-Gould, publisher; and Laura Mazer, copyeditor. Dorothy Brown helped with research and fact-checking during the final months. Wendy Harpham, Musa Mayer, Pamela Priest Naeve, Dale Ogar, Carol Somkin, John Swartzberg, Debu Tripathy, and Peter van Dernoot responded graciously and rapidly to my questions about recent studies and statistics.

I discovered Arthur Frank's books late in the writing of this manuscript. His thinking influenced my own as I completed revisions. I am indebted to his fine body of work on illness narratives.

My family and friends believed in me and contributed to my work in ways large and small, all important. I couldn't have done it without you.

Every day, I give thanks that I'm a mother and that I have a daughter who I got to see grow up into beautiful womanhood. Where children are concerned, Shira Burstein is as good as it gets.

NOTES

INTRODUCTION

1. The same difficulty of getting accurate numbers holds true for parents with other illnesses or disabilities. According to Through the Looking Glass, a national resource center on disability, "there is very little reliable data on the numbers of parents with disabilities. . . . The result is an underestimate of the numbers of families with parental disability in community needs assessments and a lack of funding for their services. It is often assumed that there are few parents with disabilities, when parents with disabilities in fact represent 15 percent of all parents of children under age eighteen." Source: www.lookingglass.org, August 13, 2005.

2. Metzger, Deena, personal communication, May 28, 2000.

3. Frank, Arthur, *The Wounded Storyteller: Body, Illness, and Ethics.* (Chicago: University of Chicago Press, 1995), 62–3, 137.

4. *Ibid.,* 25.

CHAPTER ONE

1. There were very few written resources available for parents with cancer from 1994 through 1997, when these mothers were diagnosed. The few that did exist, such as *How to Help Children Through a Parent's Serious Illness* by Kathleen McCue, were unknown to these women.

2. In general, the incidence of breast cancer is lower in African American women than in white women except in women under 45 years old. But the death rate is higher across all ages for breast cancer and most other cancers. According to the American Cancer Society Epidemiology Department, in 2002, the death rate for invasive breast

cancer in African American women was 37 percent higher than in white women, and for all cancers combined it was 20 percent higher. The reasons are complex and may include more aggressive cancers and estrogen-negative cancers, which are more likely to spread and cannot benefit from Tamoxifen. But barriers to receiving healthcare due to low income, lack of health insurance, racial bias, and stereotyping, all of which can lead to delays in diagnosis and treatment, are probable contributing causes for the disparity. There are similar implications for other racial and ethnic groups, all of whom have yet to be adequately studied. Sources: MacLean, Judy, et al, *Breast Cancer in California: A Closer Look*, California Breast Cancer Research Program, 2004; *Cancer Statistics 2005*, American Cancer Society, Inc.; Mayer, Musa, "Treatment and Outcomes for High-Risk and Metastatic Breast Cancer in California: An Inquiry into Disparities and Research Needs," in the California Breast Cancer Research Program Papers, 2003: www.cbcrp. org/publications/whitepapers/Mayer/index.php.

3. To my knowledge, in the years between 1994 and 1997, there were no resource directories or comprehensive resource organizations specifically aimed at parents with cancer. Several years later, I discovered Through the Looking Glass (www.lookingglass.org), a national organization that has pioneered research, training, and services for families in which a family member has a disability or medical issue. TLG grew out of the independent living movement, which has minimal interchange with the cancer world. Circle of Care (formerly PediatriCare), which serves ill parents in the San Francisco Bay Area, was similarly unknown to these mothers and to many medical practitioners. To this day, I am unaware of any comprehensive directories or national full-service organizations dedicated to families in which a parent has cancer. However, resources do exist; some are in the Resources section of this book.

4. According to a report of the Centers for Disease Control and Prevention and the National Cancer Institute (June 24, 2004), 9.8 million people in the United States have been diagnosed with cancer, and 64 percent of them can be expected to be living in five years. The need to provide support, services, and a high quality of life for individuals who are living long term with cancer is considered

a new healthcare challenge. See: Kolata, Gina, "New Approach About Cancer and Survival," *The New York Times*, June 1, 2004.

CHAPTER TWO

1. *Why You Should Have a Will,* Wisconsin Dividends, a publication of the University of Wisconsin Foundation, Spring 2005. Other reasons for not preparing a will, aside from fear of mortality, include procrastination, concerns about the costs of preparation, and lack of knowledge about the consequences of not having one.

2. Silence and invisibility also surround mothers living with most other illnesses. Mothers with AIDS have been more visible in research studies, articles, and services than mothers with cancer, primarily because of medical and cultural concern about transmission of the virus to their children. However, these mothers may be stigmatized not only by their association with illness and death but also by assumptions regarding lifestyle, race, class, and morals.

3. See, for example: Bray, Sharon. *A Healing Journey: Writing Together Through Breast Cancer.* (Amherst, MA: Amherst Writers and Artists Press, 2004); DeSalvo, Louise. *Writing as a Way of Healing: How Telling Our Stories Transforms Our Lives.* (Boston: Beacon Press, 1999); Martin, Chia. *Writing Your Way Through Cancer.* (Prescott, AZ: Hohm Press, 2000); Pennebaker, James. *Writing to Heal: A Guided Journal for Recovery from Trauma and Emotional Upheaval.* (Oakland, CA: New Harbinger, 2004).

4. Meyerhoff, Barbara. *Number Our Days.* (New York: Simon and Schuster, 1978), 271–2.

5. Sara Ruddick, philosopher and feminist, analyzed maternal thought and activity and defined the practices of providing protection, fostering growth, and socialization. For her original work, see: *Maternal Thinking: Toward a Politics of Peace.* (New York: Ballantine Books, 1989).

6. Frank, *op. cit.,* 55.

7. Frank, *op. cit.,* 54.

8. All of the women in the focus groups wanted to record their stories. Not all were able to do so because of the project's limited resources. Of the women in the Chapter One focus group, you will hear from Irene again in Chapter Six and read Sara's story in Chapter Eight.

CHAPTER THREE
1. CMF stands for cyclophosphamide, methotrexate, and fluorouracil.
2. 5 to 10 percent of breast cancers have a genetic component, according to the American Cancer Society Epidemiology Department, 2005. Although for most women with breast cancer there are no special implications for their offspring, for women with a strong family history of the disease, there may be an inherited predisposition. Daughters and other female relatives may be at increased risk for breast and ovarian cancer especially. Sons and brothers may be at increased risk for prostate cancer. Both male and female direct relatives may be at slightly increased risk for colon, thyroid, and pancreatic cancer. Women who have positive family histories or are very young at diagnosis should consider seeing a genetic counselor. This information was provided by Debu Tripathy, MD, Professor of Medicine at the University of Texas Southwestern Medical Center, Director of the Komen Center for Breast Cancer Research in Dallas, Texas, in a personal communication, August 14, 2005.

CHAPTER FOUR
1. Again, this pertains primarily to sons of women with strong family histories or who are very young at diagnosis.
   See Chapter Three, Note 2.
2. Frank, *op. cit.*, 75–96.
3. Frank, *op. cit.*, 115–136.

CHAPTER FIVE
1. For more about illness as a spiritual journey or turning point, see: Bolen, Jean Shinoda. *Close to the Bone: Life-Threatening Illness and the Search for Meaning.* (New York, Scribner, 1996); Duff, Kat. *The Alchemy of Illness.* (New York: Random House, 1994); LeShan, Lawrence. *Cancer as a Turning Point: A Handbook for People with Cancer, Their Families and Health Professionals.* Revised edition. (New York: Penguin Books, 1994).
2. As of this writing, there is no evidence substantiating the concern that ingredients in commercial peanut butter are a contributing factor for breast cancer. John Swartzberg, MD, Professor of Medicine,

Chair of the Editorial Board for University of California, Berkeley's *Wellness Letter,* in a personal communication, August 9, 2005.

3. Frank, *op. cit.*, 92.

4. Frank, *op. cit.*, 93.

CHAPTER SIX

1. Upponi, S. S., et al, "Pregnancy After Breast Cancer," *European Journal of Cancer,* 2003; 39 (6): 736–741. From Cambridge Breast Unit Addenbrookes Hospital, Cambridge, UK.

2. Partridge, A. and L. Schapira, "Pregnancy and Breast Cancer: Epidemiology, Treatment, and Safety Issues." *Oncology,* May 2005; 19 (6): 693–7; discussion 697–700.

3. For more information about the effects of chemotherapy on fertility, see: www.breastcancer.org/chemotherapy_infertile.html.

4. Gibbs, Nancy, "Dying to Have a Family," *Time Magazine,* March 11, 2002, 78; Benfer, Amy, "A Male Biological Clock?" See also: www.salon.com, April 13, 2001.

5. Kleinman, Arthur. *The Illness Narratives: Suffering, Healing, and the Human Condition.* (New York: Basic Books, 1998), 3–5.

6. Mayer, Musa. *Advanced Breast Cancer: A Guide to Living with Metastatic Disease.* 2nd Edition. (Sebastopol, O'Reilly, 1998), 55–72.

7. Kaplan, Louise J. *No Voice Is Ever Wholly Lost.* (New York: Simon & Schuster, 1995), 126.

8. For discussion, see: Hrdy, Sarah Blaffer. *Mother Nature: Maternal Instincts and How They Shape the Human Species* (New York: Ballantine, 1999); de Marneffe, Daphne. *Maternal Desire: On Children, Love, and the Inner Life* (New York: Little, Brown, 2004).

9. Kleinman, *op cit.*, 45.

10. Sontag, Susan. *Illness as Metaphor and AIDS and Its Metaphors.* (New York: Anchor/Doubleday, 1990), 3.

11. Charmaz, Kathy. *Good Days, Bad Days: The Self in Chronic Illness and Time.* (New Jersey: Rutgers University, 1991), 12.

12. Frank, *op. cit.*, 8–9. See also, Frank, Arthur. *At the Will of the Body: Reflections on Illness.* (New York, First Mariner Books, 2000), 138–9.

13. *Mayer, op. cit.,* 15. "This is true, but the survival rate today is much higher, both because women are diagnosed earlier today and

because treatments are better." Musa Mayer, MS, MFA, personal communication, August 17, 2005.

CHAPTER SEVEN

1. Mayer, *Advanced Breast Cancer*, 13.
2. American Cancer Society Epidemiology Department, 2005.
3. Mayer, Musa, "Treatment and Outcomes for High-Risk and Metastatic Breast Cancer in California: An Inquiry into Disparities and Research Needs," in the California Breast Cancer Research Program Papers, 2003. www.cbcrp.org/publications/whitepapers/Mayer/index.php.
4. Mayer, *op. cit.*, reports that "a survey conducted by the National Alliance of Breast Cancer Organizations in 2001 found fewer than twenty support groups across the United States to meet the specific needs of metastatic breast cancer patients, from among the nearly one thousand groups then in existence." Fewer groups exist for women with other cancers.
5. Mayer, *Advanced Breast Cancer,* 153–154. For further discussions on physician responses to advancing illness, see: Kuhl, David. *What Dying People Want: Practical Wisdom for the End of Life.* (New York: Perseus, 2002), 33–69; Nuland, Sherwin. *How We Die: Reflections on Life's Final Chapter.* (New York: Knopf, 1994), 222–269.
6. Mayer, Musa. *Holding Tight, Letting Go: Living with Metastatic Breast Cancer.* (Sebastopol, CA: O'Reilly, 1997).
7. Charmaz, *op. cit.*
8. Frank, *The Wounded Storyteller*, 59.

CHAPTER EIGHT

1. For information on communicating with children about illness, see books listed in Resources by Lea Baider et al., Wendy Harpham, Sue Heiney et al., and Kathleen McCue.

CHAPTER NINE

1. Approximately 6 percent of invasive breast cancer patients are diagnosed with Stage IV disease. The majority of women with invasive breast cancer are diagnosed at earlier stages and will survive their disease to die of other causes. Based on data in the National

Cancer Institute SEER registry for 1992–1999, reported by Musa Mayer, MS, MFA, "Treatment and Outcomes for High-Risk and Metastatic Breast Cancer in California: An Inquiry into Disparities and Research Needs," California Breast Cancer Research Program, 2003. www.cbcrp.org/publications/whitepapers/Mayer/index.php

2. Siegel, Bernie, MD. *Healing from the Inside Out.* (Carlsbad, CA: Hay House Audio Books, 1997).

3. PICC (Peripherally Inserted Central Catheter) is used to deliver IV medication directly to the bloodstream without continuously inserting needles into the patient.

4. See Dr. Arthur Frank's discussion of the loss of self through illness, especially as the body is ravaged, and the importance of reclaiming one's personal self and style. Frank, *op. cit.*, Chapter Two, 27 ff.

CHAPTER TEN

1. An ethical will is a spoken or written letter from an adult, often a parent, to children, other loved ones, or the community, transmitting the intangibles of a life: religious, spiritual, and moral beliefs and practices, lessons learned, blessings, wisdom for living, messages of forgiveness, gratitude, and love. It can be shared at any time during life or attached as a codicil to a will. For more information, see www.ethicalwill.com.

CHAPTER ELEVEN

1. The three methods currently recommended for breast cancer detection in the United States are breast self-exam (BSE), clinical breast exam (CBE), i.e., manual exam done by a healthcare professional, and mammography. All are intended to detect cancer as early as possible, improving the likelihood of successful treatment and therefore survival. According to the American Cancer Society, regular self-exam should begin by age twenty so a young woman becomes familiar with her breasts and can report unusual changes to a healthcare practitioner. CBE should begin with a woman's first gynecological exam or no later than age twenty. CBE is recommended every three years until age forty, and then every year. Annual mammograms are recommended starting at age forty for women at average risk. Women at higher risk due to family

histories, genetic tendencies, or past breast cancer should discuss the possibility of starting mammography earlier or having more frequent or additional tests, such as breast ultrasounds or MRI. For more information, see www.cancer.org.

Mammography is a detection device that neither prevents nor cures cancer. There is substantial evidence that for a certain group of women, primarily between fifty and sixty-five, mammography detects cancer that can be treated early, while it is small and before it has spread to other parts of the body. Early treatment extends survival and reduces the mortality rate. However, women should also be aware that mammograms can have false negatives (missing some cancers) and false positives (findings that are suspicious and lead to invasive testing and sometimes unnecessary treatment, stress, and health risks). MacLean, Judy, et al. *Breast Cancer in California: A Closer Look*, California Breast Cancer Research Program, 2004, 28.

Breast cancer risk for young women is relatively low and increases with age, especially after age forty.

There is currently no accurate method for detecting breast cancer in young women, and questions exist about the efficacy of both BSE and CBE. Mammography does not penetrate the denser breast tissue of pre-menopausal women and has some risk of radiation. Therefore, mammography is only recommended as a screening tool for young women at high risk, by virtue of family history, or when women are symptomatic or have particular concerns. Ideally, young women, like all women, will educate themselves about the benefits, risks, and limitations of cancer detection methods and bring questions and concerns to their healthcare providers. For more about these issues see www.youngsurvival.org and "Mammography Screening and New Technology," Breast Cancer Action website, www.bcaction.org.

2. See Chapter One, Note 2.

3. For two different views of breast cancer myths, see www.breast-cancer.org/cmn_myt_idx.html and www.bcaction.org/Pages/Get-Informed/Top10Myths.html.

4. Diana, Princess of Wales, née Lady Diana Frances Spencer, died on August 31, 1997, after a tragic car crash in Paris. She was thirty-six; her sons were fifteen and twelve.

CHAPTER TWELVE

1. CAF stands for Cytoxin, Adriamycin, and Fluorouracil.
2. Metzger, Deena, personal communication, June 1, 2000.

CHAPTER THIRTEEN

1. Inflammatory breast cancer is "an aggressive form of breast cancer, occurring in about one percent of all diagnoses, that rapidly spreads into the lymphatic channels in the breast, causing the tissue to appear reddened and swollen, resembling a rash or infection." Mayer, *Advanced Breast Cancer*, 473.
2. Marianna Cacciatore, volunteer listener.
3. The University of California, Berkeley, *Wellness Letter,* August 2001, 4, reports: "There's no evidence that emotional upset or severe stress (temporary or chronic) causes breast cancer, or causes it to recur after treatment. Or indeed that personality or attitude has any relation to breast cancer." According to John Swartzberg, MD, Chair of the Editorial Board, the same holds true for any cancer, in spite of some evidence that stress can influence the immune system. However, some women and doctors believe that having a "fighting spirit" and "positive attitude" can help, although at this point, evidence about how it helps is mainly anecdotal. Personal communication, August 18, 2005. For more about "positive attitudes," see Spiegel, David. *Living Beyond Limits.* (New York: Harper Collins, 1998), 44–65, 103–106; John, Lauren. "The Power of Negative Thinking," *Breast Cancer Action Newsletter,* May/June 2002, 3–4.
4. See Chapter Seven, Note 5.
5. 27 percent (73,000) will die of lung and bronchus cancers, 15 percent (40,000) of breast cancer, followed by colorectal disease. Cancer Facts and Figures, American Cancer Society, 2005. The death rate for invasive breast cancer has been decreasing since 1990 at an average annual rate of 2.3 percent. The death rate for many, but not all, cancers (e.g., breast, prostate, colorectal, and melanoma) has been declining, in part due to earlier detection through screening and advances in treatment. American Cancer Society Epidemiology Department, August 10, 2005.
6. National Cancer Institute Fact Book, 2004, 40. Incidence for most cancers, including breast cancer, increases with age. However, the

average age of women at first birth has also risen. Many women are mothering well into their fifties and even sixties, when cancer and other diseases are more prevalent. And breast cancer in pregnancy may increase as more women delay childbearing. Woo, Junda C., et al., "Breast Cancer in Pregnancy: A Literature Review," *Archives of Surgery*, 2003; 138 (2): 91–98.

7. U.S. Census 2000; American Cancer Society, Breast Cancer Facts and Figures, 2003–2004. Younger women struggle with complex issues regarding fertility, pregnancy, breastfeeding, and childrearing after cancer, while facing more aggressive disease and higher mortality rates. www.youngsurvival.org, 2005.

8. Mayer, *Advanced Breast Cancer*, 2–3. See also Chapter Eleven, Note 1.

9. For critical analyses about the culture of cancer, see Ehrenreich, Barbara, "Welcome to Cancerland," *Harper's*, November 2001, 43–53 and www.bcaction.org.

10. Byock, Ira. *Dying Well: The Prospect for Growth at the End of Life*. (New York: Penguin, 1997). Byock, Ira. *The Four Things That Matter Most: A Book About Living*. (New York: Free Press, 2004). For the developmental tasks of dying, see Dr. Byock's website: www.dyingwell.com/landmarks.htm.

11. Byock, *The Four Things That Matter Most: A Book About Living*.

12. Byock, Ira, personal communication, July 14, 1999.

13. Zornberg, Aviva Gottlieb. *The Beginning of Desire: Reflections on Genesis*. (New York: Doubleday, 1995), 377–378.

14. Estes, Clarissa Pinkola. *Women Who Run With the Wolves: Myths and Stories of the Wild Woman Archetype*. (New York: Ballantine, 1992), 162.

15. Metzger, Deena, personal communication, May 29, 2000.

CHAPTER FOURTEEN

1. A prayer shawl.

2. A story or commentary.

3. See Chapter Eleven, Note 4.

4. Craziness.

5. "Princes in the tower" refers to the sons of Edward IV, who were allegedly killed by Richard III.

CHAPTER SIXTEEN

1. The Neptune Society is a cremation service, devoted to cremating and dispersing the ashes of its clients in a spiritual manner.
2. Frank, *op. cit.*, 97–114.
3. Kaplan, *op. cit.*

CHAPTER SEVENTEEN

1. "You'll Never Walk Alone," from the musical *Carousel*. Music by Richard Rodgers, lyrics by Oscar Hammerstein II, 1945. Though Dorothy remembered the song the following way:

   When you walk through a storm
   Hold your head up high
   And don't be afraid of the dark
   At the end of the storm is a golden sky
   And the sweet silver song of the lark.

   The original wording is:

   When you walk through a storm
   Hold your chin up high
   And don't be afraid of the dark
   At the end of the storm is a golden sky
   And the sweet silver song of the lark.

CHAPTER EIGHTEEN

1. See "For Parents Living with Illness or Disability" in the Resources section. For example, the Children's Treehouse Foundation lists support groups for children who have an ill parent: www.childrenstreehousefdn.org.
2. See Resources section for specifics, including books by Beth Hawkins, Geralyn Lucas, and Beth Murphy et al., and websites www.youngsurvival.org and www.sharsheret.org, the latter for Jewish women under forty.
3. See "For Parents Living with Illness or Disability" in the Resources section.
4. See, for example, books by Kristine Breese, Jill Lacefield, Ruth

Picardie, and Kaethe Weingarten, listed in Resources section.

5. See Chapter One, Note 4, and Chapter Thirteen, Note 5.

6. An estimated 15.6 percent of the population or 45 million people were without health-insurance coverage in 2003, up from 15.2 percent or 43.6 million in 2002. This is the third straight year in which the percentage rose. U.S. Census Bureau, "Insurance, Poverty, and Health Insurance Coverage in the United States, 2003," issued August 2004. Lack of medical insurance affects disease detection, treatment, and survival rates. Uninsured women are 40 percent more likely to be diagnosed at a later stage of breast cancer. Uninsured women ages 35–49 are 60 percent more likely to die as privately insured women. Kaiser Commission on Medicaid and the Uninsured, "Uninsured in America: A Chart Book," Second Edition, May 2000.

7. Gafni, Marc. *Soul Prints: Your Path to Fulfillment.* (New York: Simon & Schuster, 2001), 222, 217.

8. Metzger, Deena, personal communication, June 1, 2000.

9. Some early groundbreaking books analyzing motherhood include: Bernard, Jesse. *The Future of Motherhood.* (New York: Penguin, 1975); Lazarre, Jane. *The Mother Knot.* (New York: McGraw-Hill, 1976); Rich, Adrienne. *Of Woman Born* (New York: W.W. Norton, 1976).

10. For contemporary books and resources on motherhood, see: www.literarymama.com, www.mothermovement.org, www.brainchildmag.com, www.hipmama.com, and www.mothersandmore.org.

11. See Crittenden, Ann. *The Price of Motherhood: Why the Most Important Job in the World is Still the Least Valued.* (New York: Henry Holt, 2001).

12. Childhood poverty in the United States is lower today than a decade ago (22 percent peak in 1993), but for children under eighteen years old, both the poverty rate and the percentage in poverty rose between 2002 and 2004, from 16.7 percent to 17.6 percent, from 12.1 million to 12.9 million, respectively. The hardest hit are children under six years of age and children of single-parent households. U.S. Census Bureau, "Insurance, Poverty, and Health Insurance Coverage in the United States, 2003," issued August 2004.

EPILOGUE

1. I'm grateful to Susan Rothbaum for this insight. Personal communication, April 13, 1987.

2. Ulanov, Ann & Barry. *Cinderella and Her Sisters: The Envied and the Envying.* (Philadelphia: The Westminster Press, 1983), 139–141. The Ulanovs discuss the "healing that comes in the great change from wholes to parts" when "we can consent to bits and pieces as they move in and among ourselves."

Resources

Books for Parents Living with Illness or Disability

Baider, Lea, Caryl Cooper, and Atara Kaplan De-Nour (eds.). *Cancer and the Family*, 2nd Ed. New York: John Wiley and Sons, 2000.

Breese, Kristine. *Cereal for Dinner: Strategies, Shortcuts, and Sanity for Moms Battling Illness*. New York: St. Martin's Press, 2004.

Grollman, Earl. *Talking About Death: A Dialogue Between Parent and Child*. Boston: Beacon Press, 3rd Ed., 1991.

Harpham, Wendy Schlessel. *When a Parent Has Cancer: A Guide to Caring for Your Children*. New York: Harper Paperbacks, 2004. Includes a special book for children, *Becky and the Worry Cup*.

Hawkins, Beth. *I'm Too Young to Have Breast Cancer!* Washington, DC: Lifeline Press, 2004.

Heiney, Sue, Ed., Joan Hermann, Katherine Bruss, and Joy Fincannon. *Cancer in the Family: Helping Children Cope with a Parent's Illness*. American Cancer Society, 2001.

Kramp Tierney, E. and D. Kramp. *Living with the End in Mind*. NY: Three Rivers Press, 1998.

Lacefield, Jill. *A Little Cancer on the Side: A Survivor's Book of Laughter and Inspiration*. 2003. Order from www.jilllacefield.com.

Lucas, Geralyn. *Why I Wore Lipstick to My Mastectomy*. New York: St. Martin's Press, 2004.

Mayer, Musa. *Advanced Breast Cancer: A Guide to Living with Meta-static Disease*, 2nd Edition. Sebastopol, CA: O'Reilly and Associates, 1998.

McCue, Kathleen. *How to Help Children Through a Parent's Serious Illness*. New York: St. Martin's Press, 1994.

Murphy, Beth, Ann Curry, and George Sledge. *Fighting for Our Future: How Young Women Find Strength, Hope, and Courage While Taking Control of Breast Cancer*. New York: McGraw Hill, 2002.

Picardie, Ruth. *Before I Say Goodbye: Recollections and Observations from One Woman's Final Year*. Penguin UK, 1999.

Peterson, Paula. *Penitent, with Roses: An HIV+ Mother Reflects*. Hanover, N.J.: Middlebury College Press, 2000.

Rogers, Judith. *The Disabled Woman's Guide to Pregnancy and Birth*. New York: Demo Medical Publishing, 2005.

Rolland, John S., *Families, Illness, and Disability: An Integrative Treatment Model*. New York: Basic Books, 1994.

Russell, Neil. *Can I Still Kiss You? Answering Your Children's Questions About Cancer*. Dearfield Beach, FL: Health Communications, 2001.

Van Dernoot, Peter. *Helping Your Children Cope with Your Cancer: A Guide for Parents*. Long Island City, NY: Hatherleigh Press, 2002.

Wates, Michele and Rowan Jade (eds.). *Bigger Than the Sky: Disabled Women on Parenting*. London, England: Women's Press, 1999.

Weingarten, Kathy. *The Mother's Voice: Strengthening Intimacy in Families*. New York: Guilford Press, 1997.

VIDEOS FOR PARENTS

We Can Cope: When a Parent Has Cancer
Inflexxion, Inc., Newton, MA
800-848-3895
www.wecancope.com

Talking about Your Cancer: A Parent's Guide to Helping Your Children Cope
Fox Chase Center, Department of Social Services, Philadelphia, PA
215-728-2668

My Mom Has Breast Cancer (free)
Kidscope
www.kidscope.org
Also available through Community Service Sections of many Blockbuster video stores

BOOKS FOR CHILDREN

Compassion Books has many books and resources on illness, grief, loss, and death for children of all ages as well as for parents and professionals. Order through Compassion Books by calling 800-970-4220, or visit the company's website at www.compassionbooks.com.

WEBSITES

www.kidskonnected.org
www.kid-support.org
www.siblinks.org
www.riprap.org
www.childrenstreehousefdn.org
www.gildasclub.org
www.thewellnesscommunity.org
www.cancercare.org
www.youngsurvival.org
www.sharsheret.org

www.lookingglass.org
www.gillettecancerconnect.org

FREE RESOURCES

American Cancer Society
www.cancer.org
510-832-7012 or 800-227-2345

Kidscope
404-233-0001
www.kidscope.com

National Cancer Institute
www.nci.nih.gov
800-4-CANCER

BOOKS FOR CAREGIVERS

Babcock, Elise NeeDell. *When Life Becomes Precious: Essential Guide for Patients, Loved Ones, and Friends of Those Facing Illness.* New York: Bantam, 1997.

Capossela, Cappy and Sheila Warnock. *Share the Care: How to Organize a Group to Care for Someone Who is Seriously Ill.* New York: Simon and Schuster, 1995.

Garfield, Charles. *Sometimes My Heart Goes Numb.* Orlando: Harcourt Brace, 1997.

Halpern, Susan P. *The Etiquette of Illness: What to Say When You Can't Find the Words.* New York: Bloomsbury, 2004.

Hope, Lori. *Help Me Live: 20 Things People with Cancer Want You to Know.* San Francisco: Celestial Arts, 2005.

Silver, Marc. *Breast Cancer Husband: How to Help Your Wife (and*

Yourself) during Diagnosis, Treatment, and Beyond. New York: Rodale Books 2004.

FOR ASSISTANCE WITH RECORDING A LIFE STORY, ETHICAL WILL, OR OTHER LEGACY PROJECT

www.personalhistorians.org
www.ethicalwill.com
www.thelegacycenter.net

About the Author

Linda Blachman, MPH, MA has been a writer and health professional for twenty-five years, specializing in the fields of maternal and child health and community mental health. The abiding passion of her professional and personal life has been mothering—its value, meaning, challenge, and opportunity in contemporary culture. While recovering from a disabling back injury when her own daughter was seventeen, Blachman became concerned about the plight of others struggling to raise children while dealing with far more serious illnesses. In 1995, she founded the Mothers Living Stories Project, an award-winning non-profit project that brings compassion, dignity, and support in parenting to mothers who have cancer by helping them record their life stories as living legacies. *Another Morning* is based on her work with the Project. Blachman lives in Berkeley, Calif., where she has a private practice as a personal historian, public health consultant, and counselor. She can be reached at www.lindablachman.com.

For more than twenty-five years, Seal Press has published groundbreaking books. By women. For women. Visit our website at www.sealpress.com.

Literary Mama: Reading for the Maternally Inclined edited by Andrea J. Buchanan and Amy Hudock. $14.95. 1-58005-158-8. From the best of literarymama.com, this collection of personal writing includes creative nonfiction, fiction, and poetry.

Hungry for More: A Keeping-It-Real Guide for Black Women on Weight and Body Image by Robyn McGee. $13.95. 1-58005-149-9. This straightforward book addresses the obesity epidemic in the black community and tells the story of the death of the author's sister from gastric bypass surgery.

Planet Widow: A Mother's Story of Navigating a Suddenly Unrecognizable World by Gloria Lenhart. $14.95. 1-58005-168-5. This book chronicles the events after the unexpected death of a spouse, and offers support for other young widows.

I Wanna Be Sedated: 30 Writers on Parenting Teenagers edited by Faith Conlon and Gail Hudson. $15.95. 1-58005-127-8. With hilarious and heartfelt essays, this anthology will reassure any parent of a teenager that they are not alone in their desire to be comatose.

The Truth Behind the Mommy Wars: Who Decides What Makes a Good Mother? By Miriam Peskowitz. $15.95. 1-58005-129-4. A groundbreaking book that reveals the truth behind the "wars" between working mothers and stay-at-home moms.

It's a Boy: Women Writers on Raising Sons edited by Andrea J. Buchanan. $14.95. 1-58005-145-6. Seal's edgy take on what it's really like to raise boys, from toddlers to teens and beyond.